Advanced Topics in Anemia

Advanced Topics in Anemia

Edited by **Rudy Willis**

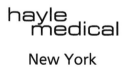

New York

Published by Hayle Medical,
30 West, 37th Street, Suite 612,
New York, NY 10018, USA
www.haylemedical.com

Advanced Topics in Anemia
Edited by Rudy Willis

International Standard Book Number: 978-1-63241-019-1 (Hardback)

Contents

Permissions

List of Contributors

Preface

This book has been a concerted effort by a group of academicians, researchers and scientists, who have contributed their research works for the realization of the book. This book has materialized in the wake of emerging advancements and innovations in this field. Therefore, the need of the hour was to compile all the required researches and disseminate the knowledge to a broad spectrum of people comprising of students, researchers and specialists of the field.

Anemia is a common blood disorder. This book presents a complete summary of many developments in the field of anemia, including its reasons and pathogenesis, and techniques of analysis related to it. Dietary reasons of anemia, particularly in rising nations are discussed. Hence, this book gives a comprehensive summary of anemia and will be helpful for readers interested in this field.

At the end of the preface, I would like to thank the authors for their brilliant chapters and the publisher for guiding us all-through the making of the book till its final stage. Also, I would like to thank my family for providing the support and encouragement throughout my academic career and research projects.

Editor

Anemia Caused by Oxidative Stress

Yoshihito Iuchi
Yamaguchi University
Japan

1. Introduction

Anemia is considered to be one of the major health problems. According to the World Health Organization, about 30 percent of people throughout the world suffer from anemia. The most common cause of anemia is iron deficiency; however, recent work has shown that reactive oxygen species (ROS) of erythrocytes are one of the principal causative factors of anemia. Elevation of ROS in erythrocytes could occur either by activation of ROS generation or by suppression of antioxidative/redox system. When erythrocytes experience an excessive elevation of ROS, oxidative stress develops. ROS are known to contribute to the pathogenesis of several hereditary disorders of erythrocytes, including sickle cell anemia, thalassemia, and glucose-6-phosphate dehydrogenase (G6PD) deficiency. Deficiency of antioxidant enzymes such as superoxide dismutase 1 (SOD1) or peroxiredoxin II (Prx II) induces elevation of oxidative stress in erythrocytes and causes anemia, while deficiency of catalase or glutathione peroxidase does not. In addition to the abnormalities of antioxidant enzymes, some transcription factors such as p45NF-E2 or Nrf2 can cause anemia. In this chapter, I provide some evidence of the involvement of oxidative stress in anemia.

2. Oxidative stress-mediated destruction of erythrocytes

2.1 Cellular oxidative stress and anti-oxidative system

Under normal physiological conditions, there is a balance between the ROS and the defense system of antioxidant enzymes and antioxidants, which prevents or limits oxidative damage. ROS are produced as a result of intracellular metabolic activity. During this process, ROS such as superoxide ($\bullet O_2^-$), hydrogen peroxide (H_2O_2), and hydroxyl radical ($\bullet OH$) are produced, even in healthy individuals. Oxidative stress is the result of an imbalance between oxidants and antioxidants. Increased pro-oxidants and/or decreased antioxidants trigger a cascade of oxidative reactions. Oxidative stress can damage specific molecular targets (lipids, proteins, nucleotides, etc.), resulting in cell dysfunction and/or death. Enzymes that participate in ROS production include xanthine oxidase (XO), nicotinamide adenine dinucleotide phosphate (NADPH) oxidase, nitric oxide synthase (NOS), cytochrome P450, cyclo-oxygenase (COX), and lipoxygenase. Major defence mechanisms against ROS include enzymatic (superoxide dismutase (SOD), catalase, glutathione peroxidase (GPx), peroxiredoxin (Prx)) as well as non-enzymatic systems (reduced glutathione (GSH), ubiquinols, uric acid, vitamins C and E, flavonoids, carotenoids).

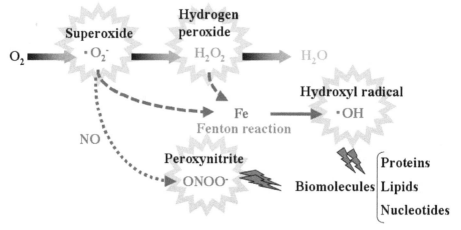

Fig. 1. Reactive oxygen species (ROS) generated in the cell.

2.2 Oxidation of erythrocyte membrane caused by ROS

During the binding of oxygen to form oxy-hemoglobin (oxy-Hb), one electron is transferred from iron to the bound oxygen forming a ferric-superoxide anion complex. The shared electron is normally returned to the iron when oxygen is released during deoxygenation. However, the electrons can remain and transform oxygen into superoxide anions. In this process, iron is left in the ferric state and Hb is transformed into methemoglobin (met-Hb). The autoxidation of Hb occurs spontaneously and transforms 0.5–3% of Hb into met-Hb per day. In addition to this physiological process, met Hb can be produced by endogenous oxidants, such as H_2O_2, nitric oxide (NO), and hydroxyl radicals. Since met-Hb cannot bind oxygen, this is the first step in the formation of harmful hemichromes (Rice-Evans & Baysal, 1987). In normal conditions, spontaneous production of met-Hb from autoxidation and conversion of met-Hb back to Hb are in balance. However, in pathological conditions, increased oxidative stress or impaired antioxidant defence will enhance production of met-Hb and generation of ROS. Hemichrome formation depends on the amount of met-Hb formed and is accelerated by ROS such as superoxide or H_2O_2. Superoxide produced by one electron reduction of oxygen would reduce ferri-hemichrome to ferro-hemichrome. In the Fenton reaction, ferro-hemichrome catalyzes decomposition of H_2O_2 to hydroxyl radical. Hydroxyl radical is an extremely reactive free radical that can react with various biomolecules such as membrane lipids. Peroxidation of membrane lipids, most notably the polyunsaturated fatty acids arachidonic acid and linoleic acid, generates a wide array of molecules, such as lipid hydroperoxides, which are secondary lipid peroxidation products (for example, malondialdehyde and 4-hydroxynonenal, HNE). Lipid peroxidation products can damage membrane structure with the formation of membrane pores, alter water permeability, decrease cell deformability, and enhance IgG binding and complement activation. Finally, disruption of the normal asymmetrical distribution of membrane phospholipids occurs. This may enhance exposure of phosphatidylserine (PS) on the outer cell surface. Erythrocytes that have PS exposed on the outer surface are recognized and engulfed by macrophages with PS-specific receptors, resulting in their degradation (Carrell et al., 1975; Hebbel, 1985; Nur et al., 2011).

At the same time, ROS can be used for killing harmful microorganisms. However, ROS not only participate in pathogen killing but also induce activation of inflammatory mediators and production of adhesion molecules and membrane damage. The increased intra- and extra-erythrocytic oxidative stress induces lipid peroxidation and membrane instability, contributing to accelerated hemolysis. Increased levels of hydroperoxides cause erythrocyte membrane damage and deformity and, ultimately, lead to cell death.

2.3 Band 3-mediated erythrocyte removal

Band 3, also termed the anion exchanger, is a major erythrocyte membrane protein, constituting 25% of the total erythrocyte membrane protein. It has two independent domains: the membrane-spanning domain, which catalyzes anion exchange and contains the antigenic determinants recognized by naturally occurring antibodies (NAbs), and the cytoplasmic domain (Pantaleo et al., 2008). A very important feature of hemichrome/free heme/iron damage is its non-random occurrence in space. The highly damaging feature of hemichromes is their tight association with the cytoplasmic domain of band 3, which, following their binding, leads to band 3 oxidation and clusterization. These band 3 clusters show increased affinity for NAbs, which activate complement and finally trigger phagocytosis-mediated erythrocyte removal. This band 3/hemichrome complex was found not only in pathological conditions in which oxidative stress in erythrocytes is thought to be elevated, but also in senescent erythrocytes (Arese et al., 2005).

3. Relationship between human hereditary anemia and oxidative stress

3.1 Sickle cell disease

Sickle cell disease (SCD) is a hemoglobinopathy clinically characterized by chronic hemolysis. Chronic activation and damage of endothelial cells by sickle erythrocytes, heme, polymorphonuclear neutrophils (PMNs), and inflammatory mediators contribute to progressive microvascular damage in all organs, including the brain, lungs, and kidneys. SCD is an inherited disorder of hemoglobin synthesis. SCD has the same single base pair mutation (GAG to GTG, Glu to Val) in the β globin molecule of sickle cells (HbS).

Chronic oxidative stress constitutes a critical factor in endothelial dysfunction, inflammation, and multiple organ damage in SCD (Nur et al., 2011). There are several causes of oxidative stress in SCD. Major sources of ROS in SCD are thought to be the (i) enhanced rate of HbS auto-oxidation, (ii) increased xanthine oxidase activity in SCD aortic endothelium, and (iii) higher number of leucocytes, which produce twice the fluxes of superoxide in SCD (Wood & Granger, 2007).

Endothelial dysfunction in patients with SCD has been related to inflammation, high levels of production of ROS and reactive nitrogen species, and erythrocyte adhesion to blood vessel walls. There have been several studies showing that patients with SCD have a high level of oxidative damage, assessed through lipid peroxidation. In turn, oxidative stress is associated with chronic hemolysis. Sickle erythrocytes have a high frequency of phosphatidyl serine exposure, which is due to oxidative stress, suggesting that oxidative stress might play a role in intravascular hemolysis. Hypertension in patients with SCD was found to be related to ROS, which can directly deactivate endothelial nitric oxide synthase (eNOS), reducing nitric oxide (NO) levels, an important vasodilator (Rusanova et al., 2010).

3.2 Thalassemia

The thalassemia syndrome is one of the most common genetic disorders affecting a single gene or gene cluster. The various thalassemia disorders are caused by insufficient production of one of the two types of globin chains that constitute the hemoglobin tetramer. In α thalassemia , α globin production is reduced or absent, and in β thalassemia, β globin production is impaired. The α and β thalassemias are characterized by the presence of a pool of unpaired hemoglobin chains. While α or β hemoglobin chains are stable when part of the $\alpha_2\beta_2$ hemoglobin tetramer, the unpaired α or β hemoglobin chains are unstable and subject to high rates of auto-oxidation. The auto-oxidation of the unpaired hemoglobin chains leads to the generation of superoxide and H_2O_2, and subsequent release of globin-free heme and iron (Bunn, 1967; Shinar & Rachmilewitz, 1990). β thalassemic erythrocytes exhibit a significant decrease in the NADPH/NADP ratio similar to that seen in severe G6PD-deficiency anemia (see next chapter). As a consequence of this decrease, both catalase activity and GSH concentration are decreased (Scot, 2006). Expression of peroxiredoxin (Prx) II, an antioxidant enzyme that detoxifies H_2O_2, is increased in β thalassemic mouse erythrocytes (Matte et al., 2010). These findings indicate that this high expression of PrxII has a compensatory effect against elevated oxidative stress in thalassemic erythrocytes (Rund & Rachmilewitz, 2005).

3.3 Glucose-6-phosphate dehydrogenase (G6PD) deficiency

Glucose-6-phosphate dehydrogenase (G6PD) deficiency was first discovered in African-American subjects. The fact that it seemed to be limited to one ethnic group suggested that it has a genetic basis. Because it was shown that transmission was generally from mother to son, it became apparent that G6PD deficiency is an X-linked disorder. G6PD deficiency is one of the glycolytic enzymopathies that frequently cause hemolytic anemia. G6PD deficiency is the most common erythrocyte enzyme defect, affecting over 400 million people (Beutler, 2008).

G6PD deficiency is mainly caused by point mutations in the G6PD gene. About 140 mutations have been described: most are single base changes, leading to amino acid substitutions (Cappellini & Fiorelli, 2008). The most frequent clinical manifestations of G6PD deficiency are neonatal jaundice and acute hemolytic anemia, which is usually triggered by an exogenous agent. Some G6PD variants cause chronic hemolysis, leading to congenital non-spherocytic hemolytic anemia. The appearance of Heinz bodies both in vivo and in vitro in G6PD-deficient cells and their inability to protect their GSH against drug challenge suggested that a major component of the hemolytic process is the inability of the erythrocytes to protect sulfhydryl groups against oxidative stress (Fig. 2, Cohen & Hochstein, 1961). However, it has been shown that, in mice, targeted disruption of the gene encoding glutathione peroxidase has little effect on oxidation of hemoglobin of murine cells challenged with peroxides.

G6PD provides erythrocytes with important protection against oxidative stress. G6PD is a key regulatory enzyme of the pentose phosphate pathway (also called hexose monophosphate shunt), which is essential for the supply of reduced NADPH. NADPH enables cells to counterbalance oxidative stress that can be triggered by several oxidant agents, and to preserve the reduced form of glutathione. NADPH is pivotal to the cellular antioxidative defence systems in most organisms. Since erythrocytes do not contain mitochondria, the pentose phosphate pathway is their only source of NADPH; therefore, defence against oxidative damage is dependent on G6PD.

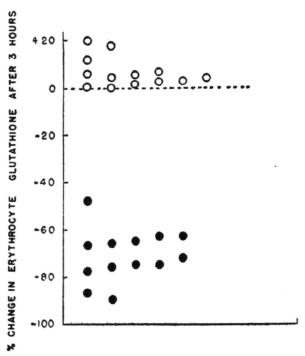

Fig. 2. Percentage change in reduced glutathione (GSH) in erythrocytes of 13 individuals with G6PD deficiency (solid circles) and 13 individuals with normal G6PD activity (open circles) after 3 hours of hydrogen peroxide diffusion (Cohen & Hochstein, 1961).

4. Animal model of anemia

4.1 Deficiency of antioxidant enzymes
4.1.1 Superoxide dismutase 1 (SOD1) deficiency

Among the known antioxidative proteins, superoxide dismutase (SOD) is thought to play a central role because of its ability to scavenge superoxide anions, the primary ROS generated from molecular oxygen in cells (Fridovich, 1995). SOD1-deficient mice have been generated by several groups. Unexpectedly, SOD1-deficient mice grow normally but develop female infertility (Ho et al., 1998; Matzuk et al., 1998), cochlear hair cell loss (McFadden et al., 1999), and vascular dysfunction (Didion et al., 2002). Adding to these phenotypes, SOD1-deficient mice exhibit severe anemia, even in infant mice (Iuchi et al., 2007; Starzyński et al., 2009). Anemia appears to be caused by shortened lifespan of erythrocytes. Increased ROS due to SOD1 deficiency makes their erythrocytes vulnerable to oxidative stress. In addition to SOD1 deficiency, GPx activity and protein levels of GPx1 were significantly lower in erythrocytes. Since GPx1 protein is prone to oxidative inactivation, oxidized GPx1 would be removed by the protease that degrades oxidized proteins in erythrocytes.

While most mammalian cells possess two intracellular SOD isoforms to protect against ROS, erythrocytes lack mitochondria and, as a result, carry only the SOD1 protein to scavenge superoxide anions. Erythrocytes of SOD1-deficient mice, therefore, face severe oxygen toxicity compared with other tissues. Erythrocytes that are hyperoxic bind oxygen in the lungs (~21%), and release oxygen in peripheral tissues, which are relatively hypoxic (~2%). Thus, erythrocytes undergo cyclic exposure to hyperoxic and hypoxic environments, generating large amounts of superoxide via auto-oxidation of hemoglobin.

The continuous destruction of oxidized erythrocytes in SOD1-deficient mice appears to induce the formation of autoantibodies against certain erythrocyte components, for example, carbonic anhydrase II, and the immune complex is deposited in the kidney glomeruli. Therefore, these mice exhibit autoimmune hemolytic anemia (AIHA)-like symptoms when they reach old age. This pathophysiological symptom is thought as a secondary effect of elevated oxidative stress in SOD1-deficient erythrocytes.

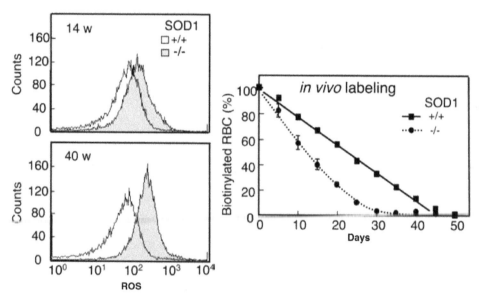

Fig. 3. Elevated ROS (left panels) and shortened lifespan (right panel) of erythrocytes in SOD1-deficient mice (Iuchi et al., 2007).

4.1.2 Catalase deficiency
Human erythrocytes contain large amounts of catalase. While the catalase and NADPH/GSH/GPx system is very important for disposal of H_2O_2 in human erythrocytes, genetic deficiencies of catalase do not predispose erythrocytes to peroxide-induced destruction (Jacob et al., 1965). Mice lacking the catalase gene develop normally (Ho et al., 2004). A link between catalase deficiency and anemia has not been reported.

4.1.3 Glutathione peroxidase-1 (GPx1) deficiency
The role of glutathione peroxidase in erythrocyte anti-oxidant defense was examined using erythrocytes from mice with genetically engineered disruption of the glutathione peroxidase-1 (GPx1) gene. Because GPx1 is the sole glutathione peroxidase in erythrocytes, all erythrocyte GSH peroxidase activity was eliminated. Oxidation of hemoglobin and membrane lipids was determined during oxidant challenge from cumene hydroperoxide and H_2O_2. As a result, no difference was detected between wild-type erythrocytes and GPx1–deficient erythrocytes,

even at high levels of H_2O_2 exposure. Thus, GPx1 appears to play little or no role in the defense of erythrocytes against exposure to peroxide (Johnson et al., 2000).

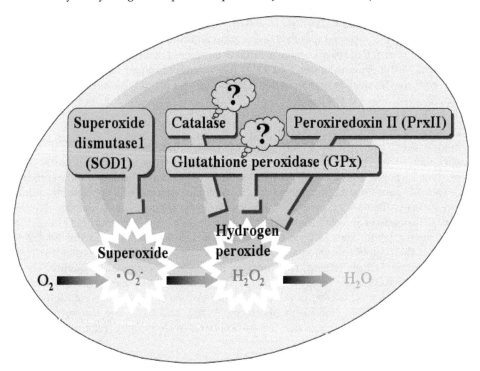

Fig. 4. Do SOD1 and PrxII actually work in erythrocytes?

4.1.4 Peroxiredoxin II (PrxII) deficiency

A number of proteins also protect cells against oxidative stress. SOD, GPx, and catalase are commonly known antioxidant enzymes and have been extensively characterized. Recently, a new family of antioxidative proteins, collectively referred to as Prxs (peroxiredoxins), have been identified. Six distinct gene products are known in the Prx family in mammals (Fujii & Ikeda, 2002). Thioredoxin-dependent peroxidase activity appears to be common to most Prx family members, and in addition, other divergent biological functions have been elucidated for individual Prx members. However, the most well-characterized function of Prx family members is the ability to modulate hydrogen peroxide signaling in response to various stimuli (Rhee et al., 2005).

Mice deficient in Prx II, which is abundantly expressed in all types of cells, were healthy in appearance and fertile. However, they had splenomegaly caused by the congestion of red pulp with hemosiderin accumulation. Erythrocytes from these mice contained markedly higher levels of ROS. The Prx II-deficient mice had significantly decreased hematocrit levels, but increased reticulocyte counts and erythropoietin levels, indicative of a compensatory action to maintain hematologic homeostasis in the mice (Lee et al., 2003).

For a long time, it was considered that catalase and GPx constitute the erythrocyte defense against H_2O_2, and there has been continuous debate about which of these is more significant

(Cohen & Hochstein, 1963; Gaetani et al., 1989; Gaetani et al., 1996). Until recently, little attention has been paid to the antioxidant role of Prxs in erythrocytes, even though Prx II is the third most abundant cytoplasmic erythrocyte protein. These mice possess fully functional catalase and GPx. Erythrocytes also possess PrxI and PrxVI, although at lower levels than PrxII. It is reported that PrxII expression and content were markedly increased in erythrocytes from β thalassemic mouse models compared with those in wild-type mice (Matte et al., 2010). This indicates that PrxII has a non-redundant function in protecting healthy erythrocytes against oxidative damage and plays a crucial role even in pathological conditions.

4.2 Deficiency of transcription factor

In many cases, transcriptional activation of genes that play an important role in detoxification of xenobiotics and defense against oxidative stress is mediated partly by the antioxidant response element (ARE). For example, AREs have been found in promoter sequences of genes including nicotinamide adenine dinucleotide phosphate–quinone oxidoreductase, heme oxygenase, glutathione-S-transferases, and glutamylcysteine synthetase (Favreau et al., 1995; Inamdar et al., 1996; Jaiswal et al., 1994; Mulcahy et al., 1995; Prestera et al., 1995). The ARE consensus sequence is very similar to the NF-E2–like sequence of the β globin locus control region, which was found to be essential for globin gene expression. Multiple proteins can interact with the NF-E2 consensus sequence. The cap 'n' collar (CNC)–bZIP factor family of proteins was identified from searches for proteins that bind and activate the NF-E2 site of the β-globin locus control region. This multiple-protein family includes p45NF-E2, NF-E2–related factor (Nrf)1, and Nrf2. The similarities among CNC family members are most notable in the basic-DNA binding region and another homology domain (Moi et al., 1994).

4.2.1 p45NF-E2 deficiency

p45NF-E2 is a member of the cap 'n' collar (CNC)-basic leucine zipper family of transcriptional activators that is expressed at high levels in various types of blood cells. It plays a crucial role in megakaryocyte maturation and platelet biogenesis. Mice with disruption of p45NF-E2 have severe platelet deficiency due to defective megakaryocyte maturation. In addition, p45NF-E2 knockout mice exhibit anemia characterized by the presence of hypochromic erythrocytes and reticulocytosis. Erythrocytes from p45NF-E2–deficient mice are sensitive to oxidative stress. Erythrocytes from p45NF-E2–deficient mice accumulated high levels of free radicals when exposed to oxidants, and this correlated with increased formation of met-Hb and loss of membrane deformability. In addition, severe anemia developed in p45NF-E2 deficient mice treated with oxidative-stress–inducing drugs, and mutant erythrocytes had decreased survival.

Because CNC factors may represent an important class of regulators of antioxidant gene expression by means of the ARE, one possibility is that p45NF-E2 is involved in regulating oxidative stress-response genes in erythrocytes. It is possible that a compensated hemolytic state contributes to the erythroid abnormalities observed in p45NF-E2 knockout mice.

4.2.2 Nrf2 deficiency

The NF-E2-related factor 2 (Nrf2) transcription factor regulates genes related to ROS scavenging and detoxification. Although Nrf2 is expressed widely and is important for cellular antioxidant potential, Nrf2 knockout mice develop and grow normally (Chan et al., 1996). Young Nrf2 knockout mice are not anemic, whereas targeted disruption of either NF-E2 or Nrf1 resulted in anemia. In aged mice, however, disruption of Nrf2 causes regenerative immune-mediated hemolytic anemia due to increased sequestration of damaged erythrocytes. Splenomegaly and spleen toxicity in Nrf2-deficient mice raised the possibility of hemolytic anemia and splenic extramedullary hematopoiesis in Nrf2-deficient mice. Nrf2-deficient erythrocytes are highly sensitive to H_2O_2-induced hemolysis in vitro, further suggesting that Nrf2-deficient erythrocytes are highly susceptible to stress. In addition, Nrf2-deficient erythrocytes showed increased met-Hb formation after incubation with high concentrations of H_2O_2, suggesting that Hb in Nrf2-deficient erythrocytes is more easily oxidized than that in Nrf2 WT erythrocytes (Lee et al., 2004). A unique feature of the Nrf2-ARE pathway (the programmed cell life pathway) (Li et al., 2002) is that it coordinately up-regulates many protective detoxification and antioxidant genes, which can synergistically increase the efficiency of the erythrocyte defense system against oxidative stress.

4.2.3 Nrf1 deficiency
Nrf1 knockout mice have also been reported to develop anemia in early stages of embryo, and they die in utero (Chan et al., 1998). Nrf1 knockout mice have abnormal fetal liver erythropoiesis as a result of a defect in the fetal liver microenvironment specific for erythroid cells. Anemic phenotype of Nrf1-deficient mice is not due to the oxidative stress in erythrocytes, but due to abnormal erythropoiesis.

5. Relationship between hereditary sideroblastic anemia and SOD2 deficiency

5.1 Hereditary sideroblastic anemia
Iron overload is a feature of human disorders including sideroblastic anemia (SA). Excess iron is toxic because it can catalyze the generation of ROS that damage cellular molecules. Some genetic lesions have been identified as causes of hereditary or acquired SA. As defined genetic lesions, dysfunction in one of the mitochondrial metabolic pathways has been observed: heme synthesis, iron homeostasis and transport, or electron transport. These lesions result in abnormal use of erythroid mitochondrial iron, causing pathologic iron deposition (Napier et al., 2005). Identified lesions affect nuclear-encoded mitochondrial proteins or the mitochondrial genome. The heme biosynthetic pathway was identified as a primary cause of SA. However, other pathways, including mitochondrial oxidative phosphorylation and iron–sulfur cluster biosynthesis, were also identified as primary defects in SAs. They may secondarily affect heme metabolism (Rouault & Tong, 2005; Martin, 2006). Two X-linked sideroblastic anemias (XLSAs) exist, one caused by mutations of an erythroid-specific form of the heme biosynthetic enzyme aminolevulinic acid (ALA)–synthase 2 (ALAS2) (Cotter et al., 1994), and one caused by mutation of a putative mitochondrial iron-transport protein, ATP-binding cassette, member 7 (ABC7) (Allikmets et al., 1999).

5.2 SOD2-deficiency anemia
SOD2-deficiency anemia is another example of mitochondrial dysfunction resulting in an erythroid-specific SA-like phenotype. Although genetically deficient mice of SOD1 have a normal lifespan along with exhibiting an anemic phenotype (Iuchi et al., 2007), inactivation of SOD2 results in embryonic or neonatal lethality. Because of its mitochondrial location, SOD2 is the principal defense against the toxicity of superoxide generated by oxidative

phosphorylation in mitochondria. The SOD2-deficient phenotype is associated with pathologic evidence of mitochondrial injury and oxidative damage to biomolecules, as well as severe damage to cardiac muscle. Hematopoietic stem cell-specific SOD2-deficient mice were generated by transplantation of SOD2-deficient mouse HSCs, and sideroblastic anemia-like symptom was the major phenotype in the transplanted animals (Friedman et al., 2001). This model suggests that oxidative stress in mitochondria affects the reduced heme biogenesis and accumulation of iron deposits in erythroid cells, and plays an important role in the pathogenesis of sideroblastic anemia.

It is interesting to note that peroxiredoxin II (Prx II), a member of the thioredoxin peroxidase family, was decreased in SOD2-deficient cells, but showed an increase with antioxidant treatment (Friedman et al., 2004). Knockout of Prx II causes hemolytic anemia (Lee et al., 2003) with evidence of increased oxidative damage to mature RBCs. This suggests that Prx II may be an important target of oxidative damage in SOD2-deficient cells. These findings suggest that mitochondrial dysfunction with excessive ROS production and with excess iron accumulation plays a critical role in causing SA.

6. Therapeutic supplementation of antioxidant for anemia

6.1 N-acetylcysteine (NAC) and its derivatives

N-acetylcysteine (NAC) is one of the precursors of GSH. In vitro and animal studies have demonstrated that treatment of blood cells with NAC increases the intracellular concentration of the reduced form of GSH and decreases oxidative stress (Amer et al., 2006; Nur et al., 2011). Treatment of sickle cell patients with NAC at a dose of 2,400 mg per day increased intracellular GSH and reduced dense cell formation (Pace et al., 2003). NAC is also effective for antioxidant enzyme-deficient mice. Administration of NAC (1.0% in drinking water) to SOD1-deficient mice significantly suppressed ROS in erythrocytes and partly improved the anemia (Iuchi et al., 2007).

Recently, several new derivatives of NAC have been developed. Among these new agents, the amide form of NAC, N-acetylcysteine amide (AD4), in which the carboxylic group is neutralized, is more lipophilic and has better membrane permeability than NAC. AD4 is also effective for its antioxidant effects. In vitro treatment of blood cells from β thalassemic patients with AD4 elevated the reduced glutathione (GSH) content of erythrocytes, platelets, and polymorphonuclear leukocytes, and reduced their ROS. These effects resulted in significantly reduced sensitivity of thalassemic erythrocytes to hemolysis and phagocytosis by macrophages. Intra-peritoneal injection of AD4 to β thalassemic mice reduced the parameters of oxidative stress. The superiority of AD4, compared with NAC, in reducing oxidative stress markers in thalassemic cells both in vitro and in vivo has been demonstrated (Amer, J. et al., 2008).

6.2 Vitamin E

Vitamin E, a fat-soluble antioxidant, has been identified as an essential erythropoietic factor for certain species of animals. Treatment with vitamin E increased the number of colony forming units of erythroid precursors, enhanced erythropoiesis, and thus corrected the experimentally induced anemia in an animal model. Results of some of clinical trials suggested that vitamin E might prevent some types of human anemia due to its putative role in promoting erythropoiesis, enhancing the stability of erythrocyte membrane proteins and lipids, and reducing oxidative stress-induced erythrocyte injury. Supplementation of vitamin E was tried for patients with some types of inherited hemolytic anemia. Some of these trials have shown that there was an improvement in hemolysis, as evidenced by longer erythrocyte lifespan, in elevated hemoglobin level, and decreased reticulocyte count (Corash et al., 1980; Hafez et al., 1986). On the other hand, some groups indicated no change in hematologic status after treatment with high doses of vitamin E (Newman et al., 1979; Johnson et al., 1983).

In patients suffering from homozygous β thalassemia, supplementation of vitamin E was effective in reducing plasma levels of lipid peroxidation end products and a significant improvement in the hemoglobin levels (Das et al., 2004). A 4- to 8-week-long supplementation with vitamin E given to children with various types of thalassemia was shown to decrease H_2O_2-mediated erythrocyte hemolysis and increase the resistance to oxidative damage. Supplementation with vitamin E in children suffering from sickle cell anemia was shown to reduce the percentage of sickled erythrocytes, increased resistance of erythrocytes to lysis, and enhanced blood hemoglobin concentration (Jilani & Iqbal, 2011).

7. Conclusion

In recent years, many studies have implicated oxidative stress in anemia complicated with some infectious diseases. For example, malaria infection results in decreased antioxidant enzymes and substances such as catalase, GPx, SOD, GSH, ascorbate, and plasma tocopherol. The development of new antioxidant drugs with a function based on ROS reduction might constitute a promising tool not only for hereditary anemia but also for the control of the infection-mediated anemia.

8. References

Allikmets, R., Raskind, W. H., Hutchinson, A., Schueck, N. D., Dean, M., & Koeller, D. M. (1999) Mutation of a putative mitochondrial iron transporter gene (ABC7) in X-linked sideroblastic anemia and ataxia (XLSA/A). Hum. Mo.l Gene.t 8, 743–749.

Amer, J., Atlas, D. & Fibach, E. (2008) N-acetylcysteine amide (AD4) attenuates oxidative stress in beta-thalassemia blood cells. Biochim. Biophys. Acta 1780, 249–255.

Amer, J., Ghoti, H., Rachmilewitz, E et al. (2006) Red blood cells, platelets and polymorphonuclear neutrophils of patients with sickle cell disease exhibit oxidative stress that can be ameliorated by antioxidants. Br. J. Haematol. 132, 108-113.

Arese, P., Turrini, F. & Schwarzer, E. (2005) Band 3/Complement-mediated recognition and removal of normally senescent and pathological human erythrocytes. Cell. Physiol. Biochem. 16, 133-146.

Bunn, H. F. & Jandl, J. H. (1967) Exchange of heme among hemoglobins and between hemoglobin and albumin. J. Biol. Chem. 243, 465–475.

Carrell, R.W., Winterbourn, C. C. & Rachmilewitz, E. A. (1975) Activated oxygen and hemolysis. Br. J. Hematol. 30, 259-264.

Chan, J. Y., Kwong, M., Lo, M., Emerson, R., Kuypers, F. A. (2001) Reduced oxidative-stress response in red blood cells from p45NFE2-deficient mice. Blood, 97, 2151-2158.

Chan, J. Y., Kwong, M., Lu, R., Chang, J., Wang, B., Yen, T. S., Kan, Y. W. (1998) Targeted disruption of the ubiquitous CNC-bZIP transcription factor, Nrf-1, results in anemia and embryonic lethality in mice. EMBO J, 17, 1779–1787.

Chan, K., Lu, R., Chang, J. C. & Kan, Y. W. (1996) NRF2, a member of the NFE2 family of transcription factors, is not essential for murine erythropoiesis, growth, and development. Proc. Natl. Acad. Sci. USA 93, 13943–13948.

Cohen, G. & Hochstein, P. (1963) Glutathione peroxidase: primary agent for elimination of hydrogen peroxide in erythrocytes. *Biochemistry.* 2, 1420-1428.

Corash, L., Spielberg, S. & Bartsocas, C. (1980) Reducedchronichaemo- lysisduring high-dosevitamin E administration in Mediterranean type glucose-6-phosphate dehydrogenase deficiency. *N. Engl. J. Med.* 303, 416-420.

Cotter, P. D., Rucknagel, D. L. & Bishop, D. F. (1994) X-linked sideroblastic anemia: identification of the mutation in the erythroid- specific delta-aminolevulinate synthase gene (ALAS2) in the original family described by Cooley. *Blood* 84, 3915-3924.

Das, N., Das Chowdhury, T., Chattopadhyay, A . & Datta, A. G. (2004) Attenuation of oxidative stress-induced changes in thalassemic erythrocytes by vitamin E. *Pol. J. Pharmacol.*, 56, 85-96.

Didion, S. P., Ryan, M. J., Didion, L. A., Fegan, P. E., Sigmund, C. D. & Faraci, F. M. (2002) Increased superoxide and vascular dysfunction in CuZnSOD- deficient mice. *Circ. Res.* 91, 938-944.

Favreau, L. V., Pickett, C. B. (1995) The rat quinone reductase antioxidant response element: identification of the nucleotide sequence required for basal andinducible activity and detection of antioxidant response element-binding proteins in hepatoma and non-hepatoma cell lines. *J Biol Chem.* 270, 24468-24474.

Friedman, J. S., Rebel, V. I., Derby, .R, Bell, K., Huang, T. T., Kuypers, F. A., Epstein, C. J. & Burakoff, S. J. (2001) Absence of mitochondrial superoxide dismutase results in a murine hemolytic anemia responsive to therapy with a catalytic antioxidant. *J. Exp. Med.* 193(8), 925-934.

Friedman, J. S., Lopez, M. F., Fleming, M. D., Rivera, A., Martin, F. M., Welsh, M. L., Boyd, A., Doctrow, S. R. & Burakoff, S. J. (2004) SOD2-deficiency anemia: protein oxidation and altered protein expression reveal targets of damage, stress response, and antioxidant responsiveness. *Blood* 104(8), 2565-73.

Fridovich, I. (1995) Superoxide radical and superoxide dismutases. *Annu. Rev. Biochem.* 64, 97-112.

Fujii, J. & Ikeda, Y. (2002) Advances in our understanding of peroxiredoxin, a multifunctional, mammalian redox protein. *Redox Rep.* 7(3), 123-130.

Gaetani, G. F., Ferraris, A. M., Rolfo, M., Mangerini, R., Arena, S. & Kirkman, H. N. (1996) Predominant role of catalase in the disposal of hydrogen peroxide within human erythrocytes. *Blood.* 87, 1595-1599.

Gaetani, G. F., Galiano, S., Canepa, L., Ferraris, A. M. & Kirkman, H. N. (1989) Catalase and glutathione-peroxidase are equally active in detoxification of hydrogen- peroxide in human-erythrocytes. *Blood.* 73, 334-339.

Hafez, M., Amar, E. S., Zedan, M., Hammad, H., Sorour, A. H., el-Desouky, E. S. &Gamil, N. (1986) Improved erythrocyte survival with combined vitamin E and selenium therapy in children with glucose-6-phosphate dehydrogenase deficiency and mild chronic hemolysis. *J. Pediatr.* 108(4), 558-561.

Hebbel, R. P. (1985) Auto-oxidation and a membrane-associated "Fenton reagent": A possible explanation for development of membrane lesions in sickle erythrocytes. *Clinics in Hematol* 14, 129-140.

Ho, Y. S., Gargano, M., Cao, J., Bronson, R. T., Heimler, I. & Hutz, R. J. (1998) Reduced fertility in female mice lacking copper-zinc superoxide dismutase. *J. Biol. Chem.* 273, 7765–7769.

Ho, Y. S., Xiong, Y., Ma, W., Spector, A. & Ho, D. S. (2004) Mice Lacking Catalase Develop Normally but Show Differential Sensitivity to Oxidant Tissue Injury. *J Biol Chem.* 279 (31), 32804–32812.

Inamdar, N. M., Ahn, Y. I., Alam, J. (1996) The heme-responsive element of the mouse heme oxygenase-1 gene is an extended AP-1 binding site that resembles the recognition sequences for MAF and NF-E2 transcription factors. *Biochem Biophys Res Commun.* 221, 570-576.

Iuchi, Y., Okada, F., Onuma, K., Onoda, T., Asao, H., Kobayashi, M. & Fujii, J. (2007) Elevated oxidative stress in erythrocytes due to an SOD1 deficiency causes anemia and triggers autoantibody production. *Biochem. J.* 402: 219-227.

Jacob, H. S., Ingbar, S. H. & Jandl, J. H. (1965) Oxidative hemolysis and erythrocyte metabolism in hereditary acatalasia. *J Clin Invest.* 44, 1187-1199.

Jaiswal, A.K. (1994) Antioxidant response element. *Biochem Pharmacol.* 48, 439-444.

Jilani, T. & Iqbal, M. P. (2011) Does vitamin E have a role in treatment and prevention of anemia's ? *Pak. J. Pharm. Sci.* 24(2), 237-242.

Johnson, G. J., Vatassery, G. R., Finkel, B. & Allen, D. W. (1983) High-dose vitamin E does not decrease the rate of chronic hemolysisin G-6-PD deficiency. *N. Engl. J. Med.* 303, 432-436.

Johnson, R. M., Goyette, G., Ravindranath, Y. & Ho, Y. (2000) Red cells from glutathione peroxidase-1-deficient mice have nearly normal defenses against exogenous peroxides. *Blood.* 96, 1985-1988.

Lee, T. H., Kim, S. U., Yu, S. L., Kim, S. H., Park, S., Moon, H. B., Dho, S. H., Kwon, K. S., Kwon, H. J., Han, Y. H. et al. (2003) Peroxiredoxin II is essential for sustaining life span of erythrocytes in mice. *Blood* 101, 5033–5038.

Lee, J. M., Chan, K., Kan, Y. W., Johnson, J. A. (2004) Targeted disruption of Nrf2 causes regenerative immune-mediated hemolytic anemia. *Proc Natl Acad Sci USA*, 101(26), 9751-9756.

Li, J., Lee, J. M., Johnson, J. A. (2002) Microarray analysis reveals an antioxidant responsive element-driven gene set involved in conferring protection from an oxidative stress-induced apoptosis in IMR-32 cells. *J. Biol. Chem.* 277, 388–394.

Martin, F. M., Bydlon, G. & Friedman, J. S. (2006) SOD2-deficiency sideroblastic anemia and red blood cell oxidative stress. *Antioxid. Redox Signal.* 8(7-8), 1217-1225.

Matte, A., Low, P. S., Turrini, F., Bertoldi, M., Campanella, M. E., Spano, D., Pantaleo, A., Siciliano, A. & De Franceschi L. (2010) Peroxiredoxin-2 expression is increased in beta-thalassemic mouse red cells but is displaced from the membrane as a marker of oxidative stress. *Free Radic Biol Med.* 2010 49(3), 457-466.

Matzuk, M. M., Dionne, L., Guo, Q., Kumar, T. R. & Lebovitz, R. M. (1998) Ovarian function in superoxide dismutase 1 and 2 knockout mice. *Endocrinology* 139, 4008–4011.

McFadden, S. L., Ding, D., Reaume, A. G., Flood, D. G. & Salvi, R. J. (1999) Age-related cochlear hair cell loss is enhanced in mice lacking copper/zinc superoxide dismutase. *Neurobiol. Aging.* 20, 1–8.

Moi, P., Chan, K., Asunis, I., Cao, A., Kan, Y. W. (1994) Isolation of NF-E2- related factor 2 (Nrf2), a NF-E2-like basic leucine zipper transcriptional activator that binds to the tandem NF-E2/AP1 repeat of the beta-globin locus control region.Proc. *Natl. Acad. Sci. USA* 91, 9926–9930.

Mulcahy, R. T., Gipp, J. J. (1995) Identification of a putative antioxidant response element in the 59-flanking region of the human gamma- glutamylcysteine synthetase heavy subunit gene. *Biochem Biophys Res Commun.* 209, 227-233.

Napier, I., Ponka, P. & Richardson, D. R. (2005) Iron trafficking in the mitochondrion: Novel pathways revealed by disease. *Blood* 105, 1867–1874.

Newman, G. J., Newman, T. B., Bowie, L. J. & Mendelsohn, J. (1979) An examinationof the role of vitamin E in G-6-PD deficiency. *Clin. Biochem.* 12, 149-151.

Nur, E., Biemond, B. J., Otten, H. M., Brandjes, D. P & Schnog, J. B. (2011) Oxidative stress in sickle cell disease; pathophysiology and potential implications for disease management. *Am. J. Hematol.* 86, 484-489.

Pace, B. S., Shartava, A., Pack-Mabien, A., Mulekar, M., Ardia, A. & Goodman, S. R. (2003) Effects of N-acetylcysteine on dense cell formation in sickle cell disease. *Am. J. Hematol.* 73(1), 26-32.

Pantaleo, A., Giribaldi, G., Mannu, F., Arese P. & Turrini, F. (2008) Naturally occurring anti-band 3 antibodies and red blood cell removal under physiological and pathological conditions. *Autoimmun. Rev.* 7(6), 457-462.

Prestera, T. & Talalay, P. (1995) Electrophile and antioxidant regulation of enzymes that detoxify carcinogens. *Proc. Nat.l Acad. Sci. USA.* 92, 8965-8969

Rhee, S. G., Kang, S. W., Jeong, W., Chang, T. S., Yang, K. S. & Woo, H. A. (2005) Intracellular messenger function of hydrogen peroxide and its regulation by peroxiredoxins. *Curr. Opin. Cell Biol.* 17, 183–189.

Rice-Evans, C. & Baysal, E. (1987) Iron-mediated oxidative stress In erythrocytes. *Biochem. J.* 244, 191-196.

Rouault, T. A. & Tong, W. H. (2005) Opinion: Iron-sulphur cluster biogenesis and mitochondrial iron homeostasis. *Nat. Rev. Mol. Cell. Biol.* 6, 345–351.

Rund, D., & Rachmilewitz, E. (2005) β-Thalassemia. *N. Engl. J. Med.* 353, 1135-1146.

Rusanova, I., Escames, G., Cossio, G., de Borace, R. G., Moreno, B., Chahboune, M., López, L. C., Díez, T. & Acuña-Castroviejo, D. (2010) Oxidative stress status, clinical outcome, and β-globin gene cluster haplotypes in pediatric patients with sickle cell disease. *Eur J Haematol.* 85(6), 529-537.

Scot, M. D. (2006) H2O2 injury in β thalassemic erythrocytes: Protective role of catalase and the prooxidant effects of GSH. *Free Radic. Biol. & Med.* 40, 1264–1272. Rund, D., & Rachmilewitz, E. (2005) β-Thalassemia. *N. Engl. J. Med.* 353, 1135-1146.

Shinar, E. & Rachmilewitz, E. (1990) Oxidative denaturation of red blood cells in thalassemia. *Semin. Hematol.* 27(1), 70-82.

Starzyński, R. R., Canonne-Hergaux, F., Willemetz, A., Gralak, M. A., Woliński, J., Styś, A., Olszak, J. & Lipiński, P. (2009) Haemolytic anaemia and alterations in hepatic iron metabolism in aged mice lacking Cu,Zn-superoxide dismutase. *Biochem. J.* 420(3), 383-390.

Wood, K. C. & Granger, D. N. (2007) Sickle cell disease: Role of reactive oxygen and nitrogen metabolites. *Clinic Exp Pharmacol Physiol* 34, 926–932.

Iron and Nitric Oxide in Anemia
of Chronic Disease (ACD)

Oluyomi Stephen Adeyemi[1], Adenike Faoziyat Sulaiman[2]
and Musbau Adewumi Akanji[2]
[1]Redeemer's University, Department of Chemical Sciences, Mowe,
[2]University of Ilorin, Department of Biochemistry, Ilorin
Nigeria

1. Introduction

Anemia of chronic disease (ACD) may also be referred to as anemia of inflammation and this develops in subjects with diseases involving acute or chronic immune activation. Anemia, which could be described as an immunopathological feature in most established infection, may also be a consequence of host response to invading pathogens. Infections with pathogens normally activate macrophages triggering a strong cytokine production among which are tumor necrosis factor (TNF), γ-interferon (IFN-γ) and nitric oxide (NO). The immune response mounted against such infections is required for parasite clearance but its persistence can cause collateral damage to the host with occurrence of anemia as the major pathology. Inflammation results as a part of this natural immune response. The inflammation triggers the release of chemicals that signal the iron regulation mechanism to adopt a defense mode. Thus this type of anemia is usually characterised by an imbalance between erythrophagocytosis and erythropoiesis, which is linked to, perturbed iron (Fe) homeostasis including altered Fe sequestration and recycling by macrophages and/or sustained and overproduction of NO. The exact mechanism of ACD is not fully understood although studies suggest that the syndrome may partly be due to the influence of hepcidin production on iron metabolism. Moreover complex relationships between Fe and NO has been demonstrated and may be linked to iron deficient anemia during infection.

Both iron and nitric oxide play important roles in the progression and outcome of ACD essentially through the promotion of free radical generation and/or altered homeostasis. Increased iron status may promote free hydroxyl radical generation in cellular systems and thus potentiate cellular damage. Subsequently continuous and sustained production of nitric oxide resulting from persistent infection could contribute to oxidative damage via the formation of peroxynitrite, a very reactive free radical, which may promote lipid peroxidation of key biomolecules and membranes. It should also be noted that production of nitric oxide during infection episodes affects iron metabolism and vice versa. This suggest that a delicate homeostatic balance exist between iron and nitric oxide in living cells such that a disruption or perturbation of this strictly regulated balance would physiologically affect the cellular system. The fact that strong link that has been demonstrated between iron and nitric oxide indicates that the duo play crucial physiological roles in cellular processes.

2. Iron metabolism

Iron metabolism may be referred to as the set of biochemical reactions maintaining the homeostasis of iron. Iron is an essential but potentially harmful nutrient. The control of this necessary but potentially toxic substance is an important part of many aspects of human health and disease. Iron contributes to many important physiologic functions in the body essentially because of its unusual flexibility to serve as both an electron donor and acceptor. Iron being critical to a number of synthetic and enzymatic processes by play unique roles in electron transfer and oxygen utilization as heme and non-heme bound proteins. Although most of the body iron is part of hemoglobin molecule where iron serves a key role in oxygen transport, it is also required for proper maintenance of immune functions affecting leukocytes, endothelial cells and cytokine production. Iron also have capacity to promote free radical generation through the Fenton and/or Haber-Weiss reactions, thereby triggering secondary chain reactions in the oxidative modification of lipids, proteins and DNA within cellular systems. Unless appropriately chelated or removed, iron, due to its catalytic action in one-electron redox reactions, plays a key role in the formation of harmful oxygen radicals that may ultimately cause oxidative damage to vital cell structures. To ensure iron availability and to eliminate the toxicity of free iron in addition to its accessibility for invading pathogens, mammals have evolved a strictly regulated system for iron homeostasis. Metabolism of iron is highly regulated within narrow limits. Iron can be recycled and thus conserved by the body. Cellular systems are equipped with exclusive mechanisms that maintain adequate amounts of iron for synthesis of physiologically functional iron-containing molecules and yet keep "free iron" at its lowest possible concentration. Many proteins, hormones and iron itself have been demonstrated to affect iron metabolism by various mechanisms at different regulatory levels. Physiologically, the cellular system acquires iron from plasma glycoprotein, transferrin (Tf). In most cases body iron is sequestered and recycled by the reticuloendothelial system, which breaks down senescent red blood cells (RBCs). Iron metabolism in mammals is a highly regulated phenomenon. This process, which ensures iron availability to meet cellular demand, is necessary in order to eliminate toxicity and free accessibility for invading pathogens.

Iron demands are met obviously through two main sources; acquisition from diet, iron is an absolute requirement for most forms of life, including humans, most microorganisms, plants and animals; therefore it is found in a wide variety of food sources. And also from destruction of heme and non-heme proteins which in most cases are being recycled for reutilization.

2.1 Iron acquisition from diet

Dietary iron represents a viable source for acquisition of iron to meet the body demands. The absorption of dietary iron is a variable and dynamic process that ensures the amount of iron absorbed compared to the amount ingested is typically low. The efficiency of iron absorption from diet depends largely on the source and demand for iron. Heme iron (obtainable from animal and plant foods) is best absorbed compared to non-heme iron (iron salts). Dietary iron is absorbed in the duodenum by enterocytes of the mucosal cells. The dietary iron must be part of a protein or be in its ferrous (Fe^{2+}) state in order to be absorbed. An enzyme, ferric reductase located on the enterocytes' brush border, Dcytb, reduces ferric Fe^{3+} to Fe^{2+} by lowering the pH. A transport protein called divalent metal transporter-1 (DMT-1 also called Nramp-2) then transport the iron across the enterocyte's cell membrane and into the cell cytosol. The mucosal cells can either store the iron as ferritin which is accomplished by oxidizing Fe^{2+} to Fe^{3+} and subsequent binding to apoferritin to form ferritin (FHC) or translocate the iron through ferroportin-1 (FPN-1) to the portal circulation, which is finally delivered to tissues and the erythroid bone marrow. Hephaestin, a ferroxidase found in the mucosal cells and capable of oxidizing Fe^{2+} to Fe^{3+} may assist ferroportin-1 in transfer of iron. Each of the steps involved in dietary iron acquisition is strictly regulated in response to body need for iron. For instance, cells in response to iron deficiency anemia produce more Dcytb, DMT-1 and ferroportin-1 thus implicating genetic involvement. Several factors including total iron stores, the extent to which bone marrow is producing new red blood cells, the concentration of hemoglobin in the blood, and the oxygen content of the blood all contribute to the rate of iron absorption through the mucosal cells. Infection or inflammation may also affect the rate of iron absorption from diet. Lesser iron is usually absorbed during inflammation and/or infection episodes leading to ACD precipitation. Dcytb is confined to iron transport across the duodenum, while ferroportin-1 is distributed throughout the body on all iron storing cells suggesting that ferroportin-1 is central to cellular iron availability. And indeed, recent discoveries have indicated inflammation leading to hepcidin-induced restriction on iron release from enterocytes via the regulation of ferroportin-1 as responsible for ACD.

2.2 Iron bound proteins

Iron is usually bound to hemoglobin, myoglobin, cytochromes, transferrin, lactoferrin and/or ferritin to restrict pathogen access to iron, although most microorganisms or pathogens have developed sophisticated iron-acquiring system that are able to compete successfully with iron-binding proteins of the host. In mammals hemoglobin of red blood cells contain more than 60% of body iron. Much of the remaining is in storage form in ferritin. In physiological conditions, tissue macrophages, in particular liver-associated Kupffer cells recover Fe^{2+} via engulfment of senescent red blood cells (RBCs) from circulation. In addition, these cells internalize the iron-containing hemoglobin; degrade it extracting Fe^{2+} through the action of heme-oxygenase-1 (HO-1) resulting in the release of ferrous iron (Fe^{2+}), carbon (II) oxide and bilverdin. Iron is then transported from the phagosome into the cytosol via the DMT-1, the main Fe^{2+} transporter, from where it can be either stored intracellularly via ferritin (FHC) or exported extracellularly via ferroportin-1(FPN-1) depending on the demand for iron. The extracellular Fe^{2+} after conversion to ferric iron (Fe^{3+}) through ceruloplasmin (CP), will bind to transferrin (Tf) and transported mainly to the bone marrow to fuel erythropoiesis. Consequently, limitations in iron (Fe^{3+}) availability may exert a strong negative impact on erythropoiesis and contribute to ACD. Hence maintaining physiological levels of RBCs relies on a subtle balance between RBC uptake and RBC generation as well as iron homeostasis.

Unique to iron homeostasis are cytosolic iron regulatory proteins (IRP1 and IRP2). These proteins, which are responsive to circulating iron levels, affect iron metabolism by binding to specific nucleotide sequences, termed iron-responsive elements (IREs). Iron-responsive elements (IREs) are usually present in mRNAs for numerous proteins involved in iron metabolism. The binding of IRP1 and IRP2 to IREs affect proteins involved in iron uptake (transferrin receptor-1; TfR1 and DMT-1), utilization (erythroid d-aminolevulinic acid synthase), storage (ferritin) and export (ferroportin-1). IRP1 is a 98-kDa bifunctional protein with mutually exclusive functions of RNA binding and aconitase activity and shares a 30%

identity with mitochondrial aconitase an enzyme of the Krebs cycle. IRP2, a second IRE-binding protein, was initially identified in rat hepatocytes, and had been cloned from a variety of mammalian tissues and cells subsequently. Recent discoveries have shown that IRP2 shares 62% amino acid sequence identity with IRP1 but differs in a unique way by possessing a 73-amino acid insertion in its N-terminal region as well as lacking the [Fe-S] cluster. IRP2 does not have aconitase activity, probably due to the absence of the [Fe-S] cluster. The Fe-S cluster in IRP1 may serve to sense iron level signals. Observations from the several investigations implicated cellular iron as an important factor in the interactions of IRPs with IREs with a consequence affecting the regulation of iron metabolism. When cellular iron becomes depleted, IRP1 and 2 acquire high affinity binding state. The binding of IRPs to the IRE in the 5`- untranslated region (UTR) of ferritin mRNA blocks the translation of ferritin, whereas the association of IRPs with IREs in the 3`- UTR of TfR mRNA stabilizes this transcript. On the other hand, when intracellular iron is abundant, IRP1 acquires aconitase activity and loses IRE binding activity, while IRP2 is degraded, resulting in efficient translation of ferritin mRNA and rapid degradation of TfR mRNA. Also contributing to the regulation of systemic iron homeostasis is the circulating peptide hormone, hepcidin. Hepcidin is usually increased during inflammatory conditions. This ensures cellular iron effluxes are limited by (i) binding to ferroportin-1 and (ii) inducing its internalization.

3. Influence of iron and nitric oxide interaction on anemia

RBCs circulate throughout the body engaged in gaseous exchange, oxygen transport, and carbon (iv) oxide removal. Erythropoiesis (Epo) must maintain steady state levels of circulating RBCs and respond to acute challenges. The bone marrow is a highly dynamic organ that produces two to three million red cells every second. These red cells are filled with haemoglobin and are replaced after 75–150 days. This process is controlled by the hypoxia sensing mechanism of the kidney, which responds by modulating the output of Epo, which in turn determines the level of erythropoietic activity. When red cell production fails to match red cell destruction, the result is anaemia.

Iron deficiency anaemia is one of the most common disorders in the world. It however remains an under managed feature of many gastroenterological conditions. About one third of inflammatory bowel disease (IBD) patients suffer from recurrent anaemia. Anaemia has significant impact on the quality of life of affected patients. Chronic fatigue, a frequent IBD symptom itself, is commonly caused by anaemia and may debilitate patients as much as abdominal pain or diarrhoea. Both iron deficiency and anaemia of chronic disease (ACD) contribute mostly to the development of anaemia in IBD. Cobalamin or folate deficiency and various other causes of anaemia such as haemolysis occur infrequently. IBD associated anaemia has been successfully controlled with a combination of iron sucrose and erythropoietin, which then positively affect the misled immune response in IBD.

NO is known to increase the affinity of the intracellular iron-regulatory protein for iron-responsive elements in transferrin receptor and ferritin mRNAs, and a recent study has indicated that NO may affect iron metabolism through disruption of the iron-sulfur complex of iron-regulatory protein 1.

The effects of NO on the regulation of cellular iron metabolism and on the erythropoiesis in anemia of chronic disease has been described extensively; however, there are few studies on the NO production during the various stages of iron deficiency anemia and during iron supplementation. Moreover, data for correlation coefficients between NO production and erythropoiesis in iron deficiency anemia are limited.

3.1 Infection influences iron homeostasis leading to anemia

Infections or inflammation conditions in most cases are characterized by anemia (ACD) with profound changes in iron homeostasis usually mediated by cytokines. Following n exposure to a wave of pathogen particles, the host immune system becomes activated leading to the production of cytokines initially by the T-helper cells type-1 (Th-1) and subsequently by T-helper cells type-2 (Th-2). The initial activation of macrophages promotes largely the production of pro-inflammatory cytokines. These cytokines including mainly tumor necrosis factor (TNF), γ-interferon (IFN-γ) and nitric oxide (NO) are key to host defence against the invading pathogens but on the other hand are crucial to promoting inflammatory condition. Inflammation, being a major pathogenic feature during chronic infection may ensue secondary to release of these pro-inflammatory signals by activated macrophages. Also noteworthy is the fact that though the released cytokines are meant to provide an environment necessary for parasite clearance but may also have some physiological effects which include the alteration of iron and subsequently nitric oxide homeostasis with far reaching consequence to the initiation and progression of ACD.

Central to iron homeostasis is the activation of macrophages essentially following exposure to infection. Macrophages are normally responsible for the processing of hemoglobin iron from senescent red blood cells (RBCs) and subsequent supply to the bone marrow for erythropoiesis. As explained earlier, the intracellular iron homeostasis is under the control of cytoplasmic iron regulatory proteins (IRP1 and IRP2), which regulate the expression of several proteins by binding to iron-responsive elements (IREs) on the respective mRNA. Furthermore in addition to its activity being regulated by cellular iron, cytokines also modulate the binding activity of IRP. Cytokines are produced by activated macrophages following contact with infectious agent. The immune cells so activated release cytokines among which is the nitric oxide (NO), tumor necrosis factor-alpha (TNF-α) and interleukin-1 (IL-1) amongst others. The T-helper cells type-1 (Th-1)-derived cytokines have been demonstrated to also affect iron homeostasis by different mechanisms. Interleukin-1 (IL-1) and tumor necrosis factor (TNF) are able to induce hypoferramia by modulating iron metabolism. Pro-inflammatory and anti-inflammatory cytokines produced by T-helper cells type-1 and 2 respectively are major contributors to development of ACD by influencing iron homeostasis. Cytokines do not only affect iron metabolism, but also have inhibitory effects on erythropoiesis by blocking proliferation and differentiation of erythroid progenitor cells limiting their ability to respond to erythropoietin as well as causing deficiency in the production of erythropoietin.

The mononuclear phagocytes acquire iron as a result of erythrophagocytosis during the normal process of removal of senescent blood red cells (RBCs). However the mechanisms involved in the liberation of iron by these cells in order for it to be returned to the circulation is yet to be understood clearly. It is assumed that during inflammatory disease or infection, there is tendency for macrophages to retain more iron in order to restrict pathogen access and this can eventually lead to anemia (ACD).

However, the ability of macrophage-produced nitric oxide (NO) in aiding the release of iron taken up by macrophages through phagocytosis and thereby contributing greatly to the maintenance of iron homeostasis have been demonstrated by several investigators. The role of NO in such scenario involving the reduction of ferritin synthesis and mobilization for intracellular iron seem to oppose the effect of other cytokines such as tumor necrosis factor-alpha (TNF-α) and interleukin-1 (IL-1) which promote iron retention through increased ferritin synthesis. NO production by macrophages is inducible upon introduction of foreign or infectious agent. The implication is that, when an active infection leading to activated macrophages stimulate the production of cytokines in order to get rid of the infectious agent and/or infection, NO acts in opposition to the other cytokines with a resultant effect of maintaining iron homeostasis. Whereas the other cytokines such as tumor necrosis factor-alpha (TNF-α) and interleukin-1 (IL-1) act in a concerted manner to ensure iron sequestration and retention by macrophages so as to minimise the iron level available to invading parasites and by so doing disrupt iron homeostasis, the NO counterbalances these effects by ensuring that iron deficit is minimal essentially through increasing the expression of transferrin receptor (TfR), reduction of ferritin synthesis and activation of IRP1.

4. Iron sequestration during infection

Regulating iron balance is necessary especially during infection. Invading pathogens require iron for replication and establishment of infection. Thus it is essential to regulate iron balance such that there is sufficient iron to meet body demands without making too much available to the invading parasites. Although divergent views and conflicting data exist as to the relationship between iron deficiency and infection, recent discoveries have demonstrated that iron depletion protects against and could control infection as well as minimise inflammatory related conditions. Beyond this, the interaction between host and infectious agent is an exciting and complex phenomenon. Yet no theory or experimental model has fully explained it. Several lines of evidence existing illustrate the unique role that iron plays in modulating the battle for survival between mammalian host and the invading pathogens with each organism displaying a unique and competitive mechanism for iron acquisition and maintenance. These mechanisms, which involve enormous genetic investments, are iron responsive and thus able to adapt to the different phases of infection with a variety of tactics on both sides. For instance, in response to poor iron availability in host, pathogens produce siderophores to take the element from host proteins. In response, the mammalian protein lipocalin-2 binds to several kinds of siderophores preventing the pathogen from accessing siderophores-bound iron. However, to evade this strategy, some pathogens produce a glycosylated form of the siderophores preventing its sequestration by lipocalin-2.

5. Role of nitric oxide in modulating iron regulatory proteins

In Biological systems, Nitric Oxide (NO), a small free-radical molecule, has been implicated in a vast array of cellular activities, which ranges from acting as a cytotoxic host defence molecule to being an intercellular signal. Two major routes of NO delivery to cells and tissues have being identified; this could be via Nitric oxide donors as: S-nitroso-N-acetyl Penicillamine (SNAP) and sodium nitroprusside (SNP) or via L-arginine in a reaction catalyzed by nitric oxide synthase.

The activity of iron regulatory protein (IRP), is modulated by both NO donors, SNAP and SNP. This may consequently affect iron uptake through transferrin receptor expression. IRP-

1 and IRP-2 are used by cells, to adjust intracellular iron concentration to levels that are adequate for their metabolic needs, but below the toxicity threshold. The proteins therefore, not only sense the status of cytoplasmic iron but also controls Ferritin and transferrin receptor.

The element regulated by the two IRPs, Fe, is essential for all fundamental and vital activities in the cells, so much so that, its deprivation threatens cell survival. While low iron body stores results in iron deficiency, a number of disease states have been pathogenically linked to excess body iron stores. These include acquired or genetic iron overload as well as delocalization of intracellular iron as seen in inflammation and atherosclerosis.

The Two-sided element can be of an advantage or disadvantage to the cell, depending on whether it serves as a micronutrient (advantage) or as a catalyst of free radical reactions (disadvantage). Oxygen radical generation is not the only type of cellular free radical known; the production of nitrogen radicals has also being established. The capacity of readily exchanging electrons makes iron not only essential for fundamental cell functions, but also a potential catalyst for chemical reactions involving free-radical formation and subsequent oxidative stress and cell damage. Cellular iron levels are therefore carefully regulated not only to maintain the body's required concentrations but also to minimize the pool of potentially toxic 'free iron'.

Iron and nitric oxide are intimately associated in various biological processes. Nitric oxide is one of the major pathophysiological stimuli that modulate the activity of IRP-1, a key effector molecule involved in the regulation of intracellular iron metabolism. IRP-1 is a cytoplasmic aconitase (converting citrate into isocitrate) when it contains a [4Fe-4S] cluster, and an RNA-binding protein after complete removal of the metal center. By binding to specific mRNA sequences, the iron responsive elements (IREs), IRP-1 modulates ferritin mRNA translation and transferrin receptor stability.

Contrarily, IRP-2 does not assemble a cluster nor possess aconitase activity, despite structural and functional similarities to IRP-1, it however possess a distinct pattern of tissue expression and is modulated via proteasome-mediated degradation. NO preferentially targets [Fe-S] clusters and the inhibition of aconitase is involved in the cytotoxic effect of NO. Its involvement in a variety of physiological and pathological processes necessitates establishing the role it plays in the IRP-mediated regulation of iron metabolism. The loss of IRP-2 is highly expressed in macrophages even when IRP-1 is activated, this may not be unconnected with the fact that, the improved ferritin synthesis and a decreased transferrin receptor mRNA is accompanied by cytokine-mediated activation of macrophages. While down-regulation of IRP-1 protein levels by NO may have a role to play, IRP-2 has a greater affinity for target IREs.

NO has a number of effects on the key regulators of cellular iron homoeostasis, IRP-1 and IRP-2 in response to fluctuations in the level of the 'labile iron pool', as a result various agents and conditions may affect IRP activity, thereby modulating iron and oxygen radical levels in different patho-biological states. The number of mRNAs regulated through IRE-IRP interactions is on the increase, thereby expanding the role of IRPs from just being iron-regulatory proteins to other roles in essential metabolic pathways.

For instance, the concentration of NO is regulated in the respiratory chain (RC) by a balance between its production and its utilization. This in turn regulates mitochondrial oxygen uptake and energy supply. Cell damage resulting from high concentrations of NO involves inhibition of a number of cellular processes, such as DNA synthesis and mitochondrial respiration.

While some of these effects may be direct, others arise from the reaction of NO with O_2 to form peroxynitrite (ONOO-). NO and ONOO- can cause damage thereby disrupting cellular functions. To differentiate the sites at which both interact with the respiratory chain from the mechanism of inhibition, NO binds to cytochrome c oxidase, the terminal member of the mitochondrial respiratory chain, and NO, as recently reported, may act as an inhibitor of this enzyme at physiological concentrations in a reversible and competitive reaction with oxygen.

ONOO- however has little or no effect on cytochrome C oxidase, but inhibits respiratory complexes I–III in an apparently reversible manner. Reaction of NO with molecular oxygen results in oxidation products that can react with low molecular weight and protein-associated thiols, such as cysteine, glutathione, and albumin, to form S-nitrosothiols. It is now established that NO shows antioxidant properties, contrary to the deleterious effects of the reactive nitrogen oxide species formed from NO and oxygen.

Since NO biochemistry is dominated by free-radical reactions, its interaction with other free-radical species could lead to either inhibition or potentiation of oxidative damage effect. Iron–sulfur clusters have long been recognized as molecular targets of NO.

Several reports have shown that NO does increase IRP-1 activity and two possible mechanism or hypothesis of such activation have been suggested for the NO effect: The first is the induction of cytoplasmic aconitase's disassembly and switching to IRP-1 when NO bind to its Fe–S cluster, while the second is NO induction of cellular iron release and reduction of the labile iron pool, effects that would be compensated by spontaneous disassembly of the aconitase cluster or by the synthesis of cluster-free IRP-1. A decrease in aconitase activity may not always be accompanied by a consistent increase in IRP-1 activity, as this is dependent on the iron status of the cell. Iron depleted cells, for instance, may respond to nitrogen reactive species by increasing their IRP-1 activity, a process reflecting disassembly of the aconitase cluster by NO or ONOO-.

IRP-2 is invariably inactivated by NO or ONOO- or in macrophages committed to the formation of reactive nitrogen species after stimulation with cytokines. This effect is attributed to redox modifications of –SH residues exposed by the cluster-free IRP-2, and to redox modifications followed by proteasome-mediated protein degradation. Thus, IRP-2 degradation may account for the enhanced ferritin synthesis and reduced TfR mRNA content observed in cytokine-stimulated macrophages producing NO and ONOO-. The effect of nitrogen reactive species on IRP may therefore explain the iron sequestration pattern that characterizes macrophages under inflammatory conditions. Current on-going patho-physiological studies across the globe will in the nearest future reveal how to use this mechanism to minimize formation and release of free radicals in diseased tissues.

6. Concluding remark

The pathophysiology of ACD may largely be attributed to iron homeostasis, which is affected by several factors. The foregoing discussion has clearly depicted the faces of underlying and intriguing factors that work independently or interdependently to contribute to the initiation and progression of ACD. These factors among which are cytokines produced mainly by activated macrophages in response to prevailing cellular condition at a particular time, more often are responsible for ACD development and also may predict its outcome. In normal physiological state, abundance of iron limits its acquisition from diet and promotes ferritin synthesis while nitric oxide working in concert with iron proteins increases mobilization for intracellular iron. However, all of these processes become perturbed secondary to introduction of other factors. For instance, in the presence of an infection, production of pro-inflammatory cytokines will promotes ACD while an early skewing toward producing anti-inflammatory signals may reverse the situation. In this regard, iron sequestration and retention by macrophages play key role in ACD. In such cases there is abundance of iron stored away in ferritin and not accessible by erythroid cells hence increased erythrophagocytosis without a commensurate erythropoiesis may precipitate anemia. Of crucial importance are the roles played by intracellular iron levels and nitric oxide in affecting iron homeostasis and eventually ACD. In the absence of an infection however, anemia may develop following inadequate iron supply to meet cellular demands.

7. References

Adeyemi O.S., Akanji M.A., Johnson T.O., Ekanem J.T. (2011). Iron and nitric oxide balance in African Trypanosomosis: Is there really a link? *Asian J. Biochem.* 6(1): 15 - 28.

Barisani, D., Cairo, G., Ginelli, E., Marozzi A. and Conte D. (2003). Nitric Oxide Reduces Nontransferrin-Bound Iron Transport in HepG2 Cells. *Hepatology*, Volume 29, Issue 2

Beckman, J.S., Beckman, T.W., Chen, J., Marshall, P.A. and Freeman, B.A. (1990). Apparent hydroxyl radical production by peroxynitrite: implications for endothelial injury from nitric oxide and superoxide. *Proc. Natl. Acad. Sci.* USA 87, 1620–1624.

Bolanos, J.P., Heales, S.J.R., Land, J.M. and Clark, J.B. (1995). Effect of peroxynitrite on the mitochondrial respiratory chain: differential susceptibility of neurons and astrocytes in primary culture. *J. Neurochem.* 64, 1965–1972.

Boveris, A., Lores Arnaiz, S., Alvarez, S., Costa, L.E. and Valdez, L. (2000). The mitochondrial production of free radicals. In: Yoshikawa, T., Toyokumi, S., Yamamoto, Y., Naito, Y. (Eds.), *Free Radicals in Chemistry, Biology and Medicine.* OICA International, London, pp. 256–261.

Brown, G.C. and Cooper, C.E. (1994). Non-molar concentrations of nitric oxide reversibly inhibit synaptosomal respiration by competing with oxygen at cytochrome oxidase. *FEBS Lett.* 356, 295–298.

Brudvig, G.W., Stevens, T.H., Morse, R.H. and Chan, S.I. (1980). Reactions of nitric oxide with cytochrome c oxidase. *Biochemistry*:19, 5275–5285.

Cairo G., and Pietrangelo, A. (2000). Iron regulatory proteins in pathobiology. Review Article. *Biochem. J.* 352, 241-250.

Cairo, G. and Pietrangelo, A. (2000). Iron regulatory proteins in pathobiology. *Biochem. J.* 352, 241–250.

Cairo, G., Castrusini, E., Minotti, E. and Bernelli-Zazzera, A. (1996). Superoxide and hydrogen peroxide-dependent inhibition of iron regulatory protein activity: a protective stratagem against oxidative injury. *FASEB J.* 10, 1326–1335.

Cairo, G., Recalcati, S., Pietrangelo, A. and Minotti, G. (2002). The iron regulatory protein: targets and modulators of free radical reactions and oxidative damage. *Free Radic. Biol. Med.* 32, 1237–1243.

Cleeter, M.W.J., Cooper, J.M., Darley-Usmar, V.M., Moncada, S. and Schapira, A.H.V. (1994). Reversible inhibition of cytochrome c oxidase, the terminal enzyme of the mitochondrial respiratory chain by nitric oxide. *FEBS Lett.* 345, 50–54.

Drapier, J. C. and Bouton, C. (1996). Modulation by nitric oxide of metalloprotein regulatory activities. *BioEssays:* 18, 549-556.

Fritsche, G., Larcher, C., Schennach, H. and Weiss, G. (2001). Regulatory interactions between iron and nitric oxide metabolism for immune defense against Plasmodium falciparum infection. *J. Infect. Dis.* 183:1388–1394.

Galleano, M., Aimo, L., Borroni, M.V. and Puntarulo, S. (2001). Nitric oxide and iron overload. Limitations of ESR detection by DETC. *Toxicology.* 167, 199–205.

Galleano, M., Simontacchi, M., and Puntarulo, S. (2004). Nitric oxide and iron: effect of iron overload on nitric oxide production in endotoxemia. Review Article. *Molecular Aspects of Medicine.* 25: 141–154.

Giulivi, C., Poderoso, J.J., Boveris, A., (1998). Production of nitric oxide by mitochondria. *J. Biol. Chem.* 273, 11038–11043.

Gow, A.J. and Stamler, J.S. (1998). Reactions between nitric oxide and haemoglobin under physiological conditions. *Nature:* 391, 169–173.

Hanson, E.S. and Leibold, E.A. (1999). Regulation of the iron regulatory proteins by reactive nitrogen and oxygen species. *Gene. Expr.* 7, 367–376.

Hida, A.I., Kawabata, T., Minamiyama, Y., Mizote, A. and Okada, S. (2003). Saccharated colloidal iron enhances lipopolysaccharide-induced nitric oxide production *in vivo*. *Free Radic. Biol. Med.* 34, 1426–1434.

Kagan, V.E., Kozlov, A.V., Tyurina, Y.Y., Shvedova, A.A. and Yalowich, J.C. (2001). Antioxidant mechanisms of nitric oxide against iron-catalized oxidative stress in cells. Antiox. *Redox Signal* 3, 189–202.

Kim, S., and Ponka, P. (2000). Effects of interferon-gamma and lipopolysacharide on macrophage iron metabolism are mediated by nitric oxide-induced degradation of iron regulatory protein 2. *J. Biol. Chem.* 275, 6220–6226.

Knowles, R.G. (1997). Nitric oxide, mitochondria and metabolism. *Biochem. Soc. Trans.* 25, 895–901.

Knowles, R.G. and Moncada, S. (1994). Nitric oxide synthases in mammals. *Biochem. J.* 298, 249–258.

Komarov, A.M., Kramer, J.H., Tong Mak, I. and Weglicki, W.B. (1997a). EPR detection of endogenous nitric oxide in postischemic heart using lipid and aqueous-soluble dithiocarbamate-iron complexes. *Mol. Cell. Biochem.* 175, 91–97.

Komarov, A.M., Mattson, D.L., Tong Mak, I. and Weglicki, W.B. (1998). Iron attenuates nitric oxide level and iNOS expression in endotoxin-treated mice. *FEBS Lett.* 424, 253–256.

Komarov, A.M., Tong Mak, I. and Wegliki, W.B. (1997b). Iron potentiates nitric oxide scavenging by dithiocarbamates in tissue of septic shock mice. *Biochim. Biophys. Acta.* 1361, 229–234.

Kubrina, L.N., Mikoyan, V.D., Mordvintcev, P.I. and Vanin, A.F. (1993). Iron potentiates bacterial lipopolisaccharide-induced nitric oxide formation in animal organs. *Biochim. Biophys. Acta.*1176, 240– 244.

Lipinski P., Drapier, J.C., Oliveira L., Retmanska H., Sochanowicz B. and Kruszewski M. (2000). Intracellular iron status as a hallmark of mammalian cell susceptibility to oxidative stress: a study of L5178Y mouse lymphoma cell lines differentially sensitive to H$_2$O$_2$. *Blood;* 95: 2960–6.

Lizasoain, I., Moro, M.A., Knowles, R.G., Darley-Usmar, V. and Moncada, S. (1996). Nitric oxide and peroxynitrite exert distinct effects on mitochondrial respiration, which are differentially blocked by glutathione or glucose. *Biochem. J.* 314, 887–898.

Mikoyan, V.D., Kubrina, L.N., Serezhenkov, V.A., Stukan, R.A., and Vanin, A.F. (1997). Complexes of Fe$_2$ with diehyldithiocarbamate or N-methyl-D-glucamine dithiocarbamate as traps of nitric oxide in animal tissues: comparative investigations. *Biochim. Biophys. Acta.* 1336, 225–234.

Mikoyan, V.D., Voevodskaya, N.V., Kubrina, L.N., Malenkova, I.V. and Vanin, A.F. (1995). The influence of antioxidants and cicloheximide on the level of nitric oxide in the livers of mice *in vivo. Biochim. Biophys. Acta.* 1269, 19–24.

Moncada, S. and Higgs, E.A. (1995). Molecular mechanisms and therapeutic strategies related to nitric oxide. *FASEB J.* 9, 1319–1330.

Moncada, S., Palmer, R.M.J. and Higgs, E.A. (1991). Nitric oxide: physiology, pathophysiology and pharmacology. *Pharmacol. Rev.* 43, 109–142.

Nathan, C., and Xie, Q.W. (1994). Nitric oxide synthases: roles, tolls, and controls. *Cell:* 78, 915–918.

Obolenskaya, M.Y., Vanin, A.F., Mordvintcev, P.I., Meulsch, A., and Decker, K. (1994). EPR evidence of nitric oxide production by regenerating rat liver. *Biochem. Biophys. Res. Commun.* 202, 571–576.

Pippard, M.J. (1994). Secondary iron overload. In: Powell, L.W. (Ed.), *Iron Metabolism in Health and Disease.* W.B. Saunders, London, pp. 271–309.

Proudfoot, L., Nikolaev, A.V., Feng, G.J., Wei, W Q., Ferguson, M.A., Brimacombe, J.S., and Liew, F.Y. (1996). Regulation of the expression of nitric oxide synthase and leishmanicidal activity by glycoconjugates of Leishmania lipophosphoglycan in murine macrophages. *Proc. Natl. Acad. Sci.* USA 93, 10984–10989.

Radi, R., Rodriguez, M., Castro, L., and Telleri, R. (1994). Inhibition of mitochondrial electron transport by peroxinitrite. *Arch. Biochem. Biophys.* 308, 89–95.

Recalcati, S., Taramelli, D., Conte, D. and Cairo, G. (1998). Nitric oxide-mediated induction of ferritin synthesis in J774 macrophages by inflammatory cytokines: Role of selective iron regulatory protein-2 down-regulation. *Blood.* 91, 1059–1066

Rubbo, H., Radi, R., Trujillo, M., Telleri, R., Kalyanaraman, B., Barnes, S., Kirk, M., and Freeman, B.A. (1994). Nitric oxide regulation of superoxide and peroxynitrite-dependent lipid peroxidation. Formation of novel nitrogen-containing, oxidized lipid derivatives. *J. Biol. Chem.* 269, 26066–26075.

Starzynski, R.R., Gonçalves, A.S., Muzeau, F., Tyrolczyk, Z., Smuda, E., Drapier, J.C., Beaumont, C., and Lipinski, P. (2006). STAT5 proteins are involved in down-regulation of iron regulatory protein 1 gene expression by nitric oxide. *The Biochemical Journal,* 400(2): 367-75.

Stuehr, D.J., (1999). Mammalian nitric oxide synthases. *Biochim. Biophys. Acta* 1411, 217–230.

Taha, Z., Kiechle, F., and Malinski, T. (1992). Oxidation of nitric oxide by oxygen in biological systems monitored by porphyrinic sensor. *Biochem. Biophys. Res. Commun.* 188, 734–739.

Takenaka, K., Suzuki, S., Sakai, N., Kassel, F., and Yamada, H. (1995). Transferrin induces nitric oxide synthase mRNA in rat cultured aortic smooth muscle cells. *Biochem. Biophys. Res. Commun.* 213, 608–615.

Tiesjema, R.H., and van Gelder, B.F. (1974). Biochemical and biophysical studies on cytochrome c oxidase. XVI. Circular dichroic study of cytochrome c oxidase and its ligand complexes. *Biochim. Biophys. Acta.* 347, 202–214.

Torres, J., Darley-Usmar, V., and Wilson, M.T. (1995). Inhibition of cytochrome c oxidase in turnover by nitric oxide: mechanism and implications for control of respiration. *Biochem. J.* 312, 169–173.

Vanin, A.F. (1999). Iron diethyldithiocarbamate as spin trap for nitric oxide detection. *Meth. Enzymol.* 301, 269–279.

Weinberg, E.D. (2000). Modulation of intramacrophage iron metabolism during microbial cell invasion. *Microbes. Infect.* 2, 85–89.

Weiss, G., Werner-Felmayer, G., Werner, E. R., Grunewald, K., Wachter, H. and Hentze, M. W. (1994). Iron regulates nitric oxide synthase activity by controlling nuclear transcription. *J. Exp. Med.* 180, 969-976

Wink, D.A., Nims, R.W., Darbyshire, J.F., Christodoulou, D., Hanbauer, I., Cox, G.W., Laval, F., Cook, J.A., and Krishna, M.C. (1994). Reaction kinetics for nitrosation of cysteine and glutathione in aerobic nitric oxide solutions at neutral pH. Insights into the fate and physiological effects of intermediates generated in the NO/O_2 reaction. *Chem. Res. Toxicol.* 7, 519–525.

3

Morbidity and Mortality in Anemia

Fawzia Ahmed Habib, Intessar Sultan and Shaista Salman
Taibah University-College of Medicine-Al Madinah Al Munawara
Kingdom of Saudi Arabia

1. Introduction

A growing body of research suggests that anemia is independently associated with morbidity and mortality in the general population as well as in patients with chronic diseases where the prevalence of anemia is high (1-4). Anemia prognosis depends on the underlying cause of the anemia. However, the severity of the anemia, its etiology, and the rapidity with which it develops can each play a significant role in the prognosis. Similarly, the age of the patient and the existence of other co-morbid conditions influence outcome. Higher mortality rates are almost always observed in patients with anemia. Many studies (5-11) identified anemia as an independent factor impacting mortality and provided the evidence that management of anemia, independent of other risk factors, improves mortality rates. In one study (3), independent of the underlying disease, anemia was associated with increased mortality in chronic kidney disease, congestive heart failure and acute myocardial infarction patients; increased morbidity in chronic kidney disease, congestive heart failure and cancer radiotherapy patients; and decreased quality of life in chronic kidney disease and cancer patients. In addition to its impact upon mortality, anemia also significantly influences morbidity. Multiple studies support this assertion especially in patients with chronic kidney disease and heart failure (12-17).

2. Morbidity and mortality among patients with certain types of anemia

2.1 Aplastic anemia

In the early 1930s aplastic anemia was considered almost inevitably fatal. However, the morbidity and mortality of this disease have decreased dramatically since the introduction of bone marrow transplantation and immunosuppressive therapy. Survival figures in aplastic anemia from several studies have shown biphasic curves, with the highest mortality rates within the first 6 months after diagnosis. Five-year survival rates have been described to range from 70% to 90% and to be similar among patients treated with either bone marrow transplantation or immunosuppression (18). Patients who undergo bone marrow transplantation have additional issues related to toxicity from the conditioning regimen and graft versus host disease (19). With immunosuppression, approximately one third of patients does not respond. For the responders, relapse and late-onset clonal disease, such as paroxysmal nocturnal hemoglobinuria, myelodysplastic syndrome, and leukemia, are risks (20). In one retrospective institutional analysis, predictors for response to immmunosuppresion at 6 months were younger age, higher baseline absolute reticulocyte, lymphocyte, and neutrophil counts with the five-year survivals ranging from 92 in the responders to 53% in the non responders (21). Two factors determines the clinical outcome in aplastic anemia, the severity of the pancytopenia and patient age. In a retrospective review from the European Group for Blood and Marrow Transplantation (EBMT), the relative risk for a poor outcome following immunosuppressive treatment was 3.4 for patients with very severe anemia and 1.5 in those with severe anemia compared with less severe cases. In the EBMT, the 5-year survival rate varied inversely and significantly with age. Also, at any degree of severity, the outcome was worse in older patients. The increase in mortality in the older patients was mainly due to infection or bleeding. Most infections were acquired from endogenous microbial flora of the skin and gastrointestinal tract (22).

2.2 Vitamin B12 deficiency anemia

Pernicious anemia is associated with a two- to threefold excess risk of intestinal-type gastric cancer but, the actual degree of risk varies with the duration of disease and geographic location. Pernicious anemia is also associated with an increased risk of gastric carcinoid tumors, presumably due to prolonged achlorhydria with compensatory hypergastrinemia, and argyrophilic cell hyperplasia. There is also a suggested excess of oesophageal cancer among these patients (23). In the analysis of the Oxford Vegetarian Study (24), low vitamin B12 intake could explain the increased death rate (2.2 times) from mental and neurological diseases among vegetarians compared to non-vegetarians. Specific neurologic problems associated with vitamin B12 deficiency consist of subacute combined degeneration of the dorsal (posterior) and lateral spinal columns, axonal degeneration of peripheral nerves and central nervous system symptoms including memory loss, irritability, and dementia (25).

In some cases, B12-deficient dementia may be misdiagnosed as Alzheimer's disease (26). The cognitive decline in older subjects associated with subclinical vitamin B12 deficiency is difficult to explain but a role for increased homocysteine level is possible. People with Alzheimer's disease were found to have elevated homocysteine, reduced B12, or reduced folate levels (27). On the other hand studies found elevated homocysteine to be associated with risk of Alzheimer's disease (26). Selhub et al. (27) analyzed data from 8,083 people, including whites, blacks, and Hispanics. They found that elevated homocysteine levels (> 11.4 µmol/l for men, > 10.4 µmol/l for women) were associated with B12 levels less than 338 pg/ml. A level of 430 pg/ml provides a safety factor for homocysteine and other potential problems. Elevated homocysteine is associated with increased mortality, with an increased risk of 33% per 5 µmol/l increase in homocysteine (28,29) with increased risk for coronary artery, cerebrovascular, and peripheral vascular diseases and venous thrombosis (30). A 2008 meta-analysis of vitamin supplementation and cognitive function found little benefit to people already diagnosed with dementia, but did improve cognition in elderly people with elevated homocysteine but who were not diagnosed with dementia (31). Another 2008 study found that vitamin supplementation did not slow cognitive decline in people with mild to moderate Alzheimer's disease (32).

Vitamin B12 deficiency appears to be associated with an increased risk of osteoporosis (33,34), and hip and spine fractures (35), possibly due to suppression of osteoblast activity (36,37). Even subtle degrees of B12 deficiency may be associated with bone loss (38), although this has not been shown in all studies (39). Supplementation with vitamin B12 and folate has been shown to reduce hip fractures in a group of elderly Japanese patients with residual hemiplegia after an ischemic stroke. However, there is insufficient data to recommend this therapeutic approach in other populations at high risk for fracture.

2.3 Folic acid deficiency anemia

Studies found that both maternal plasma folate and vitamin B12 are independent risk factors for neural tube defects (40). In a literature review, Ray et al examined 8 studies that demonstrated that folate deficiency was a risk factor for placental abruption/infarction (41). Several observational and controlled trials have shown that neural tube defects can be reduced by 80% or more when folic acid supplementation is started before conception (42). In countries like the United States and Canada, the policy of widespread fortification of flour with folic acid has proved effective in reducing the number of neural tube defects (43). Although the exact mechanism is not understood, a relative folate shortage may exacerbate an underlying genetic predisposition to neural tube defects. Diminished folate status is associated with enhanced carcinogenesis. A number of epidemiologic and case-control studies have shown that folic acid intake is inversely related to colon cancer risk (44). With regard to the underlying mechanism, Blount et al showed that folate deficiency can cause a massive incorporation of uracil into human DNA leading to chromosome breaks (45). Another study by Kim et al suggested that folate deficiency induces DNA strand breaks and hypomethylation within the *p53* gene (46). Low folate and high homocysteine levels are a risk factor for cognitive decline in high-functioning older adults (47) and high homocysteine level is an independent predictor of cognitive impairment among long-term stay geriatric patients (48). Despite the association of high homocysteine level and poor cognitive function, homocysteine-lowering therapy using supplementation with vitamins B-12 and B-6 was not associated with improved cognitive performance after two years in a double-blind, randomized trial in healthy older adults with elevated homocysteine levels (49).

2.4 Thalassemia

Iron excess in patients with thalassemia is associated with early death if untreated. Several publications provide evidence that the heart is unquestionably the most critical organ affected by iron jeopardizing survival of thalassemia patients. In a study of 97 thalassemia patients (50), 36% of patients between the ages of 15 and 18 showed detectable cardiac iron, the risk of cardiac disease increases as patient's age increases. For the full cohort, the estimated survival without cardiac disease was 80% after 5 years of chelation therapy, 65% after 10 years and only 55% after 15 years. At the New York Academy of Sciences, Seventh Symposium on Thalassemia (51), the causes of death reported in 240 thalassemia major patients in Italy born between 1960-1984 were cardiac disease (71%), infections (12%), liver (6%) and other causes (11%). Another review of information available to the Cooley's Anemia Foundation shows that 11% of its 724 registered patients (77 total) died over the time period January 1999 – July 31, 2008. The data demonstrate that heart disease in these young patients remains the leading cause by far.

Since 1999, there has been a marked improvement in survival in thalassaemia major in the UK (52), similar change with improved survival has been reported from Italy (53,54) and Cyprus (55). This improvement has been mainly driven by a reduction in deaths due to cardiac iron overload. The most likely causes for this include the introduction of T2* cardiac magnetic resonance imaging technique to quantify myocardial iron overload and appropriate intensification of iron chelation treatment, alongside other improvements in clinical care. With a reduction in deaths from iron overload, infection may become a leading cause of death in thalassaemia in the future. Splenectomy increases risk of infection with Pneumococcus and Haemophilus influenzae and deferoxamine therapy increases risk of infection with Yersinia enterocolitica, and there have been at least 3 deaths from these infections. However, the most frequently isolated organism was Klebsiella. An increased risk of Klebsiella infection in thalassaemia has previously been reported from South East Asia (56,57), and some forms of Klebsiella can use deferoxamine as an iron source (58), but it remains to be clarified whether Klebsiella infection is related to iron chelation therapy. Hepatocarcinoma is also a growing problem for hepatitis C positive patients, and improved antiviral treatments are needed. Fortunately, transmission of hepatitis C by blood transfusion is now very rare, so this risk may be limited to older patients (52).

2.5 Sickle cell anemia

The greatest burden of sickle cell anemia (SCA) is in sub-Saharan Africa (SSA), and estimates suggest that 50–80% of these patients will die before adulthood (59). Identification of risk factors has led to improved survival through targeted interventions. In the West, reported risk factors for death include infections, low hemoglobin and fetal hemoglobin (HbF), high white blood cell count and hemolysis (60-62). Comprehensive care includes prompt treatment of acute events and prophylaxis against infections, mainly with oral penicillin and vaccination against *Streptococcus pneumoniae*. Countries that have introduced these interventions have achieved significant reductions in mortality; with up to 94% surviving to 18 years in the USA (63) and 99% to 20 years in the UK (64). In most African countries, the lack of an evidence-base has led to inertia in terms of implementation of these interventions, such as penicillin prophylaxis. In Africa, available mortality data are sporadic and incomplete. Many children are not diagnosed, especially in rural areas, and death is often attributed to malaria or other comorbid conditions (65). The mortality rates in SCA amongst a hospital-based cohort in Tanzania (66) was 1.9 per 100 PYO which is similar to 3 per 100 PYO reported from the USA before use of penicillin prophylaxis (67), with the highest incidence of death was in the first 5 years of life. Evidence from previous research suggests that infection is the most likely cause of death in this period, with the proportion of deaths from infection reported to be 50% in the USA (60, 68), 28% in Jamaica (69) and 20% in Dallas (63). The prevention of pneumococcal infection with penicillin and the introduction of pneumococcal conjugate vaccine has been shown to be effective in reducing mortality (70) with improved survival rates of 84% in Jamaica (69), 86% by 18 years in Dallas (64) and 99% in London (65). One review reported 42% reduction in mortality in SCA in USA, 0 to 3 years old, between two eras, 1995–1998 and 1999–2002 (71). There is compelling justification for implementation of these interventions in Africa to prevent deaths due to infections (65,66).

Sudden death is not uncommon among SCA patients. A retrospective/prospective review of 21 autopsy cases from sickle cell patients who died suddenly between 1990 and 2004 demonstrated higher-than-expected percentages of acute and chronic sickle cell-related lung injury such as fat embolism (33.3%) and pulmonary hypertension (33.3%), with right ventricular hypertrophy (33.3%) (72). In Sickle cell trait (SCT) under unusual circumstances serious morbidity or mortality can result from complications related to polymerization of deoxy-hemoglobin S. Although rare, sudden death is the most serious complication of sickle cell trait. SCT has a substantially increased age-dependent risk of exercise-related sudden death as in military basic training and civilian organized sports. A retrospective review of all soldiers in basic training found that those with SCT had a 40-fold increased risk of sudden exertional death (73). Sudden death may occur in susceptible persons when poor physical conditioning, dehydration, heat stresses or hypoxic states precipitate sickling of the abnormal erythrocytes. Most of the death mechanisms are related to the biological consequences of diffuse microvascular occlusion due to sickling, although a significant number of such sudden deaths remain unexplained after thorough autopsy. Rare mechanisms encountered include acute splenic sequestration (74). Other problems may also be encountered in SCT patients including increased urinary tract infection in women, gross hematuria, complications of hyphema, splenic infarction with altitude hypoxia or exercise and life-threatening complications of exertional heat illness (exertional rhabdomyolysis, heat stroke, or renal failure). In addition, some disease associations have been noted with sickle cell trait which might not result from polymerization of hemoglobin S but from linkage to a different gene mutation. There is an association with renal medullary carcinoma, early end stage renal failure in autosomal dominant polycystic kidney disease, and surrogate end points for pulmonary embolism (75).

2.6 Paroxysmal nocturnal hemoglobinuria

Most patients with paroxysmal nocturnal hemoglobinuria (PNH) die from venous thrombotic events. Stroke is a common cause of morbidity and mortality in PNH and it is almost exclusively a result of cerebral venous thrombosis. Case reports of ischemic stroke complicating PNH have implicated a similar propensity for arterial events caused by the disease. PNH is a rare cause of arterial stroke with reported 9 cases but it should be considered in young stroke patients with abnormal blood findings (76).

3. Morbidity and mortality of anemia in high risk groups

3.1 Effect of anemia on maternal mortality and morbidity

Maternal anemia is a ubiquitous pregnancy complication, and has been associated with an array of adverse perinatal and reproductive outcomes. It is estimated that 20% of maternal deaths in Africa can be attributed to anemia. In combination with obstetric hemorrhage, anemia is estimated to be responsible for 17–46% of cases of maternal death (77). A review of symptoms associated with maternal deaths in Bangladesh led researchers to conclude that anemia had played a secondary role in nearly all cases (78). Estimates of maternal mortality resulting from anemia range from 34/100,000 live births in Nigeria to as high as 194/100,000 in Pakistan (79). The risk of death is greatly increased with severe anemia. There is little evidence of increased risk associated with mild or moderate anemia. Viteri (80) reported that anemic pregnant women are at greater risk of death during the perinatal period and that anemia is the major contributory or sole cause of death in 20–40% of the 500 000 maternal deaths/year. A study from Indonesia illustrated the much higher risk of maternal death in anemic women from rural areas than from urban areas, possibly as a result of problems with timely access to obstetric care (81). On the basis of the evidence available, it seems reasonable to assume that the risk of maternal mortality is greatly increased with severe anemia. The data available only confirm an associative – not a causal – relationship. Nevertheless, the strength of this relationship makes it appropriate to presume that it is causal. It must also be noted that there are currently no agreed international standards or sets of criteria for attributing death to anemia (82). Except in South Asia and Papua New Guinea, the reported rates of severe anemia do not appear to exceed 10% of pregnant women (79). In a large Indonesian study, the maternal mortality rate for women with a hemoglobin concentration <100 g/L was 70.0/10000 deliveries compared with 19.7/10000 deliveries for non-anemic women (81). However, the authors believed that the relation of maternal mortality with anemia reflected a greater extent of hemorrhage and late arrival at admission rather than the effect of a prenatal anemic condition. In another study, approximately one-third of the anemic women had megaloblastic anemia due to folic acid deficiency and two-thirds had hookworm. The cutoff for anemia was extremely low (<65 g hemoglobin/L), and the authors stated that although anemia may have contributed to mortality, it was not the sole cause of death in many of the women (83). It has been suggested that maternal deaths in the puerperium may be related to a poor ability to withstand the adverse effects of excessive blood loss, an increased risk of infection, and maternal fatigue; however, these potential causes of mortality have not been evaluated systematically (84).

Maternal morbidity resulting from anemia includes diminished work capacity and physical performance have been reported as a result mostly of iron deficiency anemia. Anemia leads to abnormalities in host defense and neurological dysfunction. Increased risks of premature labor and low birth weight have also been reported in association with anemia in pregnancy (80).

3.2 Effect of anemia on infant mortality and morbidity

There is substantial evidence that maternal iron deficiency anemia increases the risk of preterm delivery and subsequent low birth weight, and accumulating information suggests an association between maternal iron status in pregnancy and the iron status of infants postpartum. Preterm infants are likely to have more perinatal complications, to be growth-stunted, and to have low stores of iron and other nutrients. Lower birth weights in anemic women have been reported in several studies (85-87). In one study, the odds for low birth weight were increased across the range of anemia, increasing with lower hemoglobin in an approximately dose-related manner (88). Welsh women who were first diagnosed with anemia (hemoglobin <104 g/L) at 13–24 wk of gestation had a 1.18–1.75-fold higher relative risk of preterm birth, low birth weight, and prenatal mortality (89). After controlling for many other variables in a large Californian study, Klebanoff et al., (90) showed a doubled risk of preterm delivery with anemia during the second trimester but not during the third trimester. In Alabama, low hematocrit concentrations in the first half of pregnancy but higher hematocrit concentrations in the third trimester were associated with a significantly increased risk of preterm delivery (91). When numerous potentially confounding factors were taken into consideration, analysis of data from low-income, predominantly young black women in the United States showed a risk of premature delivery (<37 wk) and subsequently of having a low-birth-weight infant that was 3 times higher in mothers with iron deficiency anemia on entry to care (92). Similar relations were observed in women from rural Nepal, in whom anemia with iron deficiency in the first or second trimester was associated with a 1.87-fold higher risk of preterm birth, but anemia alone was not (88). In an analysis of 3728 deliveries in Singapore, 571 women who were anemic at the time of delivery had a higher incidence of preterm delivery than did those who were not anemic (93). An association between maternal anemia and lower infant Apgar scores was reported in some studies. In 102 Indian women in the first stage of labor, higher maternal hemoglobin concentrations were correlated with better Apgar scores and with a lower risk of birth asphyxia (94). In the Jamaican Perinatal Mortality Survey of >10000 infants in 1986, there was an ≈50% greater chance of mortality in the first year of life for those infants whose mothers had not been given iron supplements during pregnancy (95). Trials that included large numbers of iron-deficient women showed that iron supplementation improved birth weight (86,96) and Apgar scores (97). In rural populations in China antenatal supplementation with iron-folic acid was associated with longer gestation and a reduction in early neonatal mortality compared with folic acid. Multiple micronutrients were associated with modestly increased birth weight compared with folic acid, but, despite this weight gain, there was no significant reduction in early neonatal mortality (98).

3.3 Effect of anemia on children and adolescents mortality and morbidity

Apart from previously mentioned morbidity and mortality from hereditary anemia among children, by far the most common cause of anemia in this age group is chronic iron deficiency anemia (IDA). There is reasonably good evidence that mental and motor developmental test scores are lower among infants with IDA. Although some aspects of cognitive function seem to change with iron therapy, lower developmental IQ and achievement test scores have still been noted after treatment. A variety of non-cognitive alterations during infant developmental testing has also been observed, including failure to respond to test stimuli, short attention span, unhappiness, increased fearfulness, withdrawal from the examiner, and increased body tension. Exploratory analyses suggest that such behavioral abnormalities may account for poor developmental test performance in infants with IDA. There has been a steady accumulation of evidence that IDA limits maximal physical performance, sub-maximal endurance, and spontaneous activity in the adult, resulting in diminished work productivity with attendant economic losses. However, it is important to consider that studies that attempt to separate indicators of malnutrition, such as iron deficiency, from other types of environmental deprivation may be inappropriately separating factors that occur together naturally and that therefore cannot be differentiated (99). The behavioral effects of IDA may be due to changes in neurotransmission. In a recent review that focuses on human studies, short- and long-term alterations associated with iron deficiency in infancy can be related to major dopamine pathways (100). It is widely accepted that long-term consequences of iron deficiency are often irreversible. Several studies have found that reversal of the anemia did not improve standardized test scores (101,102). One study (103) examined a group of Costa Rican children at five years of age. Children who had moderately severe IDA (hemoglobin less than 10 g per dL [100 g per L]) in infancy scored significantly lower on standardized tests at five years of age, despite a return to normal hematologic status and growth.

However, there is accumulating evidence for the potential benefits of preventing iron deficiency in infancy and treating it before it becomes chronic or severe. A recent study (104) of the preschool-aged Chinese children found that children who had chronic IDA in infancy displayed less positive social and emotional development. In contrast, the behavior and affect of children whose anemia was corrected before the age of 24 months were comparable to those of children who were non-anemic throughout infancy. The persistence of poorer cognitive, motor, affective, and sensory system functioning during childhood highlights the need to prevent iron deficiency in infancy and to find interventions that lessen the long-term effects of this widespread nutrient disorder.

Iron deficiency is also implicated in such neurologic sequelae as irritability, lethargy, headaches, and infrequently papilledema, pseudotumor cerebri, and cranial nerve abnormalities. Although only a few cases (30 cases) in the literature support the association between IDA and increased intracranial tension, it may be more common than previously thought. The underlying mechanisms remain unknown, but cerebral venous thrombosis should be carefully excluded (105). Rarely has iron deficiency been recognized as a significant cause of stroke in the adult or pediatric populations (106,107). One case series reported 6 children, 6 to 18 months of age, who presented with an ischemic stroke or venous thrombosis after a viral prodrome. All patients had iron deficiency as a consistent finding among the group, and other known etiologies of childhood stroke were excluded (108)

3.4 Effect of anemia on mortality and morbidity in elderly people
In the past decade, anemia has been associated with a number of negative outcomes in elderly people. In a report from the Netherlands, community-dwelling subjects older than 85 years with anemia had higher 5-year mortality rates than subjects with normal hemoglobin levels (109,110). In a cohort of older women with mild-to-moderate physical disability, Chaves et al noted an increase in mortality associated with hemoglobin levels less than 110 g/L (111). In a study of 1744 community-dwelling persons aged 71 years or older, anemia is independently associated with increased mortality over 8 years for both races and sex. Anemia also is a risk factor for functional and cognitive decrease (1).

In an analysis of 5888 community-dwelling older adults enrolled in the Cardiovascular Health Study (2), anemia was associated with increased risk for hospitalization and mortality in older adults. In another community-based study of more than 17 000 older adults more than 66 years (4), anemia was significantly associated with risk for all-cause hospitalization, hospitalization secondary to cardiovascular disease, and all-cause mortality. In both studies, the association between hemoglobin and mortality was not linear; with the risk for death increased at both extremes of hemoglobin. As this risk occurs at hemoglobin levels that are currently considered normal, consideration should be given to refining the current definition of anemia in older adults to reflect this continuum of risk (2, 4).

Not only anemia in elderly is a strong predictor of death, it has also been associated with various conditions such as decreased physical performance, disability in daily living, mobility disabilities, cognitive impairment, depression, falls and fractures, frailty, admission to hospital and diminished quality of life (112-114). However in the presence of common comorbidities among elderly, anemia could be considered as a risk marker rather than a risk factor. In the Leiden 85-plus Study (115), a population-based prospective follow-up study of 562 people aged 85 years, anemia in very elderly people was found to be associated with an increased risk of death, independent of comorbidity. However, the associated functional decline appears to be attributed mainly to comorbidity.

3.5 Effect of anemia on mortality and morbidity in patients with cancer
Anemia is common in cancer patients, although the prevalence is influenced both by the type of malignancy and the choice of treatment. Individual studies have compared the survival of patients with and without anemia and have shown reduced survival times in patients with various malignancies associated with anemia including carcinoma of the lung, cervix, head and neck, prostate, lymphoma, and multiple myeloma. A systemic, quantitative review in 2001 (116) estimated the overall increase in risk of death with anemia to 65% (CI: 54-77%). In addition, an intriguing association has also been observed between anemia and disease progression among patients undergoing radiotherapy, particularly in those with

cervical carcinoma or with squamous cell carcinoma of the head and neck. Harrison et al found that two thirds of women with cervical carcinoma are anemic at baseline, and 82% are anemic during radiotherapy (117). Correlations between anemia, tumor tissue oxygenation, local recurrence, and survival have been demonstrated in other studies (118,119). In one study including cases of head and neck cancer, 75% of patients undergoing combined chemotherapy and radiotherapy become anemic (120) and anemia has been associated with worse local regional control and survival rates (121). However, there is presently little evidence that anemia treatment per se impacts the tumor response to chemotherapy alone.

3.6 Effect of anemia on mortality and morbidity in patients with cardiac diseases

Substantial evidence suggests that anemia is an independent risk factor for worse outcomes in patients with heart failure (CHF) and ischemia heart disease including myocardial infarction. Anemia is a common comorbidity in CHF. Compared with nonanemic patients the presence of anemia also is associated with worse cardiac clinical status, more severe systolic and diastolic dysfunction, a higher beta natriuretic peptide level, increased extracellular and plasma volume, a more rapid deterioration of renal function, a lower quality of life, and increased medical costs (122-129).

In a systematic review and meta-analysis published in 2008, after a minimal follow-up of 6 months, 46.8% of anemic patients died compared with 29.5% of non-anemic patients irrespective to the cause of CHF. In studies that analyzed hemoglobin as a continuous variable, a 1-g/dL decrease in hemoglobin was independently associated with significantly increased mortality risk (130).

The associations between hemoglobin and outcomes was studied in 2653 patients randomized in the CHARM Program in the United States and Canada. Anemia was common in heart failure, regardless of left ventricular ejection fraction (LVEF). Lower hemoglobin was associated with higher LVEF yet was an independent predictor of adverse mortality and morbidity outcomes (131). On the contrary, a large nationally representative study of older patients in the United States hospitalized with HF demonstrated no graded relationship between lower hematocrit values and increased mortality and suggest that although anemia is an independent predictor of hospital readmission, its relationship with increased mortality in HF patients is largely explained by the severity of comorbid illness. The authors suggest that anemia may be predominantly a marker rather than a mediator of increased mortality risk in older patients with HF (132).

In heart failure, the causes of anemia and the associations between anemia and outcomes are probably multiple and complex. The anemia in CHF mainly is caused by a combination of renal failure and CHF-induced increased cytokine production, and these can both lead to reduced production of erythropoietin (EPO), resistance of the bone marrow to EPO stimulation, and to cytokine-induced iron-deficiency anemia caused by reduced intestinal absorption of iron and reduced release of iron from iron stores. The use of angiotensin-converting enzyme inhibitor and angiotensin receptor blockers also may inhibit the bone marrow response to EPO. Hemodilution caused by CHF also may cause a low hemoglobin level (129). The potential mechanisms linking anemia to increased mortality risk in CHF have not been characterized but may be related to changes in ventricular loading conditions and cardiac structure, altered neurohormonal activation, or reduced free radical scavenging capacity. It is also possible that anemia is a marker of more severe underlying myocardial disease (133).

In several controlled and uncontrolled studies, correction of the anemia with subcutaneous erythropoietin (EPO) or darbepoetin in conjunction with oral and intravenous iron has been associated with an improvement in clinical status, number of hospitalizations, cardiac and renal function, and quality of life. However, larger, randomized, double-blind, controlled studies still are needed to verify these initial observations. The effect of EPO may be related partly to its nonhematologic functions including neovascularization; prevention of apoptosis of endothelial, myocardial, cerebral, and renal cells; increase in endothelial progenitor cells; and anti-inflammatory and antioxidant effects (129).

In ischemic heart disease, both advanced age and the presence of flow-limiting coronary stenosis markedly impaired cardiac compensatory response to anemia, even without concomitant acute myocardial injury. These conditions, among other limits to the patients' physiologic reserve, may explain why levels of hemoglobin tolerated by younger individuals would not be tolerated by the elderly. They may also explain why elderly patients with acute myocardial infarction represent a group at extremely high risk for death, despite infarct sizes similar to those of younger patients (3).

The clinical utility of blood transfusion in anemic cardiovascular disease populations is controversial. According to the guidelines from the American College of Physicians and the American Society of Anesthesiology, the "transfusion threshold" for patients without known risk factors for cardiac disease is a hemoglobin level in the range of 6 to 8 g/dL. In one study, patients hospitalized with acute myocardial infarction, blood transfusion was associated with a significantly lower 30-day mortality rate among patients with a hematocrit <30% on admission (134). But in 838 critically ill patients (26% with cardiovascular disease), maintaining hemoglobin at 10 to 12 g/dL did not provide additional benefits on 30-day mortality compared with maintaining hemoglobin at 7 to 9 g/dL (135). Blood transfusion may be associated with other adverse effects including immunosuppression with increased risk of infection, sensitization to HLA antigens, and iron overload. Given this profile of risks and benefits, transfusion may be considered as an acute treatment for severe anemia on an individualized basis but does not appear to be a viable therapeutic strategy for the long-term management of chronic anemia in CHF (135,136).

Pilot studies have found that in a large number of HF patients it's safe to raise hemoglobin with erythropoietin-stimulating therapies and there is a suggestion that raising hemoglobin in anemic HF patients may lead to improved outcomes (136). A prospective, randomized trial studied the treatment of anemia in patients with moderate-to-severe CHF (NYHA class III to IV) whose left ventricular ejection fraction was less than 40% of normal. Patients who received treatment had a 42.1% improvement in NYHA class, compared with the control cohort who had a decrease of 11.4%. Number of hospital days, need for diuretic therapy, and renal function impairment were all significantly greater in the control group than in the treated group (137).

The Study of Anemia in Heart Failure Trial (STAMINA-HeFT) is a large multicenter, randomized, double-blind, placebo-controlled trial. In this study treatment of anemia with erythropoiesis-stimulating agents (ESAs) (darbepoetin alfa) was not associated with significant clinical benefits. But in the post hoc analysis of outcomes among the treated group, an increase of 1.0 g/dL or more in hemoglobin is required to achieve benefit in reduction of all-cause mortality or heart failure-related hospitalization (138). However, further observational and experimental studies are needed to help identify optimal treatment algorithms for both ESAs and iron that maximize clinical benefit while minimizing adverse outcomes. A pragmatic approach to the care of patients with HF needs definitive anemia treatment goals that are dynamic and disease specific, rather than those that adopt a more simplistic hemoglobin-specific approach.

3.7 Effect of anemia on mortality and morbidity in patients with end stage renal diseases

Anemia is associated with higher mortality rates and possibly heart disease in patients with kidney disease. However, the available evidence is limited as concluded in a systematic literature review published in 2006 (139). In a retrospective review (140) of nearly 20 000 of patients undergoing maintenance hemodialysis, hemoglobin levels of 8.0 g/dL or less were associated with a 2-fold increase in odds of death when compared with hemoglobin levels ranging between 10.0 and 11.0 g/dL. A similar study (141) of nearly 100 000 hemodialysis patients confirmed that a hematocrit higher than 30% was associated with a lower mortality. Compared with patients with a hematocrit higher than 30%, the overall relative risk of death was between 33% and 51% higher for the group with a hematocrit less than 27%, and between 12% and 20% higher for the group with a hematocrit of 27% to 30%, with and without adjustments for severity of disease. Subsequent analyses have determined that hematocrit levels maintained between 33% and 36% were associated with the lowest risk of death (142). Another study showed that in patients undergoing maintenance hemodialysis, the risk of hospitalization declines with hematocrit improvement, with a 16% to 22% lower hospitalization rate for patients with hematocrit values between 36% and 39% compared with patients with hematocrits between 33% and 36% (12). Also, prospective clinical trials of patients with end-stage renal disease have demonstrated a relationship among hematocrit, left ventricular dilatation, and left ventricular hypertrophy (LVH) (13-17,143).

The optimal management of anemia in patients with end-stage renal disease is controversial. Appropriate use of ESAs and intravenous iron can effectively manage the anemia of chronic kidney disease and end-stage renal disease (ESRD) (144-146), several randomized trials have reported an increased risk of mortality and cardiovascular events in patients treated to achieve higher hematocrit levels (145-147). A large cohort of incident US hemodialysis patients found that dialysis units that treated severe anemia more aggressively with ESAs and intravenous iron had a one-year mortality rate that was 5 percent lower than in units that treated more conservatively. But the same aggressive treatment for milder anemia brought a 10 percent increase in the rate of mortality (147).

3.8 Effect of anemia on mortality and morbidity in patients with end stage renal diseases and heart failure

Anemia also may play a role in increasing cardiovascular morbidity in chronic kidney insufficiency, diabetes, renal transplantation, asymptomatic left ventricular dysfunction, left ventricular hypertrophy, acute coronary syndromes including myocardial infarction and chronic coronary heart disease, and in cardiac surgery. Renal failure, cardiac failure, and anemia therefore all interact to cause or worsen each other--the so-called cardio-renal-anemia syndrome (129). The reciprocal relationships among these 3 components of cardiorenal anemia have been the subject of a number of trials with inconsistent and sometimes paradoxic results (148). Cardiovascular disease (CVD) is a significant complication in chronic kidney disease (CKD) and a major cause of death in dialysis patients. Clinical studies have shown that anemia is associated with reduced survival in patients with renal disease, heart failure or both. Low haemoglobin (Hb) has been identified as an independent risk factor for LV growth in CKD patients, suggesting that there is a direct link between anemia and adverse cardiac outcomes. This suggests that correction of anemia may improve prognosis. In patients with chronic kidney disease and CHF, treatment of anemia improves many of the abnormalities seen in CHF: it reduces LVH (149-151);

prevents left ventricular dilatation (152); and increases left ventricular ejection fraction, (153-154), stroke volume, and cardiac output (153).

The evidence for an association between anemia and an increased risk of adverse cardiovascular outcomes in patients with CKD is strong. The relationship between anemia and adverse outcomes is complex. While it is likely to be indirect to some extent, evidence also suggests that there may be a causal link between low hemoglobin levels and the development of CVD. Treatment of anemia with epoetin has been shown to improve cardiac function and to produce regression of LVH in CKD patients, whether or not they are receiving dialysis. Furthermore, consistent treatment with epoetin before the initiation of dialysis is associated with a reduced risk of developing cardiac disease in patients with CKD. Normalizing Hb levels in patients with advanced CVD has a limited effect on changes in LV geometry, however, and – at least under certain circumstances –may increase their risk of death. The degree of CVD could affect other factors, such as vascular reactivity, which may determine whether partial or full correction of anemia is appropriate for a particular individual (154).

4. References

[1] Denny SD, Kuchibhatla MN, Cohen HJ. Impact of anemia on mortality, cognition, and function in community-dwelling elderly. Am J Med.2006;119(4):327-334.
[2] Zakai NA, Katz R, Hirsch C, et al. A prospective study of anemia status, hemoglobin concentration, and mortality in an elderly cohort: the Cardiovascular Health Study. Arch Intern Med. 2005;165(19):2214-2220.
[3] Nissenson AR, Goodnough LT, Dubois RW. Anemia: not just an innocent bystander? Arch Intern Med. 2003;163(12):1400-1404.
[4] Culleton BF, Manns BJ, Zhang J, et al. Impact of anemia on hospitalization and mortality in older adults. Blood 2006;107(10): 3841-3846 .
[5] Ma J, Ebben J, Xia H, et al. Hematocrit levels and associated mortality in hemodialysis patients. J Am Soc Nephrol. 1999;10:610-619.
[6] Collins A, Xia H, Ebben J, et al. Change in hematocrit and risk of mortality. J Am Soc Nephrol. 1998;9(suppl A):204A.
[7] Collins AJ, Li S, St Peter W, et al. Death, hospitalization, and economic associations among incident hemodialysis patients with hematocrit values of 36 to 39%. J Am Soc Nephrol.2001;12: 2465-2473.
[8] Maeda K, Tanaka Y, Tsukano Y, et al. Multivariate analysis using a linear discriminate function for predicting the prognosis of congestive heart failure. Jpn Circ J. 1982;46:137-142.
[9] Carson JL, Duff A, Poses RM, et al. Effect of anemia and cardiovascular disease on surgical mortality and morbidity. Lancet. 1996;348:1055-1060.
[10] Hebert PC, Wells G, Sweeddale M, et al. Does transfusion practice affect mortality in critically ill patients? Am J Respir Crit Care Med. 1997;155:1618-1623.
[11] McClellan WM, Flanders WD, Langston RD, et al. Anemia and renal insufficiency are independent risk factors for death among patients with congestive heart failure admitted to community hospitals: a population-based study. J Am Soc Nephrol. 2002;13:1928-1936.
[12] Besarab A, Bolton WK, Browne JK, et al. The effects of normal as compared with low hematocrit values in patients with cardiac disease who are receiving hemodialysis and epoetin.N Engl J Med. 1998;339:584-590.

[13] Foley RN, Parfrey PS, Harnett JD, Kent GM, Murray DC, Barre PE. The impact of anemia on cardiomyopathy, morbidity, and mortality in end stage renal disease. Am J Kidney Dis.1996;28:53-61.

[14] Levin A, Thompson CR, Ethier J, et al. Left ventricular mass index increase in early renal disease: impact of decline in hemoglobin. Am J Kidney Dis. 1999;34:125-134.

[15] Levin A, Singer J, Thompson CR, Ross H, Lewis M. Prevalent left ventricular hypertrophy in the predialysis population: identifying opportunities for intervention. Am J Kidney Dis.1996;27:347-354.

[16] Silverberg JS, Rahal DP, Patton R, Sniderman AD. Role of anemia in the pathogenesis of left ventricular hypertrophy in end-stage renal disease. Am J Cardiol. 1989;64:222-224.

[17] Canella G, LaCanna G, Sandrini M, et al. Reversal of left ventricular hypertrophy following recombinant human erythropoietin treatment of anaemic dialysed uraemic patients. Nephrol Dial Transplant. 1991;6:31-37.

[18] Young, NS. Aplastic anaemia. Lancet 1995; 346:228.

[19] Kojima S, Matsuyama T, Kato S, Kigasawa H, Kobayashi R, Kikuta A, et al. Outcome of 154 patients with severe aplastic anemia who received transplants from unrelated donors: the Japan Marrow Donor Program. Blood. Aug 1 2002;100(3):799-803.

[20] Orazi A, Czader MB. Myelodysplastic syndromes. Am J Clin Pathol. Aug 2009;132(2):290-305.

[21] Scheinberg, P, Wu, CO, Nunez, O, Young, NS. Predicting response to immunosuppressive therapy and survival in severe aplastic anaemia. Br J Haematol 2009; 144:206.

[22] Tichelli, A, Socie, G, Henry-Amar, M, et al. Effectiveness of immunosuppressive therapy in older patients with aplastic anemia: A report from the European Blood and Marrow Transplant (EBMT) Severe Aplastic Anaemia Working Group. Ann Intern Med 1999; 130:193. NS.

[23] Ye W and Nyrén O. Risk of cancers of the oesophagus and stomach by histology or subsite in patients hospitalised for pernicious anaemia. Gut. 2003 July;52(7): 938–941.

[24] Appleby PN, Key TJ, Thorogood M, Burr ML, Mann J. Mortality in British vegetarians. Public Health Nutr. 2002 Feb;5(1):29-36.

[25] Green, R, Kinsella, LJ. Editorial: Current concepts in the diagnosis of cobalamin deficiency. Neurology 1995; 45:1435.

[26] Van Dam F, Van Gool WA. Hyperhomocysteinemia and Alzheimer's disease: A systematic review. Arch Gerontol Geriatr. 2009 May-Jun;48(3):425-30. Epub 2008 May 13. Review.

[27] Selhub J, Bagley LC, Miller J, Rosenberg IH. B vitamins, homocysteine, and neurocognitive function in the elderly. Am J Clin Nutr. 2000 Feb;71(2):614S-620S.

[28] Hoogeveen EK, Kostense PJ, Jakobs C, Dekker JM, Nijpels G, Heine RJ, Bouter LM, Stehouwer CD. Hyperhomocysteinemia increases risk of death, especially in type 2 diabetes: 5-year follow-up of the Hoorn Study. Circulation. 2000 Apr 4;101(13):1506-11.

[29] Vollset SE, Refsum H, Tverdal A, Nygard O, Nordrehaug JE, Tell GS, Ueland PM. Plasma total homocysteine and cardiovascular and non cardiovascular mortality: the Hordaland Homocysteine Study. Am J Clin Nutr. 2001 Jul;74(1):130-6.

[30] Humphrey LL, Fu R, Rogers K, Freeman M, Helfand M. Homocysteine level and coronary heart disease incidence: a systematic review and meta-analysis. Mayo Clin Proc. 2008 Nov;83(11):1203-12

[31] Malouf R, Grimley Evans J. Folic acid with or without vitamin B12 for the prevention and treatment of healthy elderly and demented people. Cochrane Database Syst Rev. 2008 Oct 8;(4):CD004514.

[32] Aisen PS, Schneider LS, Sano M, Diaz-Arrastia R, van Dyck CH, Weiner MF, Bottiglieri T, Jin S, Stokes KT, Thomas RG, Thal LJ; Alzheimer Disease Cooperative Study. High-dose B vitamin supplementation and cognitive decline in Alzheimer disease: a randomized controlled . JAMA. 2008 Oct 15;300(15):1774-83.

[33] Dhonukshe-Rutten, RA, Lips, M, de Jong, N, et al. Vitamin B-12 status is associated with bone mineral content and bone mineral density in frail elderly women but not in men. J Nutr 2003; 133:801.

[34] Tucker, KL, Hannan, MT, Qiao, N, et al. Low plasma vitamin B12 is associated with lower BMD: the Framingham Osteoporosis Study. J Bone Miner Res 2005; 20:152.

[35] Goerss, JB, Kim, CH, Atkinson, EJ, et al. Risk of fractures in patients with pernicious anemia. J Bone Miner Res 1992; 7:573.

[36] Carmel, R, Lau, KH, Baylink, DJ, et al. Cobalamin and osteoblast-specific proteins. N Engl J Med 1988; 319:70.

[37] Kim, GS, Kim, CH, Park, JY, et al. Effects of vitamin B12 on cell proliferation and cellular alkaline phosphatase activity in human bone marrow stromal osteoprogenitor cells and UMR106 osteoblastic cells. Metabolism 1996; 45:1443.

[38] Stone, KL, Bauer, DC, Sellmeyer, D, Cummings, SR. Low serum vitamin B-12 levels are associated with increased hip bone loss in older women: a prospective study. J Clin Endocrinol Metab 2004; 89:1217.

[39] Cagnacci, A, Baldassari, F, Rivolta, G, et al. Relation of homocysteine, folate, and vitamin B12 to bone mineral density of postmenopausal women. Bone 2003; 33:956. Kumar, N. Copper deficiency myelopathy (human swayback). Mayo Clin Proc 2006; 81:1371.

[40] Afman LA, Van Der Put NM, Thomas CM, Trijbels JM, Blom HJ. Reduced vitamin B12 binding by transcobalamin II increases the risk of neural tube defects. QJM. 2001 Mar;94(3):159-66.

[41] Ray JG, Laskin CA. Folic acid and homocyst(e)ine metabolic defects and the risk of placental abruption, pre-eclampsia and spontaneous pregnancy loss: A systematic review. Placenta. Sep 1999;20(7):519-29.

[42] Wolff T, Witkop CT, Miller T, Syed SB. Folic acid supplementation for the prevention of neural tube defects: an update of the evidence for the U.S. Preventive Services Task Force. Ann Intern Med. May 5 2009;150(9):632-9.

[43] Honein MA, Paulozzi LJ, Mathews TJ, et al. Impact of folic acid fortification of the US food supply on the occurrence of neural tube defects. JAMA. Jun 20 2001;285(23):2981-6

[44] Gatof D, Ahnen D. Primary prevention of colorectal cancer: diet and drugs. Gastroenterol Clin North Am. Jun 2002;31(2):587-623, xi..

[45] Blount BC, Mack MM, Wehr CM, et al. Folate deficiency causes uracil misincorporation into human DNA and chromosome breakage: implications for cancer and neuronal damage. Proc Natl Acad Sci U S A. Apr 1 1997;94(7):3290-5..

[46] Kim YI, Pogribny IP, Basnakian AG, et al. Folate deficiency in rats induces DNA strand breaks and hypomethylation within the p53 tumor suppressor gene. Am J Clin Nutr. Jan 1997;65(1):46-52..

[47] Kado DM, Karlamangla AS, Huang MH, Troen A, Rowe JW, Selhub J. Homocysteine versus the vitamins folate, B6, and B12 as predictors of cognitive function and

decline in older high-functioning adults: MacArthur Studies of Successful Aging. Am J Med. Feb 2005;118(2):161-7.

[48] Adunsky A, Arinzon Z, Fidelman Z, Krasniansky I, Arad M, Gepstein R. Plasma homocysteine levels and cognitive status in long-term stay geriatric patients: a cross-sectional study. Arch Gerontol Geriatr. Mar-Apr 2005;40(2):129-38. x

[49] McMahon JA, Green TJ, Skeaff CM, Knight RG, Mann JI, Williams SM. A controlled trial of homocysteine lowering and cognitive performance. N Engl J Med. Jun 29 2006;354(26):2764-72.

[50] Borgna-Pignatti C, Rugolotto S, DeStefano P, Zhao H, Cappellini MD, Del Vecchio GC, et al. Survival and complications in patients with thalassemia major treated with transfusion and deferoxamine. Haematologica 2004;89:1187-93.

[51] Borgna-Pignatti C, Rugolotto S, Piga, A, DiGregorio F, Gamberi M.R., Sabato V, Melevendi C, Cappellini MD, Verlato G; Survival and Disease Complications in Thalassemia Major. Annuals of the New York Academy of Sciences, Volume 850, 1998

[52] Modell B , Khan M, Darlison M, Westwood MA, Ingram D and Pennell DJ. Improved survival of thalassaemia major in the UK and relation to T2* cardiovascular magnetic resonance. Journal of Cardiovascular Magnetic Resonance 2008, 10:42

[53] Piga A, Gaglioti C, Fogliacco E, Tricta F: Comparative effects of deferiprone and deferoxamine on survival and cardiac disease in patients with thalassemia major: a retrospective analysis. Haematologica 2003, 88:489-96.

[54] Borgna-Pignatti C, Cappellini MD, De Stefano P, Del Vecchio GC, Forni GL, Gamberini MR, Ghilardi R, Piga A, Romeo MA, Zhao H, Cnaan A: Cardiac morbidity and mortality in deferoxamine- or deferiprone-treated patients with thalassemia major. Blood 2006, 107:3733-7.

[55] Telfer P, Coen PG, Christou S, Hadjigavriel M, Kolnakou A, Pangalou E, Pavlides N, Psiloines M, Simamonian K, Skordos G, Sitarou M, Angastiniotis M: Survival of medically treated thalassemia patients in Cyprus. Trends and risk factors over the period 1980–2004. Haematologica 2006, 91:1187-92.

[56] Chung BH, Ha SY, Chan GC, Chiang A, Lee TL, Ho HK, Lee CY, Luk CW, Lau YL: Klebsiella infection in patients with thalassemia. Clin Infect Dis 2003, 36:575-9.

[57] Wang SC, Lin KH, Chern JP, Lu MY, Jou ST, Lin DT, Lin KS: Severe bacterial infection in transfusion-dependent patients with thalassemia major. Clin Infect Dis 2003, 37:984-8.

[58] Khimji PL, Miles AA: Microbial iron-chelators and their action on Klebsiella infections in the skin of guinea-pigs. Br J Exp Pathol 1978, 59:137-47.

[59] Weatherall D, Akinyanju O, Fucharoen S, Olivieri N, Musgrove P (2006) Inherited Disorders of Hemoglobin. In: Jamison D, editor. Disease Control Priorities in Developing Countries 2nd ed. New York: Oxford University Press. pp. 663–80.

[60] Leikin SL, Gallagher D, Kinney TR, Sloane D, Klug P, et al. (1989) Mortality in children and adolescents with sickle cell disease. Cooperative Study of Sickle Cell Disease. Pediatrics: 84(3): 500–8.

[61] Platt OS, Brambilla DJ, Rosse WF, Milner PF, Castro O, et al. (1994) Mortality in sickle cell disease. Life expectancy and risk factors for early death. N Engl J Med: 330(23): 1639–44.

[62] Kato GJ, McGowan V, Machado RF, Little JA, Taylor Jt, et al. (2006) Lactate dehydrogenase as a biomarker of hemolysis-associated nitric oxide resistance,

priapism, leg ulceration, pulmonary hypertension, and death in patients with sickle cell disease. Blood: 107(6): 2279–85.

[63] Quinn CT, Rogers ZR, Buchanan GR (2004) Survival of children with sickle cell disease. Blood: 103(11): 4023–7.

[64] Telfer P, Coen P, Chakravorty S, Wilkey O, Evans J, et al. (2007) Clinical outcomes in children with sickle cell disease living in England: a neonatal cohort in East London. Haematologica: 92(7): 905–12.

[65] Obaro S (2009) Pneumococcal Disease in Sickle Cell Disease in Africa: Does Absence of Evidence Imply Evidence of Absence? Arch Dis Child.

[66] Makani J, Cox SE, Soka D, Komba AN, Oruo J, et al. (2011) Mortality in Sickle Cell Anemia in Africa: A Prospective Cohort Study in Tanzania. PLoS ONE 6(2): e14699

[67] Powars D, Chan LS, Schroeder WA (1990) The variable expression of sickle cell disease is genetically determined. Semin Hematol: 27(4): 360–76

[68] http://www.plosone.org/article/info%3Adoi%2F10.1371%2Fjournal.pone.0014699 - pone.0014699-Leikin1

[69] Lee A, Thomas P, Cupidore L, Serjeant B, Serjeant G (1995) Improved survival in homozygous sickle cell disease: lessons from a cohort study. BMJ: 311(7020): 1600–590

[70] Vichinsky EP (1991) Comprehensive care in sickle cell disease: its impact on morbidity and mortality. Semin Hematol: 28(3): 220–6

[71] Yanni E, Grosse SD, Yang Q, Olney RS (2009) Trends in pediatric sickle cell disease-related mortality in the United States, 1983-2002. J Pediatr: 154(4): 541–5.

[72] Graham JK, Mosunjac M, Hanzlick RL, Mosunjac M. Sickle cell lung disease and sudden death: a retrospective/prospective study of 21 autopsy cases and literature review. Am J Forensic Med Pathol. 2007 Jun;28(2):168–72.

[73] Murray MJ, Evans P. Sudden exertional death in a soldier with sickle cell trait. Mil Med. 1996 May;161(5):303-5.

[74] Mitchell BL. Sickle cell trait and sudden death--bringing it home. J Natl Med Assoc. 2007 Mar;99(3):300-5.

[75] John N. A Review of Clinical Profile in Sickle Cell Traits. OMJ. 25, 3-8 (2010)

[76] Audebert H; Planck J; Eisenburg M; Schrezenmeier H; Haberl RL. Cerebral Ischemic Infarction in Paroxysmal Nocturnal Hemoglobinuria: Report of 2 Cases and Updated Review of 7 Previously Published Patients. Journal Of Neurology 2005, 252(11),1379-1386.

[77] World Bank, WHO, UNFPA. Preventing the tragedy of maternal deaths. A report on the International Safe Motherhood Conference Nairobi, Kenya, 1987. Geneva: WHO.

[78] Alauddin M. Maternal mortality in rural Bangladesh. The Tangail District. Stud Fam Plann 1986; 17: 13–21.

[79] World Health Organization. Prevention and Management of Severe Anaemia in Pregnancy. Geneva: WHO; 1993.

[80] Viteri FE, Torun B. Anemia and physical work capacity. In: Garby L (ed) Clinics in Haematology, vol. 3, WB Saunders, 1974; 609–26

[81] Chi I, Agoestina T, Harbin J. Maternal mortality at twelve teaching hospitals in Indonesia: an epidemiologic analysis. Int J Gynaecol Obstet 1992; 39: 87–92

[82] Llewellyn-Jones D. Severe Anemia in pregnancy (as seen in Kuala-Lumpur, Malaysia). Aust N Z J. Obstet Gynaecol 1965;5:191-7.

[83] Rush D. Nutrition and maternal mortality in the developing world. Am J Clin Nutr 2000; 72 (Suppl.): 212–40.

[84] Broek NV. Anaemia and micronutrient deficiencies. Reducing maternal death and disability during pregnancy Br Med Bull (2003) 67 (1): 149-160.

[85] Hemminki E, Rimpela U. Iron supplementation, maternal packed cell volume, and fetal growth. Arch Dis Child 1991;66:422–5.

[86] Agarwal KN, Agarwal DK, Mishra KP. Impact of Anemia prophylaxis in pregnancy on maternal hemoglobin, serum ferritin and birth weight. Indian J Med Res 1991;94:277–80.

[87] Singla PN, Tyagi M, Kumar A, Dash D, Shankar R. Fetal growth in maternal anemia. J Trop Pediatr 1997;43:89–92.

[88] Dreyfuss M. Anemia and iron deficiency during pregnancy: etiologies and effects on birth outcomes in Nepal. PhD dissertation. Johns Hopkins University, Baltimore, 1998.

[89] Murphy JF, O'Riordan J, Newcombe RJ, Coles EC, Pearson JF. Relation of hemoglobin levels in first and second trimesters to outcome of pregnancy. Lancet 1986;1:992–5.

[90] Klebanoff MA, Shiono PH, Selby JV, Trachtenberg AI, Graubard BI. Anemia and spontaneous preterm birth. Am J Obstet Gynecol 1991;164:59–63.

[91] Lu ZM, Goldenberg RL, Cliver SP, Cutter G, Blankson M. The relationship between maternal hematocrit and pregnancy outcome. Obstet Gynecol 1991;77:190–4.

[92] Scholl TO, Hediger ML, Fischer RL, Shearer JW. Anemia vs iron deficiency: increased risk of preterm delivery in a prospective study. Am J Clin Nutr 1992;55:985–8.

[93] Singh K, Fong YF, Arulkumaran S. Anemia in pregnancy—a cross-sectional study in Singapore. Eur J Clin Nutr 1998;52:65–70

[94] Rusia U, Madan N, Agarwal N, Sikka M, Sood S. Effect of maternal iron deficiency Anemia on foetal outcome. Indian J Pathol Microbiol 1995;38:273–9.

[95] Greenwood R, Golding J, McCaw-Binns A, Keeling J, Ashley D. The epidemiology of perinatal death in Jamaica. Paediatr Perinat Epidemiol 1994;8:143 57.

[96] Hemminki E, Starfield B. Routine administration of iron and vitamins during pregnancy: review of controlled clinical trials. Br J Obstet Gynaecol 1978;85:404–10.

[97] Preziosi P, Prual A, Galan P, Daouda H, Boureima H, Hercberg S. Effect of iron supplementation on the iron status of pregnant women: consequences for newborns. Am J Clin Nutr 1997;66:1178–82.

[98] Zeng L, Dibley MJ, Cheng Y, Dang S, Chang S, Kong L, Yan H. Impact of micronutrient supplementation during pregnancy on birth weight, duration of gestation, and perinatal mortality in rural western China: double blind cluster randomised controlled trial. BMJ. 2008;337:a2001.

[99] Lozof B. Iron and learning potential in childhood. Bull N Y Acad Med. 1989;65(10):1050–1088

[100] Lozoff B. Early Iron Deficiency Has Brain and Behavior Effects Consistent with Dopaminergic Dysfunction. J. Nutr. 2011; 141:4 740S-746S

[101] Mackler B, Person F, Miller LR. Iron-deficiency in the rat: biochemical studies of brain metabolism. Pediatr Res 1978;12:217–20.

[102] Voorhess ML, Stuart MJ, Stockman JA, et al. Iron-deficiency and increased urinary norepinephrine excretion. J Pediatr 1975;86: 542–7.

[103] Oski FA, Honig AS. The effects of therapy on the developmental score of iron-deficient infants. J Pediatr 1978;92:21–4.

[104] Chang S, Wang L, Wang Y, Brouwer ID, Kok FJ, Lozoff B, Chen C. Iron-Deficiency Anemia in Infancy and Social Emotional Development in Preschool-Aged Chinese Children. PEDIATRICS Vol. 127 No. 4 April 1, 2011

[105] Biousse V, Rucker JC, Vignal C, Crassard I, Katz BJ, Newman NJ. Anemia and papilledema. American Journal of Ophthalmology 135(4),437-446, 2003

[106] Habis A, Hobson WL, Greenberg R. Cerebral sinovenous thrombosis in a toddler with iron deficiency anemia. Pediatr Emerg Care. 2010 Nov;26(11):848-51).

[107] Maguire JL, deVeber G, Parkin PC. Association between iron-deficiency anemia and stroke in young children. Pediatrics. 2007 Nov;120(5):1053-7.

[108] Hartfield DS, Lowry NJ, Keene DL, Yager JY. Iron deficiency: a cause of stroke in infants and children. Pediatr Neurol. 1997 Jan;16(1):50-3).

[109] http://bloodjournal.hematologylibrary.org/content/107/10/3841.

[110] Izaks GJ, Westendorp RG, Knook DL. The definition of anemia in older persons. JAMA 1999;281:1714-7.

[111] Chaves PH, Xue QL, Guralnik JM, et al. What constitutes normal hemoglobin concentration in community-dwelling disabled older women?J Am Geriatr Soc 2004; 52:1811-6.

[112] Beghé C, Wilson A, Ershler WB. Prevalence and outcomes of anemia in geriatrics: a systematic review of the literature. Am J Med 2004;116 (Suppl 7A):3S-10S.

[113] Eisenstaedt R, Penninx BW, Woodman RC. Anemia in the elderly: current understanding and emerging concepts. Blood Rev 2006;20:213-26.

[114] Lipschitz D. Medical and functional consequences of anemia in the elderly. J Am Geriatr Soc 2003;51(Suppl 3):S10-3.

[115] Paltiel O, Clarfield AM "Anemia in elderly people: Risk marker or risk factor?" CMAJ 2009

[116] Caro JJ, Salas M, Ward A, et al: 2001; Anemia as an independent prognostic factor for survival in patients with cancer: A systemic, quantitative review. Cancer 91:2214-2221,

[117] Harrison LB, Shasha D, White C, Ramdeen B. Radiotherapy-associated anemia: the scope of the problem. Oncologist. 2000;5(suppl 2):1-7.

[118] Bush RS. The significance of anemia in clinical radiation therapy. Int J Radiat Oncol Biol Phys. 1986;12:2047-2050.

[119] Grogan M, Thomas GM, Melamed I, et al. The importance of hemoglobin levels during radiotherapy for carcinoma of the cervix. Cancer. 1999;86:1528-1536.

[120] Lee JS, Scott C, Komaki R, et al. Concurrent chemoradiation therapy with oral etoposide for locally advanced inoperable non-small-cell lung cancer: radiation therapy oncology group protocol 91-06. J Clin Oncol. 1996;14:1055-1064.

[121] Fein DA, Lee WR, Hanlon L, et al. Pretreatment hemoglobin level influences local control and survival of T1-T2 squamous cell carcinomas of the glottic larynx. J Clin Oncol.1995;13:2077-2083.

[122] Kalra PR, Bolger AP, Francis DP, Genth-Zotz S, Sharma R, Ponikowski PP, Poole-Wilson PA, Coats AJ, Anker SD. Effect of anemia on exercise tolerance in chronic heart failure in men. Am J Cardiol 2003;91:888-891.

[123] Ezekowitz JA, McALister FA, Armstrong PW. Anemia is common in heart failure and is associated with poor outcomes. Insights form a cohort of 12 065 patients with new-onset heart failure. Circulation 2003;107:294-299.

[124] Anand IS, Kuskowski MA, Rector TS, Florea VG, Glazer RD, Hester A, Chiang YT, Aknay N, Maggioni AP, Opasich C, Latini R, Cohn JN. Anemia and change in hemoglobin over time related to mortality and morbidity in patients with chronic heart failure: results from Val HeFT. Circulation 2005;112:1121-1127.

[125] Sharma R, Francis DP, Pitt B, Poole-Wilson PA, Coats AJ, Anker SD. Haemoglobin predicts survival in patients with chronic heart failure: a substudy of the ELITE II trial.Eur Heart J 2004;25:1021-1028.

[126] Horwich TB, Fonarow GC, Hamilton MA, Maclellan WR, Borenstein J. Anemia is associated with worse symptoms, greater impairment in functional capacity and a significant increase in mortality in patients with advance heart failure. J Am Coll Cardiol 2002;39:1780-1786.

[127] Mozaffarian D, Nye R, Levy WC. Anemia predicts mortality in severe heart failure. The prospective randomized amlodipine survival evaluation (PRAISE). J Am Coll Cardiol 2003;41:1933-1939.

[128] Anand I, McMurray JV, Whitmore J, Warren M, Pham A, McCamish MA, Burton PBJ. Anemia and its relationship to clinical outcome in heart failure. Circulation2004;110:149-154.

[129] Silverberg DS, Wexler D, Iaina A, Schwartz D. The interaction between heart failure and other heart diseases, renal failure, and anemia. Semin Nephrol. 2006 Jul;26(4):296-306.

[130] Groenveld HF, Januzzi JL, Damman K, Wijngaarden J, Hillege HL, van Veldhuisen DJ, and Meer PV, Anemia and Mortality in Heart Failure Patients. A Systematic Review and Meta-Analysis. J Am Coll Cardiol, 2008; 52:818-827

[131] Swedberg K, Pfeffer M, Granger C, Held P, McMurray J, Ohlin G, Olofsson B, Ostergren J, Yusuf S. Candesartan in heart failure--assessment of reduction in mortality and morbidity (CHARM): rationale and design. Charm-Programme Investigators. J Card Fail. 1999 Sep;5(3):276-82.

[132] Kosiborod M, Curtis JP, Wang Y, Smith GL, Masoudi FA; Foody; Havranek EP; Krumholz HM. Anemia and Outcomes in Patients With Heart Failure. A Study From the National Heart Care Project. Arch Intern Med. 2005;165:2237-224.

[133] Mitka M. Researchers probe anemia-heart failure link. JAMA. 2003;290:1835-1838.

[134] Wu WC, Rathore SS, Wang Y, Radford MJ, Krumholz HM. Blood transfusion in elderly patients with acute myocardial infarction. N Engl J Med. 2001;345:1230 -1236.

[135] Hebert PC, Wells G, Blajchman MA, Marshall J, Martin C, Pagliarello G, Tweeddale M, Schweitzer I, Yetisir E. A multicenter, randomized, controlled clinical trial of transfusion requirements in critical care: Transfusion Requirements in Critical Care Investigators, Canadian Critical Care Trials Group. N Engl J Med. 1999;340:409-417.

[136] Tang Y and Katz SD. Anemia in Chronic Heart Failure: Prevalence, Etiology, Clinical Correlates, and Treatment Options. Circulation 2006, 113:2454-2461.

[137] Silverberg OS, Wexler D, Sheps D, et al. The effect of correction of mild anemia in severe, resistant congestive heart failure using subcutaneous erythropoietin and intravenous iron: a randomized controlled study. J Am Coll Cardiol. 2001;37:1775-1780

[138] Ghali JK, Anand I, Abraham WT, et al. Randomized, double-blind, placebo-controlled trial to assess the impact of darbepoetin alfa treatment on exercise tolerance in anemic patients with symptomatic heart failure: results from STAMINA-HeFT. European Society of Cardiology Heart Failure 2006 Congress; June 17-20, 2006; Helsinki, Finland. Abstract 549

[139] Volkova N, Arab L. Evidence-based systematic literature review of hemoglobin/hematocrit and all-cause mortality in dialysis patients. Am J Kidney Dis. 2006 Jan;47(1):24-36.

[140] Ma J, Ebben J, Xia H, et al. Hematocrit levels and associated mortality in hemodialysis patients. J Am Soc Nephrol. 1999;10:610-619.

[141] Collins A, Xia H, Ebben J, et al. Change in hematocrit and risk of mortality. J Am Soc Nephrol. 1998;9(suppl A):204A.

[142] Collins AJ, Li S, St Peter W, et al. Death, hospitalization, and economic associations among incident hemodialysis patients with hematocrit values of 36 to 39%. J Am Soc Nephrol.2001;12: 2465-2473.

[143] Collins A, Ma JZ, Ebben J, et al. Impact of hematocrit on morbidity and mortality. Semin Nephrol. 2000;20:345-349.

[144] Eschbach JW, Abdulhadi MH, Browne JK, et al. Recombinant human erythropoietin in anemic patients with end-stage renal disease: results of a phase III multicenter clinical trial. Ann Intern Med. 1989;111(12):992-1000.

[145] Singh AK, Szczech L, Tang KL, et al; CHOIR Investigators. Correction of anemia with epoetin alfa in chronic kidney disease. N Engl J Med. 2006;355(20):2085-2098.

[146] Pfeffer MA, Burdmann EA, Chen CY, et al; TREAT Investigators. A trial of darbepoetin alfa in type 2 diabetes and chronic kidney disease. N Engl J Med. 2009; 361(21):2019-2032.

[147] Brookhart MA, Schneeweiss S, Avorn J, Bradbury BD, Liu J; Winkelmayer WC. Comparative Mortality Risk of Anemia Management Practices in Incident Hemodialysis Patients. JAMA. 2010;303:857-864

[148] Kazory A and Ross EA, Anemia: The Point of Convergence or Divergence for Kidney Disease and Heart Failure? J Am Coll Cardiol, 2009; 53:639-647.

[149] Low I, Grutzmacher P, Bergmann M, Schoeppe W. Echocardiographic findings in patients on maintenance hemodialysis substituted with recombinant human erythropoietin. Clin Nephrol. 1989;31:26-30.

[150] Low-Friedrich I, Grutzmacher P, Marz W, Bergmann M, Schoeppe W. Therapy with recombinant human erythropoietin reduces cardiac size and improves heart function in chronic hemodialysis patients. Am J Nephrol. 1991;11:54-60.

[151] Goldberg N, Lundin AP, Delano B, Friedman EA, Stein RA. Changes in left ventricular size, wall thickness, and function in anemic patients treated with recombinant human erythropoietin. Am Heart J. 1992;124:424-427.

[152] Foley RN, Parfrey PS, Morgan J, et al. A randomized controlled trial of complete vs partial correction of anemia in hemodialysis patients with asymptomatic concentric LV hypertrophy or LV dilatation. J Am Soc Nephrol. 1998;9:208.

[153] Linde T, Wikstrom B, Andersson LG, Danielson BG. Renal Anemia treatment with recombinant human erythropoietin increases cardiac output in patients with ischemic heart disease. Scand J Urol Nephrol. 1996;30:115-120.

[154] Eckardt KU. Managing a fateful alliance: Anemia and cardiovascular outcomes. Nephrol Dial Transplant. 2005 Jun;20 Suppl 6:vi16-20.

4

Erythrocyte: Programmed Cell Death

Daniela Vittori, Daiana Vota and Alcira Nesse
Department of Biological Chemistry, School of Sciences, University of Buenos Aires,
and IQUIBICEN - National Council of Scientific and Technical Investigation
Argentina

1. Introduction

Erythrocytes are produced by a complex and finely regulated process of erythropoiesis. It starts with a pluripotential stem cell that, in addition of its self replication capacity, can give rise to separate cell lineages. Erythropoiesis passes from the stem cell through the multipotent progenitor CFU-GEMM (colony-forming unit granulocyte erythroid monocyte and megakaryocyte), and then BFU-E (burst-forming unit erythroid) and CFU-E (colony-forming unit eryhtroid), to the first recognizable erythrocyte precursor in the bone marrow, the pronormoblast. This cell gives rise to a series of progressively smaller normoblasts with increasing content of hemoglobin. The nucleus is finally extruded from the late normoblast leading to mature red blood cell through the reticulocyte stage. Erythropoiesis ends with the mature circulating red cell, which is a non-nucleated biconcave disc, performing its function of oxygen delivery. In this process, the glycoprotein hormone erythropoietin has been known as the major humoral regulator of red cell production. It is now well established that erythropoietin stimulates erythropoiesis, at least in part, by protecting erythroblasts from apoptosis.

Human mature erythrocytes are terminally differentiated cells that are devoid of mitochondria, as well as of nucleus and other organelles. In circulation, the red cell is constantly tested for its capacity to undergo marked cellular deformation. This ability to change its shape is essential for optimal cell function, since the resting diameter of the human red cell far exceeds that of the capillaries and splenic endothelial slits through which it must pass (Mohandas & Groner, 1989). A two dimensional network of proteins interacting between transmembrane location and cytoplasmic surface of the plasma membrane gives the red blood cell its properties of elasticity and flexibility that allows the success of this journey.

The mature erythrocyte is unable to self-repair and has no capacity to synthesize proteins. Therefore, its lifespan is finite and is shortened further when the cell's environment becomes hostile or when the erythrocyte's ability to cope with damaging extracellular influences becomes impaired. The erythrocyte limited lifespan implies that, as in other cells, life and death are well regulated for erythrocytes, in spite of their lack of capacity for protein synthesis (Bosman et al., 2005).

In the present review, we aim to show updated information concerning erythrocyte death in order to contribute to the understanding of the physiopathological relationship of this process with the development of anemia.

2. Anemia

The term anemia is derived from ancient Greek for "bloodlessness". It is a condition involving abnormal reduction of hemoglobin content. In healthy adults, there is steady-state equilibrium between the rate of release of new red cells from the bone marrow into the circulation and the rate of removal of senescent red cells from the circulation by reticuloendothelial system. Balance disruption appears by decreased cell production, increased destruction or both, leading then to anemia. Different mechanisms which may lead to anemia are blood loss, decreased red cell lifespan, acquired or congenital defects, ineffective erythropoiesis, and impairment of red cell formation.

In this chapter we focus on anemia resulting from accelerated clearance of red blood cells from circulating blood before hemolysis.

3. Erythrocyte death

Apoptosis is a regulated process of self-destruction characterized by a series of changes affecting the nucleus, cytoplasm and plasma membrane of the cell, and leading to the rapid capture and ingestion of the dying cell by macrophages. Programmed death allows the elimination of cells without release of intracellular proteins which would otherwise cause inflammation.

It is well known that eukaryotic cells use a similar death program. Moreover, erythrocyte precursors, which are true organelle-containing cells, are susceptible to apoptosis induction. Instead, human mature erythrocytes have been considered as unable to undergo programmed cell death due to their lack of mitochondria, nucleus, and other organelles. Increasing evidence is now available to demonstrate that mature erythrocytes can undergo a rapid self-destruction process sharing several features with apoptosis, including cell shrinkage, plasma membrane microvesiculation, shape changes, cytoskeleton alterations associated with protein degradation, and loss of plasma membrane phospholipid asymmetry leading to the externalization of phosphatidylserine. As described, erythrocyte death is characterized by some features that are shared by apoptosis. To distinguish the death of erythrocytes from apoptosis of nucleated cells, some authors suggest the term "eryptosis" (Lang KS et al., 2005).

Erythrocyte lifespan is limited to approximately 120 days and is ended by a process of senescence during which aging erythrocytes suffer changes that display molecules that are recognized by macrophages leading to their clearance from peripheral blood by reticuloendothelial system (Bratosin et al., 1998). Programmed erythrocyte death prevents intravascular hemolysis and allows the elimination of cells without inflammation. Even though this is one of the processes that regulate effective erythropoiesis, a disturbance of the fine equilibrium between erythrocyte production and cell destruction may be caused by the presence of factors that create a harmful environment.

The knowledge of the mechanism of the erythrocyte death is of the highest importance since, apart from its association with anemia, it could lead to improvements of the storage conditions in blood banks by increasing the time of viability of stored red blood cells (Bratosin et al., 2002).

4. Mechanism of suicidal erythrocyte death

As mentioned above, mature erythrocytes can undergo a rapid self-destruction process leading to increased intracellular calcium content, modifications of the erythrocyte morphology, metabolic disruption, membrane protein modifications, and externalization of phosphatidylserine, thereby activating a clearance mechanism involving heterophagic removal in the reticuloendothelial system.

Data describing cell changes and mechanism involved in erythrocyte premature death are stated below.

4.1 Intracellular calcium content

It is well established that two properties of red blood cells, deformability and elasticity, are dramatically affected by calcium ions. Thus, a rise in internal Ca^{2+} leads to changes in cell shape and volume, increased cellular rigidity and hemolysis (Weed et al., 1969; Palek et al., 1974; Kirkpatrick et al., 1975). Such alterations seem to arise from Ca^{2+} interactions with various molecular targets. These include both low-affinity associations with membrane phospholipids (Chandra et al., 1987) and high-affinity ones with specific membrane proteins, especially the Ca-dependent K channel (Romero, 1976) as well as with some cytoskeletal proteins (Wallis et al., 1993). It was observed that the presence of the bivalent-cation ionophore A23187 did not induce erythrocyte death in the absence of extracellular Ca^{2+}, nor in the presence of both Ca^{2+} and the Ca^{2+} chelator EDTA, thus characterizing erythrocyte death as an active process requiring Ca^{2+} entry into the cells (Bratosin et al., 2001).

Since internal Ca^{2+} is subjected to metabolic control via an ATP-dependent extrusion mechanism (Ca pump) (Schatzmann, 1983), it is expected that the decreased ATP content attained during red cell aging should lead to raised cellular Ca^{2+}. The homeostasis of Ca^{2+} in these cells is carried out by the concerted action of just two mechanisms: the active extrusion already mentioned and the entry through defined Ca^{2+} channels (Romero & Romero, 1999). Different factors that may cause cellular stress, such as hyperosmotic shock, oxidative stress, or energy depletion, are capable of Ca^{2+} channel activation in the erythrocyte, including the nonselective cation channel TRPC, with subsequent increased entry of Ca^{2+} (Föller el al., 2008). It has been reported that free Ca^{2+} concentration, cell-shrinkage, and phospholipid scrambling were significantly lower in Cl⁻-depleted TRPC6 -/- erythrocytes than in wildtype mouse erythrocytes, which let the authors conclude that human and mouse erythrocytes express TRPC6 cation channels which participate in cation leak and Ca^{2+}-induced suicidal death (Föller el al., 2008).

The increase in erythrocyte cytosolic Ca^{2+} concentration further stimulates Ca^{2+}-sensitive K+ channel (Gardos channel). The subsequent efflux of K+ hyperpolarises the cell membrane, which drives Cl- exit in parallel to K+. The cellular loss of KCl with osmotically obliged water leads to cell shrinkage. It has been reported that cell shrinkage leads to formation of ceramide. This compound can also contribute to the triggering of cell membrane scrambling (Lang et al., 2004), one of the typical features of suicidal erythrocyte death.

Another important effect caused by a raise in intracellular Ca^{2+} concerns the activation of different enzymes, including calpain. This endogenous protease primarily cleaves the Ca pump, then band 3 protein and finally some cytoskeletal proteins.

4.2 Enzyme activity
4.2.1 Enzymes of the glycolytic pathways

Band 3, the anion-exchange protein, also binds various cytoskeletal proteins as well as hemoglobin and cytoplasmic glycolytic enzymes. It has been shown that mild oxidants, such as potassium ferricyanade, diamide, and hydrogen peroxide stimulate red blood cell glycolysis in proportion to the elevation of band 3 tyrosine phophorylation. Band 3 sequences surrounding tyrosine residues have been associated with intracellular binding of several cytosolic proteins, including hemoglobin and the glycolytic enzymes aldolase, phosphofructokinase, and glyceraldehyde-3-phosphate dehydrogenase. *In vitro*, the tyrosine phosphorylation of band 3 prevented the binding of these glycolytic enzymes. Since these enzymes are inhibited in their bound state, the functional consequence of N-terminal band 3 tyrosine phosphorylation would be an enhanced rate of glycolysis in the intact cells (Harrison et al., 1991; Mallozi et al., 1995). This mechanism of erythrocyte metabolic regulation can stimulate or reduce energy production in times of special needs, such as during a free radical attack.

4.2.2 Enzymes involved in thiol metabolism and protection against oxidative damage
Activities of some cytoplasmic enzymes decline during erythrocyte aging or when they are induced to programmed cell death. Oxidative stress as well as antioxidant depletion cause decreased activity of erythrocyte catalase (CAT), superoxide dismutase (SOD), and glutathione peroxidase (GPX). However, the enzyme behavior seems to depend on the biological model as well as the oxidant agent, since there are some reports showing activation of CAT, SOD, and GPX which has been associated with the metabolic response to cell injure.

4.2.3 Proteases
Members of the caspase family contain a cystein residue in their active center and exist as zymogens that need to be activated by proteolytic cleavage adjacent to aspartates. During apoptosis, caspases function either as initiators (e.g. caspase-8 and -9) in response to proapoptotic signals or as effectors (e.g. caspase-3) (Berg et al., 2001). Mature erythrocytes contain considerable amounts of caspase-3 and caspase-8 whereas other essential components of the mitochondrial apoptotic cascade such as caspase-9, Apaf-1 and cytochrome c are absent. Strikingly, although caspase-3 and -8 were functionally active *in vitro*, they did not become activated by various proapoptotic stimuli. Cysteine protease inhibitors prevented programmed erythrocyte death induced by Ca^{2+} influx, and allowed erythrocyte survival *in vitro* and *in vivo*. However, the cysteine proteases involved seem not to be caspases, since caspase-3, while present in erythrocytes, was not activated during cell death, and cytochrome c, a critical component of the apoptosome, was lacking. Therefore, Ca^{2+}-induced erythrocyte death appeared to proceed in the absence of caspase activation (Bratosin et al., 2001). In opposition, pretreatment of red cells with the caspase-8 or the caspase-3 specific inhibitors blocked the oxidative stress-induced inhibition of aminophospholipid translocase activity, leading to the conclusion that caspase-8 dependent caspase-3 activation could play a role in the phosphatidylserine externalization (Mandal et al., 2005). Other authors observed that treatment of erythrocytes with peroxynitrite under conditions in which the oxidant diffuses to the intracellular compartment led to phosphatidylserine translocation in parallel with activation of caspases (Pietraforte et al., 2007). Taking together, the abovementioned results suggest that the role of caspases in the mature human erythrocytes needs to be clarified.

The major Ca^{2+}-activated cysteine protease found to be involved in the process of cell death is calpain. Following an increase of cytosolic calcium, calpain translocates from the cytosol to the membrane where it undergoes autoproteolytic activation. Although caspases were found inactive in senescent erythrocytes or cells treated with calcium ionophores, activation of the cysteine protease calpain was readily induced in response to elevated calcium levels (Berg et al., 2001). Red blood cells exposed to the oxidative agent peroxynitrite also showed an increase of the active form of μ-calpain (Matarrese et al., 2005). In contrast, calpain inhibitors did not affect phosphatidylserine exposure suggesting that it is presumably a protease-independent event in erythrocytes. A possible explanation may be that increased intracellular calcium is sufficient to disrupt phospholipid asymmetry by activating an aminophospholipid scramblase and inactivating aminophospholipid translocase.

The activation of calpain in normal human erythrocytes incubated in the presence of Ca^{2+} and ionophore A23187 led to the decline of the Ca^{2+}-dependent ATPase activity of the cells, which was prevented by preloading of the erythrocyte with an anticalpain antibody. The decline of the pump activity corresponded to the degradation of the pump protein and was inversely correlated to the amount of the natural inhibitor of calpain, calpastatin, present in the cells. Results suggested that the Ca pump and band 3 were the most sensitive proteins to calpain-induced degradation (Salamino et al., 1994).

Calpain was also responsible for phosphotyrosine phosphatase 1B (PTP1B) cleavage in platelets (Frangioni et al., 1993) and in cell lines with erythroid differentiation ability (Callero et al., 2011), which was accompanied by stimulation of its enzymatic activity. Reversible oxidation of PTP1B *in vitro* strongly facilitated the association with calpain and led to greatly increased calpain-dependent cleavage (Trümpler et al., 2009). Both oxidative environment and increased intracellular Ca^{2+} may account for the altered tyrosyl phosphorylation that may have important implications in the programmed erythrocyte death.

4.3 Phosphatydilserine externalization

Alterations in the transbilayer distribution of phospholipids in erythrocyte membrane have significant physiologic consequences. Phospholipids in the plasma membrane of mammalian cells are not randomly distributed between the two leaflets of the membrane bilayer. Choline-containing phospholipids phosphatidylcholine and sphingomyelin dominate the outer leaflet, while the aminophospholipids phosphatidylethanolamine and phosphatidylserine are major components of the inner leaflet (Williamson & Schlegel, 2002). Of these phospholipids, only phosphatidylserine demonstrates an absolute distribution, and the appearance of this lipid on the external surface has significant consequences for the red blood cell (Daleke, 2008). Several functional roles for asymmetric phospholipid distribution in plasma membranes have been suggested. For instance, several regulatory and structural proteins including protein kinase C (Palfrey & Waseem, 1985), annexin (Meers & Mealy, 1994), and membrane skeletal proteins, such as spectrin (O'Toole et al., 1999), appear to localize to the cytoplasmic face of the membrane through their interaction with phosphatidylserine (Manno et al., 2002).

Although asymmetric lipid synthesis and chemical modification make some contribution, ATP-dependent directional lipid transport is the primary mechanism for generation and maintenance of lipid asymmetry. The latter transport is catalyzed by an enzyme called the aminophospholipid translocase, a P-type ATPase that specifically and rapidly transports the aminophospholipids, phosphatidylethanolamine and phosphatidylserine, from the outer to the inner leaflet of the plasma membrane (Tang et al., 1996). At least one membrane protein is required to facilitate a rapid loss of lipid asymmetry. Although no protein mediating this function has been identified they are called "phospholipid scramblases". The bivalent cation Ca^{2+} plays an important role in the regulation of lipid scrambling. In erythrocyte, once activated by Ca^{2+}, the scrambling pathway remains active for at least 2 h (Williamson et al., 1992). Scramblase creates a proteinaceous aqueous pore that facilitates migration of the polar headgroup of the lipids across the hydrophobic core of the bilayer, while keeping the acyl chain moieties in the core of the bilayer (Bevers & Williamson, 2010).

Whether triggered by injury, disease or cell activation, the movement of phosphatidylserine to the surface of the cell alters rheologic and hemostatic properties of the membrane. Erythrocytes with surface-exposed phosphatidylserine adhere to one another and to vascular endothelial cells (Daleke, 2008). Thus, the regulation and control of the distribution of phospholipid asymmetry are essential for maintenance erythrocyte mechanical stability and proper cell function. Furthermore, asymmetric distribution of aminophospholipids has significant effects on cell shape and on membrane mechanical stability. Ghosts that maintained their asymmetric lipid distribution had normal discoid morphology whereas ghosts in which asymmetric lipid distribution was lost exhibited echinocytic morphology (Manno et al., 2002). Understanding the cause of perturbations of transbilayer distribution of phospholipids and the molecular mechanism by which they are regulated is essential for ameliorating some of the consequences of erythrocyte membrane abnormalities.

In summary, phosphatidylserine translocation, now generally accepted as a hallmark of cells in apoptosis, results from the inhibition of aminophospholipid translocase activity and activation of scramblase. Surface exposure of phosphatidylserine on apoptotic cells presents a recognition and engulfment signal for removal by phagocytosis competent cells even before the development of morphological changes usually associated with death (Schlegel & Williamson, 2001).

4.4 Erythrocyte morphology

The volume of red cells decreases with cell aging and substantial amount of hemoglobin is lost from circulating erythrocytes during total lifespan. This is probably due to loss of potassium and to loss of membrane via microvesiculation, resulting in cellular dehydration, membrane protein removal, and increased density.

Vesicle formation appears to be accompanied by the breakdown of band 3 protein. It has been postulated that removal of senescent erythrocytes by macrophages is mediated by senescent cell-specific autoantigens originated on band 3, the anion exchanger and the major membrane protein of the erythrocyte (Kay, 2005). In accordance, Willekens et al. (2008) confirmed that vesiculation is not only associated with the removal of membrane-bound hemoglobin, but is associated with generation of senescent cell antigen, a neoantigen that originates from band 3 after its breakdown in senescent red blood cells. Based on results from immunological analysis of vesicles and taken into consideration the existence of an efficient body mechanism to remove these vesicles, the authors concluded that vesiculation constitutes a mechanism for the removal of erythrocyte membrane patches containing removal molecules, thereby postponing the elimination of otherwise healthy erythrocytes.

Allan and Thomas (1981) found the importance of a raised intracellular Ca^{2+} concentration in the microvesiculation process. Plasma membrane microvesiculation, induced *in vitro* by Ca^{2+}, was found identical to that expressed by the very small subpopulation of *in vivo* senescent erythrocytes purified from peripheral blood of healthy donors (Bratosin et al., 2001). Recent comparative proteomic analysis of erythrocytes and their vesicles provide new clues to the mechanisms involved in erythrocyte death (Bosman et al., 2010).

The structure and molecular interaction of proteins within the complex assembly of the erythrocyte cytoskeleton explain the particular shape and shape transformations of these cells. Spectrin, band 3, actin, ankyrin, and other cytoskeletal proteins play an important role for membrane integrity, typical discocyte form, and elasticity of red blood cells. Conversely, protein damage has been implicated in altered erythrocyte morphology.

The shape of Ca^{2+}-loaded erythrocytes changed from normal discocytes to echinocytes or spheroechinocytes with plasma membrane microvesiculation (Bratosin et al., 2001; Vota et al., 2010) (Figure 1). Morphological changes induced by A23187 in the presence of Ca^{2+} were associated with cell shrinkage, one of the characteristic features of apoptosis that distinguishes this active and regulated self-destruction process from the passive and chaotic event of necrosis induced by plasma membrane damage (Bratosin et al., 2001).

On the other hand, stomatocytes were the main morphological cell transformation associated to *in vitro* (Vota et al., 2010) and *in vivo* (Richards et al., 2007; Antonelou et al., 2011) oxidative stress (Figure 1).

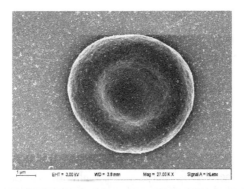

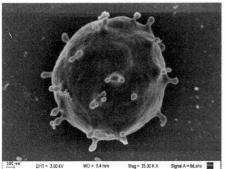 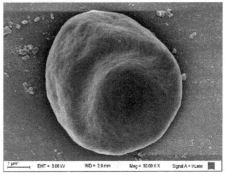

Fig. 1. Altered shapes of erythrocytes subjected to proeryptotic agents. The normal discoid biconcave shape (top) turned to spherocyte with microvesiculation due to increased intracellular calcium concentration (left bottom) or to stomatocyte induced by oxidative stress (right bottom). Results obtained in our laboratory.

4.5 Protein modifications

Erythrocyte membrane proteins are susceptible to covalent modification by the lipid peroxidation products generated by an oxygen radical attack. *In vitro* and *in vivo* assays in which erythrocyte metabolic alterations were associated to oxidant environments induced increased lipoperoxidation (Quintanar-Escorza et al., 2010; Calderón-Salinas et al., 2011).

The cytoplasmic domain of band 3 serves as a center of erythrocyte membrane organization and constitutes the major substrate of erythrocyte tyrosine kinases. Tyrosine phosphorylation of band 3 is induced by several stimuli, including malaria parasite invasion, cell shrinkage, normal cell aging, and oxidative stress (Harrison et al., 1991). Erythrocytes contain protein tyrosine kinase activity, with band 3 protein being the major substrate for the kinases (Brunati et al., 1996). Besides, phosphotyrosine phosphatase was found associated to band 3 protein. This phosphatase is normally highly active and prevents the accumulation of band 3 phosphotyrosine. However, in A23187-treated erythrocytes increased intracellular Ca^{2+} was found to promote band 3 tyrosine phosphorylation via dissociation of phosphotyrosine phosphatase from band 3 (Zipser et al., 2002).

Tyrosine phosphorylation of band 3 markedly reduced its affinity for ankyrin, leading to release of band 3 from the spectrin/actin membrane skeleton, enhancement of the lateral mobility of band 3 in the bilayer, and progressive vesiculation. Because release of band 3 from its ankyrin and adducin linkages to the cytoskeleton can facilitate changes in multiple membrane properties, the authors suggested that tyrosine phosphorylation of band 3 may produce changes in erythrocyte biology that allow the cell to respond to initial stress (Ferru et al., 2011).

Another marker of red blood cell apoptosis is band 3 clustering, which generates a cell surface epitope identified by autologous IgG antibodies and may act as a signal for the removal of erythrocytes from circulation (Kay et al., 1989).

The nitration of tyrosine residues in proteins occurs through the action of reactive oxygen and nitrogen species such as peroxynitrite, the product of the reaction between nitric oxide and superoxide anion. The nitrated peptides were able to activate *lyn*, an erythrocyte *src* tyrosine kinase. It suggested a mechanism of peroxynitrite-mediated signaling that may be correlated with upregulation of tyrosine phosphorylation (Mallozi et al., 2001).

5. Processes that induce premature erythrocyte death

Eryptosis can be triggered by different injuries such as energy depletion, osmotic shock or oxidative stress.

5.1 Energy depletion

As mentioned in Section 4.1, the reduced calcium-ATPase activity due to energy depletion leads to decreased calcium efflux and this in turn accelerates the transmembrane movement of potassium and chloride, resulting in cell dehydration.

Energy stress also impairs the replenishment of glutathione and thus weakens the antioxidative defense of erythrocytes (Bilmen et al., 2001). Accordingly, this condition similarly activates cation channels affecting calcium flux (Duranton et al., 2002). On the other hand, phosphatidylserine and phosphatidylethanolamine are maintained in the cell inner leaflet by an ATP-dependent transporter known as flippase (Williamson & Schlegel, 2002). Membrane-bound Mg^{2+}-ATPases seem to play a key role in the maintenance of the membrane lipid organization. This subfamily of ATPases has been reported to actively translocate aminophospholipids across membranes. Decreased ATP-dependent transport may be very well one of the consequences of phosphatidylserine exposure (Soupene & Kuypers, 2006). Besides, energy depletion involves activation of PKC and PKC-dependent phosphorylation of membrane proteins with subsequent stimulation of eryptosis (Föller et al., 2008).

5.2 Osmotic shock

Osmotic shock is found among the well-known inducers of apoptotic cell death. The cellular mechanisms involved in the triggering of apoptosis following cell exposure to hypertonic extracellular fluid have been deeply studied in nucleated cells. Erythrocytes have similarly been shown to bind annexin following osmotic shock.

Erythrocytes incubated in a hyperosmotic environment released prostaglandin E2 (PGE2), which in turn activated nonselective cation channels (Kaestner & Bernhardt, 2002; Lang PA et al., 2005), and increased the cytosolic Ca^{2+} concentration. Activation of the cell volume- and redox potential-sensitive cation channel and subsequent Ca^{2+} entry contributed to the development of erythrocyte cell membrane scrambling. Osmotic cell shrinkage was involved in the stimulation of sphingomyelinase which caused sphingomyelin degradation with subsequent release of ceramide in erythrocytes (Lang et al., 2004). Ceramide then activated scramblase leading to breakdown of phosphatidylserine asymmetry of the cell membrane. The ability of ceramide to induce this kind of erythrocyte death was somewhat surprising, as erythrocytes lack mitochondria, crucial elements in the ceramide-triggered signaling cascade in nucleated cells (Lang et al., 2004). Thus, at least in erythrocytes, ceramide must trigger annexin binding through a pathway distinct from that described in nucleated cells.

5.3 Oxidative stress

Increasing intracellular oxidants by altering ambient oxygen concentrations or lowering antioxidant levels accelerates the onset of erythrocyte senescence whereas lowering ambient oxygen or increasing reactive oxygen species (ROS) scavenging appears to delay senescence. In general, conditions that induce senescence often appear to be accompanied by a rise in intracellular ROS levels. Polyunsaturated fatty acids within the membrane, an oxygen rich environment, and iron rich hemoglobin make red cells susceptible to peroxidative damage. The product of membrane lipid peroxidation can affect the anion transport function and activity of enzymes of the glycolytic pathway associated to band 3 (Dumaswala et al., 1999).

By virtue of its potent oxidant and nitrating ability, peroxynitrite has been proposed as an important mediator of inflammation-induced tissue injury and dysfunction, and it is considered the most efficient nitrating species of biological relevance (Szabó et al., 2007). The red blood cells are, in fact, the major scavengers of peroxynitrite in blood and it has been calculated that at 45% hematocrit about 40–45% of peroxynitrite crosses the cell membrane and quickly reacts with hemoglobin, while the remainder reacts extracellularly with carbon dioxide (Romero & Radi, 2005). In an *in vitro* experimental system mimicking the oxidative imbalance detectable *in vivo*, peroxynitrite acted both extra- and intracellularly as a function of cell density and carbon dioxide concentration, inducing the appearance of distinct cellular biomarkers as well as modulation of metabolism (Pietraforte et al., 2007). Intracellular oxidations, due mostly to direct reactions of peroxynitrite with glutathione and hemoglobin (methemoglobin), lead to decreased ATP and the appearance of apoptotic signs, such as clustering of band 3, externalization of phosphatidylserine, and activation of caspases. Surface/membrane oxidations were principally due to indirect radical reactions causing oxidation of surface thiols, formation of membrane-associated 3-nitrotyrosine, and downregulation of glycophorins A, the latter being considered a senescence biomarker (Matarrese et al., 2005; Pietraforte et al., 2007; Metere et al., 2009).

6. *In vivo* erythrocyte death and possible prevention

Oxidative stress is a term used to describe the body's prolonged exposure to oxidative factors that cause more free radicals than the body can neutralize. Under this condition, free radical formation may play a role in the pathophysiology of several diseases. There is evidence that erythrocytes undergo oxidative changes in conditions where free radical formation is known to be high such as rheumatoid arthritis (Richards et al., 2007), diabetes (Manuel y Keenoy et al., 2001; Calderón-Salinas et al., 2011), and hemodialysis treatment (Zachee et al., 1988). Oxidative damage was also considered the cause of decreased deformability and altered rheology of erythrocytes found in individuals with chronic fatigue syndrome, a condition that may be triggered by certain infectious diseases, multiple nutrient deficiencies, food intolerance, or extreme physical or mental stress (Richards et al., 2007). Erythrocyte alterations would have the physiological effect of reducing oxygen delivery to the tissues. In several models, 2,3-diphosphoglycerate (2,3-DPG) levels were increased and this effect may be explained as a compensation since 2,3-DPG have the effect of decreasing oxygen affinity. Therefore, this would allow more oxygen to be delivered to the tissues.

Any erythrocyte disorder facilitating erythrocyte shrinkage, could, to the extent as it leads to activation of the cell volume regulatory cation channels, trigger premature apoptosis and thus accelerate erythrocyte death. Red blood cells from patients with sepsis (Kempe et al., 2007), sickle cell disease (Wood et al., 1996), thalassemia (Kuypers et al., 1998), glucose-6-phosphate dehydrogenase deficiency (Lang et al., 2002), and phosphate depletion (Birka et al., 2004) are more sensitive to apoptotic stimuli, a property correlating with the shortened erythrocyte lifespan in these disorders. Membrane lipid disorders play an important role in the pathology of hemoglobinopathies, leading to premature removal (anemia) and imbalance in hemostasis (e.g. lipid breakdown products of phosphatidylserine-exposed cells result in vascular dysfunction) (Neidlinger et al., 2006).

Altered phosphorylation of erythrocyte cytoskeletal proteins and increased ROS production result in disruption of cytoskeleton stability in healthy and sickle cell erythrocytes (George et al., 2010).

Significant modifications in red blood cell structure and membrane proteome in end stage renal disease patients were observed in the context of increased ROS accumulation. The intrinsic oxidative stimuli related to the uremic state were closely associated with membrane cytoskeleton instability, loss of surface area through vesiculation, and transformation of normal discocytes. The observed alterations might contribute to premature erythrocyte death and to the progression of anemia (Antonelou et al., 2011).

Under normal conditions, red blood cells are continuously exposed to ROS from both internal and external sources. In healthy erythrocytes, significant oxidative damage is prevented by a very efficient antioxidant system, consisting of enzymatic and nonenzymatic pathways. Enzymes for preventing oxidative denaturation in erythrocytes include superoxide dismutase, catalase, glutathione peroxidase and glutathione reductase which sustain glutathione regeneration, and NADH-methemoglobin reductase. In addition to primary antioxidant defense systems that prevent the generation of free radicals or radical chain reactions, secondary systems have been proposed. These include proteases that preferentially degrade proteins damaged by oxidation. Endogenous non-enzymatic antioxidants also provide defense against oxidative damage: they are lipophylic (vitamin E, carotenoids, melatonin) and water soluble compounds (vitamin C, gluthatione, ceruloplasmin, uric acid) (Burak Çimen, 2008).

Free radicals are produced as intermediate products of normal metabolic functions. Thus, antioxidants function as modulators of cellular homeostasis including detoxification of radicals and metals as well as potent free radical scavengers.

Erythropoietin, the hormone that is the principal regulator of red blood cell production, prevents apoptosis of erythroid progenitors, supporting their survival. It is well known that the target cells for erythropoietin are the progenitors of erythrocytes found in the hematopoietic organs. However, early works have shown prolonged red blood cell survival during treatment with recombinant human erythropoietin (Schwartz et al., 1992; Polenakovic & Sikole, 1996), suggesting a contribution to the maintenance of corrected hematocrit values. Later, other works were performed to elucidate mechanisms of action of erythropoietin upon mature erythrocytes. Myssina et al. (2003) reported that erythropoietin inhibited cell death through a direct effect via erythropoietin receptor on mature erythrocytes. Unlike the general knowledge of the absence of erythropoietin receptors in reticulocytes, the authors detected the expression of about six erythropoietin binding sites per mature red blood cell. In this work, they postulated that erythropoietin bound to erythrocytes inhibited the volume-sensitive cation channel responsible for calcium entry, and thus blocked phosphatidylserine translocation. More investigation is needed to elucidate the erythropoietin effects upon erythrocytes, since it is well known that erythropoietin induces increased intracellular Ca^{2+} concentration in human erythroid progenitors when they are activated via binding of the hormone with its specific receptor.

On the other hand, a direct effect of erythropoietin on mature erythrocytes might be possible, since erythropoietin similar to other proteins would protect red cell membranes from lipid peroxidation by scavenging hydroxyl radicals generated by oxidative stress. Chattopadhyay et al. (2000) reported that the oxidative damage brought about by copper (II) ascorbate upon red blood cells was due to generation of hydroxyl radical and that erythropoietin was able to protect the membrane from oxidative damage.

In a preliminary study, mature erythrocytes from patients with chronic renal insufficiency exhibited higher annexin binding when compared with red blood cells from healthy individuals. Moreover, the number of cells expressing phosphatidylserine externalization decreased after dialysis only when patients received erythropoietin immediately before dialysis (Myssina et al., 2003). Irrespective the erythropoietin mechanism it seems that the hormone does not only inhibit apoptosis of erythroid progenitor cells, but blunts the suicidal death of mature erythrocytes. This protective antieryptotic mechanism may ameliorate erythrocyte death *in vivo*, resulting in increased lifespan of circulating cells.

7. Conclusion

The human red blood cell, by lacking nucleus or any other subcellular organelle, represents the final differentiation stage of the erythroid series. After a limited period in circulation, aged cells become sequestered and removed by macrophages from the reticuloendothelial system. This fate implies that erythrocyte life and death should be well regulated.

Senescence of red blood cells occurs along their lifespan in the vascular system. During aging, erythrocytes display molecules that lead to recognition and removal of old damaged cells by the immune system. Current evidence indicates that neoantigens on altered band 3 and phosphatidylserine exposed at the outside of erythrocytes are the main signals for cell removal and phagocytosis. Vesicles, generated as an integral part of the aging process probably to remove damaged membrane patches, disappear rapidly from circulation. The formation of vesicles as well as changes in electrolyte movements lead to decreased cell volume. Disruption of cell metabolism, hemoglobin denaturalization, changes in cytoskeletal protein interaction, protein phosphorylation/dephosphorylation disbalance, and membrane protein modifications are among the factors responsible for the appearance of morphological alterations.

Considering that senescence represents the time-dependent induction of erythrocyte self-destruction process, premature cell death due to proeryptotic factors could greatly contribute to the development of anemia.

Energy depletion, oxidative stress, and osmotic shock are the most common events that can produce erythrocyte damage, leading to premature eryptosis (Fig. 2). The common feature is the increased intracellular calcium concentration due to either calcium channel activation or depressed calcium pump. Calcium accumulation in turn activates the potassium channel favoring this cation efflux, followed by chloride and water exit, which in conjunction generate cell shrinkage. Calpain, activated by calcium, affects cytoskeletal proteins inducing membrane destabilization and blebbling, and is involved in scramblase activation, thus facilitating phosphatydilserine translocation.

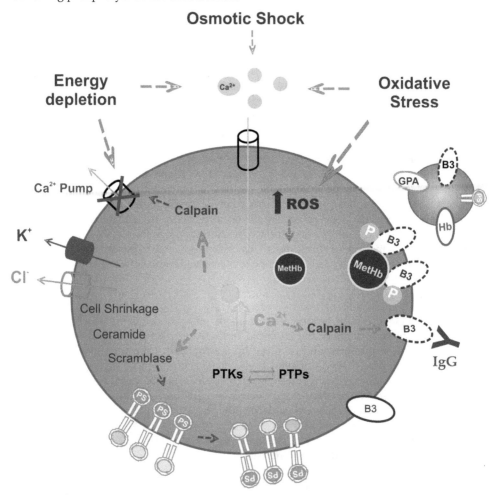

Fig. 2. Mechanisms involved in programmed erythrocyte death. B3: band 3; ROS: reactive oxygen species; Hb: hemoglobin; MetHb: methemoglobin; GPA: glycophorin A; PTKs: phosphotyrosine kinases; PTPs: phosphotyrosine phosphateses; PS: phosphatidylserine.

Additional increase in intracellular oxidants by altering ambient oxygen concentrations or lowering antioxidant levels also accelerates the onset of senescence. Concurrent effects mediated by oxidized hemoglobin and by protein phosphorylation due to disbalance in the kinase/phosphatase ratio are directed towards erythrocyte damage, and consequently to eryptosis.

It is evident that elucidation of mechanisms that regulate eryptosis is a complex issue because of technical problems in obtaining purified cell fractions of a well-defined cell age or in the correct manipulation of erythrocytes *in vitro*, and especially due to the low probability to test hypothesis of programmed erythrocyte death *in vivo*. However, to get an insight into this mechanism is essential for understanding the pathological circumstances surrounding anemia associated to many different diseases.

8. Acknowledgments

Dr. Daniela Vittori and Dr. Alcira Nesse are research scientists from the CONICET (National Council for Scientific and Technical Research, Argentina), and Lic. Daiana Vota is recipient of a fellowship from CONICET. The three authors are teachers at the Department of Biological Chemistry (School of Sciences, University of Buenos Aires, Argentina).

9. References

Allan, D. & Thomas, P. (1981). Ca2+-induced biochemical changes in human erythrocytes and their relation to microvesiculation. *Biochem J* 198, 433-440.

Antonelou, M.H., Kriebardis, A.G., Velentzas, A.D., Kokkalis, A.C., Georgakopoulou, S-C., & Papassideri I.S. (2011). Oxidative stress-associated shape transformation and membrane proteome remodeling in erythrocytes of end stage renal disease patients on hemodialysis. *J Proteom* doi:10.1016/j.jprot.2011.04.009.

Berg, C.P., Engels, I.H., Rothbart, A., Lauber, K., Renz, A., Schlosser, S.F., Schulze-Osthoff, K., & Wesselborg. S. (2001). Human mature red blood cells express caspase-3 and caspase-8, but are devoid of mitochondrial regulators of apoptosis. *Cell Death Differ* 8, 1197-1206.

Bevers, E.M. & Williamson, P.L. (2010). Phospholipid scramblase: an update. *FEBS Letters* 584, 2724-2730.

Bilmen, S., Aksu, T.A., Gümüslü, S., Korquin, D.K., & Canatan, D. (2001). Antioxidant capacity of G-6-PD-deficient erythrocytes. *Clin Chim Acta* 303, 83-86.

Birka, C., Lang, P.A., Kempe, D.S., Hoefling, L., Tanneur, V., Duranton, C., Nammi, S., Henke, G., Myssina, S., Krikov, M., Huber, S.M., Wieder, T., & Lang, F. (2004). Enhanced susceptibility to erythrocyte "apoptosis" following phosphate depletion. *Pflugers Arch* 448, 471–477.

Bosman, G.J., Willekens, F.L., & Werre, J.M. (2005). Erythrocyte aging: a more than superficial resemblance to apoptosis? *Cell Physiol Biochem* 16, 1-8.

Bosman, G.J., Lasonder, E., Groenen-Döpp, Y.A., Willekens, F.L., Werre, J.M., & Novotný, V.M. (2010). Comparative proteomics of erythrocyte aging in vivo and in vitro. *J Proteom* 73, 396-402.

Bratosin, D., Mazurier, J., Tissier, J.P., Estaquier, J., Huart, J.J., Ameisen, J.C., Aminoff, D., & Montruil, J. (1998). Cellular and molecular mechanisms of senescent erythrocyte phagocytosis by macrophages. A review. *Biochemie* 80, 173-195.

Bratosin, D., Estaquier, J., Petit, F., Arnoult, D., Quatannens, B., Tissier, J-P., Slomianny, C., Sartiaux, C., Alonso, C., Huart, J-J., Montreuil, J., & Ameisen, J.C. (2001). Programmed cell death in mature erythrocytes: a model for investigating death effector pathways operating in the absence of mitochondria. *Cell Death Differ* 8, 1143-1156.

Bratosin, D., Estaquier, J., Ameisen, J.C., & Montreuil, J. (2002). Molecular and cellular mechanisms of programmed cell death: impact on blood transfusion. *Vox Sang* 83, 307-310.

Brunati, A.M., Bordin, L., Clari, G., & Morel, V. (1996). The Lyn-catalyzed Tyr phosphorylation of the transmembrane band 3 protein of the human erythrocytes. *Eur J Biochem* 240, 394-399.

Burak Çimen, M.Y. (2008). Free radical metabolism in human erythrocytes. *Clin Chim Acta* 390, 1-11.

Calderón-Salinas, J.V., Muñoz-Reyes, E.G., Guerrero-Romero, J.F., Rodríguez-Morán, M., Bracho-Riquelme, R.L., Carrera-Gracia, M.A., & Quintanar-Escorza, M.A. (2011). Eryptosis and oxidative damage in type 2 diabetic mellitus patients with chronic kidney disease. *Mol Cell Biochem* doi: 10.1007/s11010-011-0887-1.

Callero, M.A., Vota, D.M., Chamorro, M.E., Wenker, S.D., Vittori, D.C., & Nesse, A.B. (2011). Calcium as a mediator between erythropoietin and protein tyrosine phosphatase 1B. *Arch Biochem Biophys* 505, 242-249.

Chandra, R., Joshi, P.C., Bajpai, V.K., & Gupta, C.M. (1987). Membrane phopholipid organization in calcium-loaded human erythrocytes. *Biochim Biophys Acta* 902, 253-262.

Chattopadhyay, A., Das Choudhury, T., Bandyopadhyay, D., & Datta A. (2000). Protective effect of erythropoietin on the oxidative damage of erythrocyte membrane by hydroxyl radical. *Biochem Pharmacol* 59, 419-425.

Daleke, D.L. (2008). Regulation of phospholipid asymmetry in the erythrocyte membrane. *Curr Opin Hematol* 15, 191-195.

Dumaswala, U.J., Jacobsen, D.W., Jain, S.K., & Sukalski, K.A. (1999). Protein and lipid oxidation of banked human erythrocytes: role of glutathione. *Free Radic Biol Med* 27, 1041-1049.

Duranton, B., Huber, S.M., & Lang, F. (2002). Oxidation induced a Cl(-)-dependent cation conductance in human red blood cells. *Cell Biol Toxicol* 18, 381-396.

Ferru, E., Giger, K., Pantaleo, A., Campanella, E., Grey, J., Ritchie, K., Vono, R., Turrini, F., & Low, P. (2011). Regulation of membrane-cytoskeletal interactions by tyrosine phosphorylation of erythrocyte band 3. *Blood* 117, 5998-6006.

Föller, M., Kasinathan, R. S., Koka, S., Lang, C., Shumilina, E., Birnbaumer, L., Lang, F., & Huber, S. M. (2008). TRPC6 contributes to the Ca^{2+} leak of human erythrocytes. *Cell Physiol Biochem* 21, 183–192.

Frangioni, J.V., Oda, A., Smith, M., Salzman, E., & Neel, B.G. (1993). Calpain-catalyzed cleavage amd subcellular relocation of protein phosphotyrosine phosphatase 1B (PTP-1B) in human platelets. *EMBO J* 12, 4843-4856.

George, A., Pushkaran, S., Li, L., An, X., Zheng, Y., & Mohandas, N. (2010). Altered phosphorylation of cytoskeleton proteins in sickle red blood cells: The role of protein kinase C, Rac GTPases, and reactive oxygen species. *Blood Cells Mol Dis* 45, 41-45.

Harrison, M.L., Rathinavelu, P., Arese, P., Geahlen, R.L., & Low, P.S. (1991). Role of Band 3 tyrosine phosphorylation in the regulation of erythrocyte glycolysis. *J Biol Chem* 266, 4106-4111.

Kaestner, L. & Bernhardt, I. (2002). Ion channels in the human red blood cell membrane: their further investigation and physiological relevance. *Bioelectrochemistry* 55, 71-74.

Kay, M.M., Flowers, N., Goodman, J., & Bosman, G. (1989). Alteration in membrane protein band 3 associated with accelerated erythrocyte aging. *Proc Natl Acad Sci (USA)*. 86, 5834-5838.

Kay, M. (2005). Immunoregulation of cellular life span. *Ann N Y Acad Sci* 1057, 85-111.

Kempe, D.S., Akel, A., Lang, P.A., Hermle, T., Biswas, R., Muresanu, J., Friedrich, B., Dreischer, P., Wolz, C., Schumacher, U., Peschel, A., Götz, F., Döring, G., Wieder, T., Gulbins, E., & Lang, F. (2007). Suicidal erythrocyte death in sepsis. *J Mol Med (Berl)* 85, 273-281.

Kirkpatrick, F.H., Hillman, D.G., & La Celle, P.L. (1975). A23187 and red cells: changes in deformability, K^+, Mg^{2+}, Ca^{2+} and ATP. *Experientia* 31, 653-654.

Kuypers, F.A., Yuan, J., Lewis, R.A., Snyder, L.M., Kiefer, C.R., Bunyjaratvej, A. Fucharoen, S., Ma, L., Styles, L., de Jong, K., & Schrier, S.L. (1998). Membrane phospholipid asymmetry in human thalassemia. *Blood* 91, 3044-3051.

Lang, K.S., Roll, B., Myssina, S., Schittenhelm, M., Scheel-Walter, H.G., Kanz, L., Fritz, J., Lang, F., Huber, S.M., & Wieder, T. (2002). Enhanced erythrocyte apoptosis in sickle cell anemia, thalassemia, and glucose-6-phosphate dehydrogenase deficiency. *Cell Physiol Biochem* 12, 365-372.

Lang, K.S., Myssina, S., Brand, V., Sandu, C., Lang, P.A., Berchtold, S., Huber, S.M., Lang, F., & Wieder, T. (2004). Involvemnt of ceramide in hyperosmotic shock-induced death of erythrocytes. *Cell Death Differ* 11, 231-243.

Lang, K.S., Lang, P.A., Bauer, C., Duranton, C., Wieder, T., Huber, S., & Lang, F. (2005). Mechanisms of suicidal erythrocyte death. Cell Physiol Biochem 15, 195-202.

Lang, P.A., Kempe, D.S., Myssina, S., Tanneur, V., Birka, C., Laufer, S., Lang, F., Wieder, T., & Huber S.M. (2005). PGE(2) in the regulation of programmed erythrocyte death. *Cell Death Differ* 12, 415-428.

Mallozi, C., Di Stasi, A.M., & Minetti, M. (1995). Free radicals induce reversible membrane-cytoplasm translocation of glyceraldehydes-3-phosphate dehydogenase in human erythrocytes. *Arch Biochem Biophys* 321, 345-352.

Mallozi, C., Di Stasi, A.M., & Minetti, M. (2001). Nitrotyrosine mimics phosphotyrosine binding to the SH2 domain of the *src* family tyrosine kinase *lyn*. *FEBS Letters* 503, 189-195.

Mandal, D., Mazumder, A., Das, P., Kundu, M., & Basu, J. (2005). Fas-, caspase-8, and caspase-3-dependent signaling regulates the activity of the aminophospholipid translocase and phosphatidylserine externalization in human erythrocytes. *J Biol Chem* 280, 39460-39467.

Manno, S., Takakuwa, Y., & Mohandas N. (2002). Identification of a functional role for lipid asymmetry in biological membranes: Phosphatidylserine-skeletal protein interactions modulate membrane stability. *Proc Natl Acad Sci (USA)* 99, 1943-1948.

Manuel y Keenoy, B., Vertommen, J., & De Leeuw, I. (2001). Divergent effects of different oxidants on glutathione homeostasis and protein damage in erythrocytes from diabetic patients: effects of high glucose. *Mol Cell Biochem* 225, 59-73.

Matarrese, P., Straface, E., Pietraforte, D., Gambardella, L., Vona, R., Maccaglia, A., Minetti, M., & Malomi, W. (2005). Peroxynitrite induces senescence and apoptosis of red blood cells through the activation of aspartyl and cysteinyl porteases. *FASEB J* 19, 416-8.

Meers, P. & Mealy, T. (1994). Phospholipid determinants for the annexin V binding sites and the role of tryptophan 187. *Biochemistry* 33, 5829-5837.

Metere, A., Iorio, E., Pietraforte, D., Podo, F., & Minetti, M. (2009). Peroxynitrite signaling in human erythrocytes: Synergistic role of hemoglobin oxidation and band 3 tyrosine phospsorylation. *Arch Biochem Biophys* 484, 173-182.

Mohandas, N., & Groner, W. (1989). Cell membrane and volume changes during red cell development and aging. *Ann N Y Acad Sci* 554,217-224.

Myssina, S., Huber, S.M., Birka, C., Lang, P.A., Lang, K.S., Friedrich, B., Risler, T., Wieder, T, & Lang, F. (2003). Inhibition of erythrocyte cation channels by erythropoietin. *J Am Soc Nephrol* 14, 2750-2757.

Neidlinger, N.A., Larkin, S.K., Bhagat, A., Victorino, G.P., & Kuypers, F.A. (2006). Hydrolysis of phosphatidylserine-exposing red blood cells by secretory phospholipase A2 generates lysophosphatidic acid and results in vascular dysfunction. *J Biol Chem* 28, 775-781.

O'Toole, P.J., Wolfe, C., Ladha, S., & Cherry, R.J. (1999). Rapid diffusion of spectrin bound to a lipid surface. *Biochim Biophys Acta* 1419, 64-70.

Palek, J., Stewart, G., & Lionetti, F.J. (1974). The dependence of shape of human erythrocyte ghosts on calcium, magnesium, and adenosine triphosphate. *Blood* 44, 583-597.

Palfrey, H.C. & Waseem, A. (1985). Protein kinase C in the human erythrocyte. Translocation to the plasma membrane and phosphorylation of bands 4.1 and 4.9 and other membrane proteins. *J Biol Chem* 260, 16021-16029.

Pietraforte, D., Matarrese, P., Straface, E., Gambardella, L., Metere, A., Scorza, G., Leto, T., Malorni, W., & Minetti, M. (2007). Two different pathways are envolved in peroxynitrite-induced senescente and apoptosis of human erythrocytes. *Free Radical Biol Med* 42, 202-214.

Polenakovic, M. & Sikole, A. (1996). Is erythropoietin a survival factor for red blood cells? *J Am Soc Nephrol* 7, 1178-1182.

Quintanar-Escorza, M.A., González-Martínez, M.T., Intriago-Ortega, M.P., & Calderón-Salinas, J.V. (2010). Oxidative damage increases intracellular free calcium $[Ca^{2+}]_i$ concentration in human erythrocytes incubated with lead. *Toxicol In Vitro* 24, 1338-1346.

Richards, R.S., Wang, L., & Jelinek, H. (2007). Erythrocyte Oxidative Damage in Chronic Fatigue Syndrome. *Archiv Med Res* 38, 94-98.

Romero, N. & Radi, R. (2005). Hemoglobin and red blood cells as tools for studying peroxinitrite biochemistry. *Methods Enzymol* 396, 229-245.

Romero, P.J. (1976) The role of membrane-bound Ca in ghost permeability to Na and K. *J Membrane Biol* 29, 329-343.

Romero, P.J. & Romero, E.A. (1999). The role of calcium metabolism in human red blood cell ageing: A Proposal. *Blood Cells Mol Dis* 15, 9-19.

Salamino, F., Sparatore, B., Melloni, E., Michetti, M., Vioti, P.L., Pontremoli, S., & Carafoli, E. (1994). The plasma membrane calcium pump is the preferred calpain substrate within the erythrocyte. *Cell Calcium* 15, 28-35.

Schatzmann, H.J. (1983). The red cell calcium pump. *Annu Rev Physiol* 45, 303-312.

Schlegel, R.A. & Williamson, P. (2001). Phosphatidylserine, a death knell. *Cell Death Differ* 8, 551-563.

Schwartz, A.B., Kahn, S.B., Kelch, B., Kim K.E., & Pequignot, E. (1992). Red blood cell improved survival due to recombinant human erythropoietin explained effectiveness of less frequent, low dose subcutaneous therapy. *Clin Nephrol* 38, 283-289.

Soupene, E. & Kuypers, F.A. (2006). Identification of an erythroid ATP-dependent aminophospholipid transporter. *Brit J Hematol* 133, 436-438.

Szabó, C., Ischiropoulos, H., & Radi, R. (2007). Peroxynitrite: biochemistry, pathophysiology and development of therapeutics. *Nature Rev* 6, 662-680.

Tang, X., Halleck, M.S., Schlegel, R.A., & Williamson, P. (1996). A subfamily of P-type ATPases with aminophospholipid transporting activity. *Science* 272, 1495-1497.

Trümpler, A., Schlott, B., Herrlich, P., Greer, P., & Böhmer, F-D. (2009). Calpain-mediated degradation of reversibly oxidized protein-tyrosine phosphatase 1B. *FEBS J* 276, 5622-5633.

Vota, D., Callero, M., Chamorro, M.E., Crisp, R., Nesse, A., & Vittori, D. (2010). Mechanisms involved in premature self-destruction of red blood cells under different eryptosis stimuli. *Haematologica* 95 (s2), 304.

Wallis, C.J., Babitch, J.A., & Wenegieme, E.F. (1993). Divalent cation binding to erythrocyte spectrin. *Biochemistry* 32, 5045-5050.

Weed, R.I., La Celle, P.L., & Merrill, E.W. (1969). Metabolic dependence of red cell deformability. *J Clin Invest* 48, 795-809.

Willekens, F.L., Werre, J.M., Groenen-Döpp, Y.A., Roerdinkholder-Stoelwinder, B., de Pauw, B., & Bosman, G.J. (2008). Erythrocyte vesiculation: a self-protective mechanism? *Brit J Haematol* 141, 549-556.

Williamson, P, Kulick, A., Zachowski, A., Schlegel, R.A., & Devaux, P.F. (1992). Ca^{2+} induces transbilayer redistribution of all major phospholipids in human erythrocytes. *Biochemistry* 31, 6355-6360.

Wlliamson, P. & Schlegel, R.A. (2002). Transbilayer phospholipids movement and the clearance of apoptotic cells. *Biochim Biophys Acta* 1585, 53-63.

Wood, B.L., Gibson, D.F., & Tait, J.F. (1996). Increased phosphatidylserine exposure in sickle cell disease: flow-cytometric measurements and clinical associations. *Blood* 88, 1873-1880.

Zachee, P., Emonds, M., Lins, R., & Boogaerts, M. (1988). Red blood cells, the scavengers for toxic free radicals during haemodialysis. *Nephrol Dial Transplant* 4, 104-105.

Zipser, Y., Piade, A., Barbul, A., Korenstein, R., & Kosower, N.S. (2002). Ca2+ promotes erythrocyte band 3 tyrosine phosphorylation via dissociation of phosphotyrosine phosphatase from band 3. *Biochem J* 368, 137-144.

5

Diagnostic Evaluation of Anaemia

Vikrant Kale and Abdur Rahmaan Aftab
Gastroenterology Department,
St.Luke's Hospital, Kilkenny
Ireland

1. Introduction

Anaemia is one of the major signs of disease. It is never normal and its cause(s) should always be sought.

The history, physical examination, and simple laboratory testing are all useful in evaluating the anaemic patient.

The workup should be directed towards answering the following questions concerning whether one or more of the major processes leading to anaemia may be operative:

- Is the patient bleeding (now or in the past)?
- Is there evidence for increased RBC destruction (haemolysis)?
- Is the bone marrow suppressed?
- Is the patient iron deficient? If so, why?
- Is the patient deficient in folic acid or vitamin B12? If so, why?

Depending on the provisional diagnosis, you may need special investigations like *radiologic tests, bone marrow aspiration, gastrointestinal endoscopies, molecular studies etc.* to arrive at a definite diagnosis.

2. History taking

2.1 Onset, duration and progress

Insidious onset, long duration and gradual progress of symptoms in a patient with anaemia suggests nutritional anaemia, chronic haemolytic anaemia (congenital or acquired), anaemia of chronic disease and anaemia due to chronic blood loss. Rapid onset, short duration and rapid progress of symptoms indicate acute leukaemia, acute haemolytic anaemia, hemolytic/aplastic crisis in chronic haemolytic anaemia, anaemia secondary to acute blood loss and infiltrative disorders of the bone marrow.

Presence of symptoms other than those due to anaemia is a pointer to underlying disease causing anaemia and provides clues for further work up of the patient. Inquiry should be made to uncover conditions that may cause gastro-intestinal, genito-urinary or any other blood loss.

An anaemic patient who complains of angina or symptoms of cerebral hypoxia urgently needs the oxygen carrying capacity raised by red cell transfusions and inspired oxygen, whatever may be the cause of anaemia.Passage of dark red or brown urine indicates haemoglobinuria and suggests haemolysis. History of episodes of bone pain, backache, abdominal pain in past suggests the diagnosis of Sickle Cell Disease.

2.2 Age & sex

Anaemia is more common in pregnant women, females in reproductive age and children during the phase of rapid growth. A predominantly cereal based diet which is poor in green leafy vegetables and vitamin C containing foods is a common cause of iron deficiency.

In a female patient, a detailed menstrual history and history of reproductive performance (number of deliveries and interval between deliveries), provide information about stress on iron balance and raises the possibility of iron deficiency anaemia.

Self imposed or improperly advised dietary restrictions can contribute to nutritional anaemia.

2.3 Drug ingestion

Drug ingestion can cause anaemia in several ways. Long term ingestion of aspirin (in patients of coronary artery disease) can lead to chronic blood loss and iron deficiency anaemia. Certain drugs can cause haemolysis in individuals with G-6-PD deficiency. Rifampicin and alpha methyl dopa can cause autoimmune haemolytic anaemia. Chemotherapeutic drugs can cause marrow depression and pancytopenia.

A past history of cardiac valve surgery can indicate the possibility of haemolysis.

3. Physical examination

Clinical examination can provide a wealth of diagnostic information. Although signs are not always present, they can be helpful in making a clinical diagnosis.

A smooth(bald) tongue and nail changes of koilonychia (brittle, flat or concave nails, more common in toe nails than in finger nails), and bilateral, painless parotid enlargement in a patient with anaemia suggests the diagnosis of *iron deficiency anaemia*. Skin pigmentation in the peri-oral region and over the knuckles is suggestive of *megaloblastic anaemia*. The presence of mild jaundice would suggest possibility of *haemolytic anaemia*. A generalized greyish discoloration of skin indicates *iron overload* in anaemic patients who have been given blood transfusions over several years. Skin pigmentation and various skeletal abnormalities may be present in some cases of *constitutional hypoplastic anaemia*. The presence of petechial haemorrhages would indicate a marrow infiltrative disease (leukaemia, lymphoma, myeloma, metastases, etc.), they may also be seen in megaloblastic anaemia.

Fronto-temporal bossing, malar prominence, upper jaw and teeth projecting beyond the lower jaw, flat bridge of the nose - all giving rise to typical facial appearance are characteristic of *Thalassemia syndromes*. Puffiness of lower eye lids, loss of eye brow hair and thick voice would suggest *myxedema* as the cause of anaemia; this can be confirmed by delayed relaxation of muscle after eliciting deep reflexes.

The presence of hypertension should alert the clinician to the possibility of *anaemia secondary to chronic renal failure*.

Tenderness of calf muscles suggests megaloblastic anaemia but could be present even in iron deficiency anaemia. Signs of sub-acute combined degeneration indicate *pernicious anaemia*. Lymphadenopathy suggests the possibility of *leukaemia or lymphoma*.

4. Laboratory evaluation

Lab tests in the diagnosis of Anaemia:

1.Complete Blood Count(CBC)	2. Iron supply studies

A. Red blood cell count
- Haemoglobin
- Hematocrit(HCT)
- Reticulocyte count
 	
B. Red blood cell indices
- Mean cell volume(MCV)
- Mean cell haemoglobin(MCH)
- Mean cell haemoglobin
  Concentration(MCHC)
- Red cell distribution width
  (RDW)
 	
C. White blood cell count
- Cell differential
- Nuclear segmentation of
  Neutrophils
 	
D. Platelet count
 	
E. Cell morphology
- Cell size
- Haemoglobin content
- Anisocytosis
- Poikilocytosis
- Polychromasia
	A. Serum Iron
	
	B. Total iron binding capacity
	
	C. Serum ferritin
	
	D. Marrow iron stain
	
	3. Marrow examination
	
	A. Aspirate
	- M/E ratio*
	- Cell morphology
	- Iron stain
	
	B. Biopsy
	- Cellularity
	- Morphology

M/E ratio – ratio of myeloid to erythroid precursors.
Source – Harrison's Principles of Internal Medicine, 16th edition.

4.1 Mean corpuscular volume
The normal range for MCV is from 80 to 100 femtoliters (fL). Values in excess of 115 fL are almost exclusively seen in vitamin B12 or folic acid deficiency. Even higher values can occur as an artefact when cold agglutinins are present, which causes RBCs to go through the counting aperture in doublets or triplets. Low values usually indicate a microcytic anaemia.

4.2 Mean corpuscular haemoglobin
The normal MCH ranges from 27.5 to 33.2 picograms of haemoglobin per RBC. Low values are seen in iron deficiency and thalassemia, while increased values occur in macrocytosis of any cause.

4.3 Mean corpuscular haemoglobin concentration
The mean normal value for the MCHC is 34 grams of haemoglobin per dL of RBCs. Low values occur in the same conditions that generate low values for MCV and MCH, while increased values occur almost exclusively in the presence of congenital or acquired spherocytosis or in other congenital haemolytic anaemia in which red cells are abnormally desiccated (eg, sickle cell anaemia, haemoglobin C disease, xerocytosis).

4.4 Reticulocyte count
The reticulocyte count, either as a percentage of all RBCs, the absolute reticulocyte count, the corrected absolute reticulocyte count, or as the reticulocyte production index, helps to distinguish among the different types of anaemia:
-   Anaemia with a high reticulocyte count reflects an increased erythropoietic response to continued haemolysis or blood loss.
-   A stable anaemia with a low reticulocyte count is strong evidence for deficient production of RBCs (ie, a reduced marrow response to the anaemia).
-   Haemolysis or blood loss can be associated with a low reticulocyte count if there is a concurrent disorder that impairs RBC production (eg, infection, prior chemotherapy).
-   A low reticulocyte percentage accompanied by pancytopenia is suggestive of aplastic anaemia, while a reticulocyte percentage of zero with normal white blood cell and platelet counts suggests a diagnosis of pure red cell aplasia.

4.5 White blood cell count and differential
A low total white blood cell (WBC) count (leukopenia) in a patient with anaemia should lead to consideration of bone marrow suppression or replacement, hypersplenism, or deficiencies of cobalamin(B12) or folate. In comparison, a high total WBC count (leukocytosis) may reflect the presence of infection, inflammation, or a hematologic malignancy.
Clues to the specific abnormality present may be obtained from the WBC differential, which, in conjunction with the total WBC may show increased or decreased absolute numbers of the various cell types in the circulation. Examples include:
-   An increased absolute neutrophil count in infection or steroid therapy
-   An increased absolute monocyte count in myelodysplasia
-   An increased absolute eosinophil count in certain infections
-   A decreased absolute neutrophil count following chemotherapy
-   A decreased absolute lymphocyte count in HIV infection or following treatment with corticosteroids.

4.6 Neutrophil hypersegmentation
Neutrophil hypersegmentation (NH) is defined as the presence of >5 percent of neutrophils with five or more lobes and/or the presence of one or more neutrophils with six or more lobes. This peripheral smear finding, along with macro-ovalocytic red cells, is classically associated with impaired DNA synthesis, as seen in disorders of vitamins B12 and folic acid.

4.7 Circulating nucleated red blood cells
Nucleated RBCs (NRBCs) are not normally found in the circulation. They may be present in patients with known hematologic disease (eg, sickle cell disease, thalassemia major, various

haemolytic anaemia after splenectomy), or as a part of the leukoerythroblastic pattern seen in patients with bone marrow replacement.

In patients without known hematologic disease, NRBCs may reflect the presence of a life-threatening disease, such as sepsis or severe heart failure.

4.8 Platelet count

Abnormalities in the platelet count often provide important diagnostic information. Thrombocytopenia occurs in a variety of disorders associated with anaemia, including hypersplenism, marrow involvement with malignancy, autoimmune platelet destruction (either idiopathic or drug-related), sepsis, or folate or cobalamin deficiency.

High platelet counts, in comparison, may reflect myeloproliferative disease, chronic iron deficiency, and inflammatory, infectious, or neoplastic disorders. Changes in platelet morphology (giant platelets, degranulated platelets) also may be important, suggesting myeloproliferative or myelodysplastic disease.

4.9 Pancytopenia

The combination of anaemia, thrombocytopenia, and neutropenia is termed pancytopenia. The presence of severe pancytopenia narrows the differential diagnosis to disorders such as aplastic anaemia, folate or cobalamin deficiency, or hematologic malignancy (eg, acute myeloid leukaemia). Mild degrees of pancytopenia may be seen in patients with splenomegaly and splenic trapping of circulating cellular elements(hypersplenism).

4.10 Blood smear

Many clinicians rely on the above RBC parameters and the RDW in evaluating a patient with anaemia. However, the RDW is of limited utility, and examination of the peripheral blood smear provides information not otherwise available.

As examples, the automated counter may miss the red cell fragmentation ("helmet cells", schistocytes) of microangiopathic haemolysis, microspherocytes in autoimmune haemolytic anaemia, teardrop RBCs in myeloid metaplasia, a leukoerythroblastic pattern with bone marrow replacement, the "bite cells" in oxidative haemolysis, or RBC parasites such as malaria or babesiosis.

4.11 Serial evaluation of haemoglobin and hematocrit

Measuring the rate of fall of the patient's Hb or HCT often provides helpful diagnostic information. Suppose the Hb concentration has fallen from 15 to 10 g/dL in one week. If this were due to total cessation of RBC production (ie, a reticulocyte count of zero) and if the rate of RBC destruction were normal (1 percent/day), the Hb concentration would have fallen by 7 percent over seven days, resulting a decline of 1.05 g/dL (0.07 x 15). The greater fall in Hb in this patient (5 g/dL) indicates that marrow suppression cannot be the sole cause of the anaemia and that blood loss and/or increased RBC destruction must be present.

4.12 Evaluation for iron deficiency

More complete evaluation for iron deficiency is indicated when the history (menometrorrhagia, symptoms of peptic ulcer disease) and preliminary laboratory data (low MCV, low MCH, high RDW, increased platelet count) support this diagnosis. In this setting, the plasma levels of iron, iron binding capacity (transferrin), transferrin saturation, and ferritin should be measured. This is discussed in detail below.

4.13 Evaluation for haemolysis

Haemolysis should be considered if the patient has a rapid fall in haemoglobin concentration, reticulocytosis, and/or abnormally shaped RBCs (especially spherocytes or fragmented RBCs) on the peripheral smear. The usual ancillary findings of haemolysis are an increase in the serum lactate dehydrogenase (LDH) and indirect bilirubin concentrations and a reduction in the serum haptoglobin concentration.

The combination of an increased LDH and reduced haptoglobin is 90 percent specific for diagnosing haemolysis, while the combination of a normal LDH and a serum haptoglobin greater than 25 mg/dL is 92 percent sensitive for ruling out haemolysis.

4.14 Intravascular haemolysis

Serum or plasma haemoglobin and urinary hemosiderin should be measured if intravascular haemolysis is a consideration, as with paroxysmal nocturnal haemoglobinuria.

4.15 Bone marrow examination

Examination of the bone marrow generally offers little additional diagnostic information in the more common forms of anaemia. If erythropoiesis is increased in response to the anaemia, the bone marrow will show erythroid hyperplasia, a nonspecific finding. Similarly, although the absence of stainable iron in the bone marrow had previously been considered the "gold standard" for the diagnosis of iron deficiency, this diagnosis is usually established by laboratory tests alone

Indications for examination of the bone marrow in anaemic patients include pancytopenia or the presence of abnormal cells in the circulation, such as blast forms. Such patients may have aplastic anaemia, myelodysplasia, marrow replacement with malignancy, or a myeloproliferative disease. Other findings that may be seen in the marrow in anaemic patients include megaloblastic erythropoiesis (folate or cobalamin deficiency), absence of recognizable RBC precursors (pure RBC aplasia), vacuolization of RBC precursors (alcohol or drug-induced anaemia), and increased iron-laden RBC precursors (the sideroblastic anaemia).

4.16 Multiple causes of anaemia

Multiple causes are frequently present in adults, particularly the elderly. Common examples are:

- A patient with gastrointestinal bleeding secondary to colon cancer may also have the anaemia of chronic disease, leading to a blunted reticulocyte response.
- A patient with a chronic hemolytic anaemia (eg, sickle cell anaemia, hereditary spherocytosis) may develop worsening anaemia following acute infection, particularly with parvovirus B19, which may blunt or temporarily ablate erythropoiesis and the reticulocyte response.
- A patient with autoimmune hemolytic anaemia may develop worsening anaemia from gastrointestinal blood loss following treatment with corticosteroids.
- Anaemia, renal failure, and congestive failure are often found together, a condition that has been termed "cardio-renal anaemia syndrome." Treatment of the anaemia may improve both the renal failure and heart failure.

Algorithm for diagnosing cause of anaemia

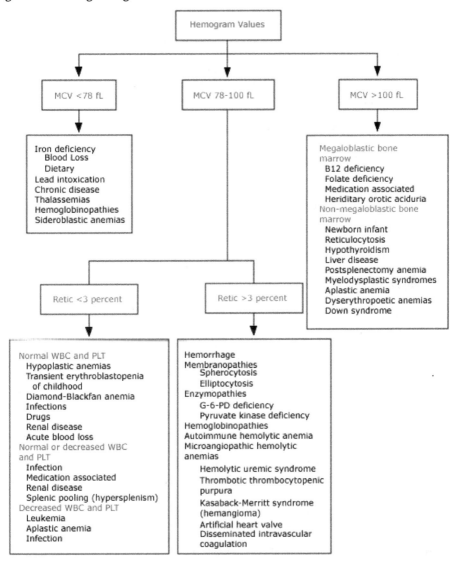

Source : Nathan, DG, Oski, FA. *Hematology of Infancy and Childhood*, 4th ed, WB Saunders, Philadelphia, PA 1993. p. 352.

5. Anaemia due to decreased red cell production

A variety of disorders are associated with anaemia due to decreased red cell production (ie, hypoproliferative anaemia). This situation is simplistically identified by the finding of a low corrected absolute reticulocyte count (reticulocytopenia).

The differential diagnosis of a hypoproliferative anaemia can often be narrowed by identification of one of the six specific presenting patterns outlined below.

5.1 Normocytic anaemia without leukopenia or thrombocytopenia

The peripheral smear in this setting demonstrates normal red blood cell (RBC) morphology. The red cell indices are normal or slightly hypochromic or microcytic. The white blood cell (WBC) count is usually normal although there may be a neutrophilic leukocytosis. The WBC are not dysplastic and blasts are not seen. The platelet count is usually normal or elevated. The platelets are not dysplastic.

The bone marrow is usually not examined in these cases. If studied, it would show normal cellularity, normal maturation of the several cell lines, and normal iron stores.

This pattern can be induced by a number of disorders-

5.1.1 Anaemia of (chronic) inflammation

This condition is most often associated with infection, inflammation, or malignancy. Initial evaluation with ESR or CRP and then focussed investigations to find a cause should be done.

5.1.2 Mild to moderate iron deficiency

Mild to moderate iron deficiency can be associated with anaemia without the classic findings of hypochromia or microcytosis.

5.1.3 Renal failure

The anaemia associated with renal failure is usually due to a marked reduction in erythropoietin (EPO) production relative to the degree of anaemia. The EPO level usually does not fall until the creatinine clearance drops below 30 mL/minute. Urinalysis for Albumin to Creatinine ratio(ACR) is helpful in detecting renal disease, especially in patients with Diabetes mellitus.

5.1.4 Endocrine disorders

A mild hypoproliferative anaemia can be seen in a number of endocrine disorders, including hypothyroidism, hyperthyroidism, panhypopituitarism, and primary or secondary hyperparathyroidism. How the anaemia occurs in these disorders is not well understood but correction of the endocrine disturbance usually corrects the anaemia.

5.2 Normocytic anaemia with low to absent reticulocytes

The presentation in this setting is similar to variant 1 with one important exception: the RBC morphology is normal but the reticulocyte count is very low, usually <10,000/microL, frequently as low as 2,000/microL, and occasionally zero.

This pattern is highly suggestive of pure red cell aplasia. The bone marrow will show normal overall cellularity and morphology except for the virtual absence of all identifiable erythroid precursors. Giant proerythroblasts may be seen in those patients with pure red cell aplasia secondary to infection with parvovirus.

There are many causes of acquired pure red cell aplasia in adults, the most common being idiopathic, drug-induced, myelodysplastic syndrome, T-cell large granular lymphocytic leukaemia, and thymoma. Regardless of the etiology, the final common pathway seems to be an immunologic attack, usually mediated by T cells, on erythroid progenitors at a maturity level between CFU-E (colony-forming units-erythroid) and proerythroblasts.

5.3 Normocytic anaemia with pancytopenia

The peripheral smear in these patients usually reveals normal RBC morphology but macrocytosis is occasionally seen. The WBC count is low with prominent neutropenia (absolute neutrophil count below 1000/microL) and, in some cases, lymphopenia (<1000/microL) as well. WBC morphology is normal. The platelet count is reduced; the platelet morphology is generally normal with occasional large platelets.

Bone marrow examination is almost always performed in patients with pancytopenia, usually in conjunction with cytogenetic studies. The marrow in most cases of hypoproliferative anaemia with pancytopenia is either profoundly hypocellular with relatively normal morphology of the remaining elements or hypocellular with dysplasia of red cell, neutrophil, and platelet precursors. In some patients, however, the marrow is totally replaced with malignant cells or fibrosis.

Pancytopenia without prominent morphologic abnormalities has a very different set of clinical implications from isolated anaemia. The major causes of this problem include:

-   Aplastic anaemia
-   Bone marrow suppression following chemotherapy and/or radiation therapy
-   Hypoplastic myelodysplastic syndrome
-   Marrow replaced by leukaemia, lymphoma, cancer, or rarely, fibrosis

Although splenomegaly can also cause pancytopenia (ie, hypersplenism), the increased peripheral destruction seen in hypersplenism is associated with enhanced erythropoiesis and a high reticulocyte count, and the bone marrow is normocellular to hypercellular, rather than aplastic or hypocellular.

5.4 Macrocytic non-megaloblastic anaemia

The peripheral smear in this disorder shows RBCs that are distinctly macrocytic with very few macroovalocytes. The mean cell volume (MCV) is generally greater than 100 fL. The WBC may be slightly low but there is no dysplasia or blasts. Few, if any, five to six lobed neutrophils are present. The platelet count may be normal or as low as 50,000/microL.

The bone marrow is usually not examined in this setting but, if performed, cellularity and maturation are normal. *Megaloblastosis*, characteristic of cobalamin or folate deficiency, is not seen.

Several disorders can produce a hypoproliferative, macrocytic anaemia without megaloblastosis-

-   Alcohol abuse
-   Therapy with zidovudine(AZT), other anti-viral agents, hydroxyurea, methotrexate, phenytoin
-   Myelodysplastic syndrome, early in its course
-   Early in the course of cobalamin or folate deficiency.

5.5 Macrocytic megaloblastic anaemia

The peripheral smear in this setting reveals macrocytic RBCs with macroovalocytes. The WBC count is normal or low, but the neutrophils show hypersegmentation with at least 5 percent of the cells having five or more lobes. The platelet count is normal or low.

These findings are highly suggestive of folate or cobalamin (vitamin B12) deficiency. Bone marrow examination is usually not necessary.

5.6 Leucoerythroblastic anaemia

The peripheral smear in a patient with a leukoerythroblastic anaemia shows abnormal RBC morphology with tear-drop forms, elliptocytes, macrocytes, and circulating nucleated RBC. The WBC count may be high, low, or normal, but there is myeloid immaturity extending back to the myeloblast stage. The platelet count is usually low with abnormal morphology, including giant platelets and even megakaryocyte fragments.

A leukoerythroblastic picture reflects replacement of the bone marrow by granulomas, cancer, fibrosis, or primary myelofibrosis (PMF). The remaining pluripotent stem cells move to the liver and spleen as they did in fetal life, resulting in extramedullary hematopoiesis. The stromal support system in the liver and spleen is not optimal, as it is in the marrow. As a result, hematopoietic cells are released prematurely or abnormally into the circulation. The reticulocyte count is of limited value in this setting because extramedullary hematopoiesis is associated with both disordered release of reticulocytes into the peripheral blood and disordered maturation of nucleated RBC to reticulocytes in the peripheral circulation.

Having recognized the virtually pathognomonic peripheral smear findings, the differential diagnosis focuses on what is replacing the marrow. Therefore, a bone marrow biopsy (aspiration may result in a dry tap) with appropriate staining (for reticulin and collagen) is necessary. There are two major causes:

-Metastatic cancer.

-Myelofibrosis, as seen in the myeloproliferative syndromes such as PMF or myelofibrosis associated with acute myeloid leukaemia, other cancer, or radiation.

The differential diagnosis of a *hypoproliferative anaemia with microcytosis*, which is most often due to iron deficiency, is discussed below.

6. Anaemia due to iron deficiency

The development of iron deficiency, and the rapidity with which it progresses, is dependent upon the individual's initial iron stores which are, in turn, dependent upon age, sex, rate of growth and the balance between iron absorption and loss.

Causes of iron deficiency are discussed below.

6.1 Blood loss

The major cause of iron deficiency in affluent countries is blood loss, either overt or occult. Overt blood loss is, by definition, obvious and not difficult for the clinician to recognize, often by history alone. Examples include severe traumatic haemorrhage, haematemesis, malena, haemoptysis, severe menorrhagia and gross haematuria.

Occult bleeding, on the other hand, may be difficult to track down. This usually occurs via the gastrointestinal tract in men. Other causes are repeated voluntary blood donations, the post-operative setting in which blood loss greatly exceeds the amount of blood transfused, or iatrogenic anaemia due to repeated and massive blood drawing in the course of workup of a complicated medical condition. Additional factors are often responsible in women, including underestimating the degree of menometrorrhagia, blood loss during delivery, and direct iron loss to the fetus during pregnancy and to the neonate during lactation.

Although reduced gastrointestinal absorption of iron and a diet deficient in iron can also cause iron deficiency, it is most reasonable to believe, as a first assumption, that *iron deficiency reflects blood loss*, in order to avoiding missing an occult malignancy or other bleeding intestinal lesion.

6.2 Decreased iron absorption

Gastrointestinal malabsorption of iron is a relatively uncommon cause of iron deficiency, although it may be observed in certain diseases associated with generalized malabsorption or achlorhydria [5]. However, the use of proton pump inhibitors, which reduce gastric acid secretion, has not been associated with clinical iron deficiency.

6.3 Foods and medications

There are a number of foods and medications that impair absorption of iron.

Absorption of haem iron is affected by:
Amount of haem iron, especially in meat
Content of calcium in the meal (calcium impairs iron absorption)
Absorption of nonhaem iron is affected by:
Iron status
Amount of potentially available nonhaem iron
Balance between positive and negative factors
Positive factors
Ascorbic acid
Meat or fish (haem iron enhances absorption of nonhaem iron)
Negative factors
Phytate (in bran, oats, rye fibre)
Polyphenols (in tea, some vegetables and cereals)
Dietary calcium
Soy protein

6.4 Coeliac disease

Iron deficiency anaemia, refractory to oral iron treatment can be seen in patients with coeliac disease, autoimmune atrophic gastritis or Helicobacter pylori infection. It is unclear whether there is a component of blood loss contributing to iron deficiency in this condition, although a component of the anaemia of chronic disease (inflammation) is seen in some individuals.

6.5 Other causes

There are several other uncommon causes of iron deficiency:

6.5.1 Intravascular haemolysis
Intravascular haemolysis, with its accompanying haemoglobinuria and hemosiderinuria can lead to significant urinary iron losses in patients with paroxysmal nocturnal haemoglobinuria and in cardiac patients with intravascular destruction of red cells secondary to malfunctioning valvular prostheses, patches, or intracardiac myxomas.

6.5.2 Pulmonary hemosiderosis
Pulmonary hemosiderosis (eg, chronic pulmonary haemorrhage in anti-glomerular basement membrane antibody disease) can appear as functional iron deficiency.

6.5.3 Response to erythropoietin
A response to treatment with erythropoietin (EPO) for the anaemia of chronic renal failure often leads to iron deficiency, since the iron requirements generated by this response can usually not be met by mobilization of the patient's iron stores alone.

6.5.4 Gastric bypass for morbid obesity
This form of surgery bypasses the duodenum, the major site of intestinal iron absorption. As a result, iron deficiency can occur following gastric bypass surgery, not only through the bypassing of the site of major iron absorption, but also as the result of decreased gastric acid availability.

6.5.5 Congenital iron deficiency
Rare families with iron deficiency anaemia unresponsive to oral iron therapy, but partially responsive to parenteral iron, have been reported.

6.6 Estimation of iron stores
The patient's history, complete blood count, red blood cell indices, and examination of the peripheral blood smear usually allow the clinician to make a presumptive diagnosis of iron deficiency anaemia. This can be followed by a therapeutic trial of iron administration to provide both confirmation of the diagnosis and therapy.

6.6.1 Therapeutic trial of iron
A presumptive diagnosis of iron deficiency anaemia is made if there is a positive response to a trial of oral iron therapy, characterized by a modest reticulocytosis beginning in about five to seven days, followed by an increase in haemoglobin at a rate of about 2 to 4 g/dL every three weeks until the haemoglobin concentration returns to normal.

The limitation of this approach occurs if there is no response, or the response is modest or incomplete. In this setting, the clinician cannot differentiate among poor patient compliance, inability to absorb the iron preparation, an incorrect diagnosis, continued bleeding, or a coexisting condition such as the anaemia of chronic disease or renal failure that blocks the full reticulocyte response.

For these reasons, laboratory tests (eg, iron studies, iron panel) are often ordered to confirm the diagnosis prior to initiation of therapy.

6.6.2 Serum or plasma ferritin
The serum or plasma ferritin concentration is an *excellent indicator of iron stores* in otherwise healthy adults and has replaced assessment of bone marrow iron stores as the gold standard

for the diagnosis of iron deficiency in most patients. There is no clinical situation other than iron deficiency in which extremely low values of serum ferritin are seen.

6.6.3 Pregnancy
Serum ferritin is useful in diagnosing iron deficiency in pregnant women, who often have an elevated serum transferrin in the absence of iron deficiency.

6.6.4 Inflammatory states
Ferritin is an acute phase reactant, with plasma levels increasing in liver disease, infection, inflammation, and malignancy.

6.6.5 Serum iron and transferrin (TIBC)
In iron deficiency anaemia, the serum iron concentration (SI) is reduced, and the level of transferrin - also measured as total iron binding capacity (TIBC) is elevated; the latter finding reflects the reciprocal relationship between serum iron and transferrin gene expression in most nonerythroid cells.
The accuracy of measurement of transferrin/TIBC for predicting the presence of iron deficiency is second only to the serum or plasma ferritin concentration. Confounding factors are pregnancy and oral contraceptives, which increase the plasma transferrin concentration.

6.6.6 Bone marrow iron
Iron in bone marrow macrophages and erythroid precursors (sideroblasts) can be detected with the Prussian Blue stain on marrow spicules. Lack of stainable iron in erythroid precursors as well as marrow macrophages is considered by most clinicians to be the "gold standard" for the diagnosis of iron deficiency. In contrast, in uncomplicated anaemia of chronic disease, iron is present in marrow macrophages but absent or reduced in erythroid precursors.
However, bone marrow sampling and testing for stainable iron is expensive, invasive, and usually unnecessary. It has been replaced in practice by measurement of serum ferritin.

6.6.7 Assessment of iron sufficiency
Serum ferritin is often ordered to assess whether the patient is iron sufficient, rather than deficient. Similarly, defining iron sufficiency for the purpose of predicting a response in anaemic patients with chronic renal insufficiency to treatment with erythropoietin requires a relatively high amount of available iron, usually stated as a serum ferritin ≥100 ng/mL and a transferrin saturation ≥20 percent.

6.6.8 Red cell morphology and indices
Despite the classic description of iron deficiency as leading to a hypochromic, microcytic anaemia, many iron deficient patients in western countries will have normal red cell morphology. Further, the finding of a hypochromic microcytic anaemia is not pathognomonic of iron deficiency, with thalassemia and, less commonly, the anaemia of chronic inflammation being the other common conditions encountered in daily practice. It is important to rule out these disorders before beginning a trial of iron therapy, since many patients with thalassemia or chronic inflammation are already iron overloaded.

7.Evaluation of anaemia due to blood loss

7.1 Upper and lower GI evaluation

Upper and lower GI investigations should be considered in all postmenopausal female and all male patients where Iron Deficiency anaemia(IDA) has been confirmed unless there is a history of significant overt non-GI blood loss.

In the absence of suggestive symptoms (which are unreliable), the order of investigations is determined by local availability, although all patients should be screened for coeliac disease with serology. Small-bowel biopsy samples should be taken at OGD if coeliac serology was positive or not performed.

If oesophago-gastro-duodenoscopy (OGD) is performed as the initial GI investigation, only the presence of gastric cancer or coeliac disease, as explained below, should deter lower GI investigation. In particular, the presence of oesophagitis, erosions and peptic ulcer disease should not be accepted as the cause of IDA until lower GI investigations have been carried out.

Colonoscopy has the following advantages over radiology: it allows biopsy of lesions, treatment of adenomas, and identification of superficial pathology such as angiodysplasia and NSAID damage. Performing gastroscopy and colonoscopy at the same session speeds investigation and saves time for both the hospital and the patient, because only one attendance for endoscopy is required.

Radiographic imaging is a sufficient alternative where colonoscopy is contraindicated. The sensitivity of CT colonography for lesions >10 mm in size is over 90%. Barium enema is less reliable, but is still useful if colonoscopy or CT colonography are not readily available.

7.2 Screening for and further investigation of coeliac disease

Ideally coeliac serology—tissue transglutaminase (tTG) antibody or endomysial antibody, if tTG antibody testing is not available—should be undertaken at presentation. But if this has not been carried out or if the result is not available, duodenal biopsy specimens should be taken. If coeliac serology is negative, small-bowel biopsies need not be performed at OGD unless there are other features, such as diarrhoea, which make coeliac disease more likely. If the tTG antibody test is negative, the post-test probability of coeliac disease is 0.3%, which is less than in the general population. If coeliac serology is positive, coeliac disease is likely and should be confirmed by small-bowel biopsy.

7.3 Further evaluation

Further imaging of the small bowel is probably not necessary unless there is an inadequate response to iron therapy, especially if transfusion dependent. In those with an inadequate response, *video capsule endoscopy or enteroscopy* may be helpful to detect angiodysplasia, Crohn's disease and small-bowel neoplasia.

Video capsule endoscopy has a diagnostic yield of 40–55% in this setting. However, it seldom results in a beneficial subsequent intervention. Many lesions detected by both enteroscopy and video capsule endoscopy are within the reach of a gastroscope, and repeat OGD should be considered before these procedures. Bleeding lesions identified by video capsule endoscopy may be amenable to treatment by push or double-balloon enteroscopy. However, the benefits of these procedures after a normal video capsule endoscopy in the context of IDA are unproven.

Small-bowel imaging (*MRI enteroclysis, CT enterography or barium studies*) should also be considered in patients with symptoms suggestive of small-bowel disease, transfusion-dependent IDA, and rapid recurrence of anaemia after normalisation of Hb concentrations. However, many small intestinal lesions that cause asymptomatic anaemia are mucosal and flat or nearly so and most small intestinal imaging modalities apart from video capsule endoscopy are only efficient at identifying mass lesions. CT has the additional advantage of being able to identify extraintestinal pathology such as renal tumours and lymphomas.

Helicobacter pylori colonisation may impair iron uptake and increase iron loss, potentially leading to iron deficiency and IDA. Eradication of *H pylori* appears to reverse anaemia in anecdotal reports and small studies. *H pylori* should be sought by non-invasive testing, if IDA persists or recurs after a normal OGD and colonoscopy, and eradicated if present. *H pylori* urease (CLO) testing of biopsy specimens taken at the initial gastroscopy is an alternative approach.

Autoimmune gastritis has been identified as a potential cause of IDA in up to a quarter of cases, but, although of interest, its diagnosis is currently of little practical value.

Giardia lamblia has occasionally been found during the investigation of IDA. If there is associated diarrhoea, then small-bowel biopsy samples will be taken anyway and may detect this. Where giardiasis is suspected, stool should be sent for ELISA, even if histology of duodenal biopsy samples is negative.

Radiological imaging of the mesenteric vessels is of limited use but may be of value in transfusion-dependent IDA for demonstrating vascular malformations or other occult lesions. There is no evidence to recommend labelled red cell imaging or Meckel's scans in patients with IDA. Faecal occult blood testing is of no benefit in the investigation of IDA, being insensitive and non-specific.

8. Evaluation of anaemia due to increased destruction

Hemolytic anaemia is defined as anaemia due to a shortened survival of circulating red blood cells (RBCs). Although the time of RBC senescent death in adults is 110 to 120 days, it is convenient to define haemolysis as a shortening of RBC survival to a value of less than 100 days.

While there are no symptoms specific for the diagnosis of hemolytic anaemia, recognizing haemolysis is not difficult in the classic patient, who may have many of the following:

- Rapid onset of pallor and anaemia
- Jaundice with increased indirect bilirubin concentration
- History of pigmented (bilirubin) gallstones
- Splenomegaly
- Presence of circulating spherocytic red cells (eg, autoimmune hemolytic anaemia, congenital spherocytosis)
- Other informative red cell shape changes (see below)
- Increased serum lactate dehydrogenase (LDH) concentration
- Reduced or absent level of serum haptoglobin
- A positive direct antiglobulin test (Coombs test)
- Increased reticulocyte percentage or absolute reticulocyte number, indicating the bone marrow's response to the anaemia

Laboratory findings, including an examination of the peripheral smear, are used to confirm the presence of haemolysis, and, if possible, the underlying cause.

Extravascular destruction of red blood cells
Intrinsic red blood cell defects
Enzyme deficiencies (eg, G6PD or pyruvate kinase deficiencies)
Haemoglobinopathies (eg, sickle cell disease, thalassemias, unstable haemoglobins)
Membrane defects (eg, hereditary spherocytosis, elliptocytosis)
Extrinsic red blood cell defects
Liver disease
Hypersplenism
Infections (eg, bartonella, babesia, malaria)
Oxidant agents (eg, dapsone, nitrites, aniline dyes)
Other agents (eg, lead, snake and spider bites)
Large granular lymphocytic leukaemia
Autoimmune hemolytic anaemia (warm- or cold-reacting, drugs)
Intravenous immune globulin infusion
Intravascular destruction of red blood cells
Microangiopathy (eg, aortic stenosis, prosthetic valve)
Transfusion reactions (eg, ABO incompatibility)
Infection (eg, clostridial sepsis, severe malaria)
Paroxysmal cold haemoglobinuria; cold agglutinin disease (on occasion)
Paroxysmal nocturnal haemoglobinuria
Following intravenous infusion of Rho(D) immune globulin
Following intravenous infusion with hypotonic solutions
Snake bites

Common causes of hemolytic anaemia in the adult

Hematologic consultation should be obtained in virtually all patients with a new onset of haemolysis, since sudden and life-threatening worsening of anaemia may occur, requiring urgent coordination between clinicians, clinical pathologists, and blood bank personnel for appropriate management.

Haemolysis may also be the first sign of an underlying systemic disorder (eg, thrombotic thrombocytopenic purpura, lupus erythematosus, chronic lymphocytic leukaemia) and may require urgent intervention to prevent death or disease-related complications.

8.1 Peripheral smear

Abnormalities suspicious for the presence of haemolysis include the following:

- Spherocytes, microspherocytes, and elliptocytes.
- Fragmented RBC (schistocytes, helmet cells) indicating the presence of microangiopathic hemolytic anaemia.
- Acanthocytes (spur cells) in patients with liver disease.
- Blister or "bite" cells due to the presence of oxidant-induced damage to the red cell and its membrane.
- RBCs with inclusions, as in Malaria, Babesiosis, and Bartonella infections.
- Teardrop RBCs with circulating nucleated RBC and early white blood cell forms, indicating the presence of marrow involvement, as in primary myelofibrosis or tumor infiltration.
- Red cell "ghosts" indicating the presence of intravascular haemolysis, most often associated with overwhelming bacterial infection (eg, Clostridium perfringens).

8.2 Serum LDH and haptoglobin

Two major tests used to diagnose the presence of haemolysis are lactate dehydrogenase (LDH), released from hemolyzed RBCs, and haptoglobin, which binds to haemoglobin released during intravascular or extravascular haemolysis or ineffective erythropoiesis with release of haemoglobin from late erythroid precursors in the bone marrow. Higher haptoglobin values in the presence of haemolysis can reflect either a lesser degree of haemolysis or concurrent inflammation, since haptoglobin is an acute phase reactant.

The combination of an increased serum LDH and a reduced haptoglobin is 90 percent specific for diagnosing haemolysis, while the combination of a normal serum LDH and a serum haptoglobin >25 mg/dL is 92 percent sensitive for ruling out haemolysis.

8.3 Reticulocyte count

The normal reticulocyte percentage is 0.5 to 1.5 percent. In patients with an otherwise intact bone marrow, the increase in erythropoietin production induced in a patient with hemolytic anaemia should raise the reticulocyte percentage above 4 to 5 percent. However, when the bone marrow is compromised (eg, following chemotherapy, infection, underlying marrow disease, cobalamin, folate, or iron deficiency), the reticulocyte response may be blunted or ablated.

8.4 Other tests

Other tests helpful in determining the presence or absence of haemolysis include:

Increased serum concentrations of indirect bilirubin from the catabolism of haemoglobin haem.

Increased mean corpuscular haemoglobin concentration (MCHC), indicating the presence of spherocytes.

Positive direct antiglobulin (Coombs') test in autoimmune hemolytic anaemia.

Tests for cold agglutinins or the Donath-Landsteiner antibody if symptoms are related to exposure to cold.

Testing for the presence of insoluble globin particles within the red blood cell (ie, Heinz bodies).

Increased blood concentration of carboxyhaemoglobin due to haemoglobin haem catabolism.

8.5 Testing for intravascular haemolysis

If intravascular haemolysis is suspected, the following additional tests are of value:

- Measurement of the PLASMA haemoglobin concentration (ie, testing for haemoglobinemia)
- Measurement of free haemoglobin in the urine supernatant (ie, testing for haemoglobinuria)
- Testing for hemosiderin in the urine sediment ≥7 days after the incident, allowing time for hemosiderin-containing tubular cells to be shed into the urine

9. Conclusion

Anaemia is a frequent clinical finding, often leading to significant ill health and always requires prompt investigation and selective treatment.

By following a simple escalation pathway from history, examination and targetted investigations, a diagnosis can usually be made and effective treatment applied.

10. References

Droogendijk J, et al, *Scand J Gastroenterol.* 2011 Jul 4.

Gehrs BC, Friedberg RC., *Am J Hematol.* 2002 Apr;69(4):258-71.

Goddard AF, James MW, McIntyre AS, Scott BB; on behalf of the British Society of Gastroenterology. *Gut. 2011 Jun 6.*

Harrison's Principles of Internal Medicine, 16th Edition.

Mehta BC. Approach to a patient with anaemia. *Indian J Med Sci* 2004;58:26-9

Nathan, DG, Oski, FA. *Hematology of Infancy and Childhood*, 4th ed, WB Saunders, Philadelphia, PA 1993.

Pierce A, Nester T; for the Education Committee of the Academy of Clinical Laboratory Physicians and Scientists. *Am J Clin Pathol.* 2011 Jul;136(1):7-12.

Powell N, McNair A. *Eur J Gastroenterol Hepatol.* 2008 Nov;20(11):1094-100.

Stanley L Schrier, MD, *Uptodate.com,* Approach to the adult patient with anaemia,

Stevens LA, Li S, Kurella Tamura M, et al, *Am J Kidney Dis.* 2011 Mar;57(3 Suppl 2):S9-16.

Trifan A, Singeap AM, et al., *J Gastrointestin Liver Dis.*2010 Mar;19(1):21-5.

Vitale G, Fatti LM, et al. *J Am Geriatr Soc.*2010 Sep;58(9):1825-7.

6

Phosphatidylserine Shedding from RBCs – A Mechanism of Membrane Modulation and Damage Control

Eitan Fibach
Hematology, Hadassah – Hebrew
University Medical Center, Jerusalem
Israel

1. Introduction

Normally, phospholipids (PLs) are distributed across the membrane of all cells, including the RBCs, asymmetrically [1]: aminophospholipids such as phosphatidylserine (PS) are mainly localized in the cytoplasmic leaflet of the membrane, whereas lipids with a choline head (e.g., phosphatidylcholine) are mainly localized in the outer leaflet [2]. The PS distribution across the cell membrane is in a dynamic equilibrium; while the enzyme aminophospholipid translocase inserts it inward, the scramblase causes its externalization. Some of this external PS is shed into the extracellular medium either as membrane-bound vesicles [3] or as membrane-free PS [4]. In RBCs, exposed PS is one of the signals of senescence, mediating the removal of old or damaged RBCs from the circulation [5]. Shedding of PS may reduce this signal and thus function to moderate RBC removal [6]. PS externalization and shedding are also associated with development of RBCs in the bone marrow, fulfilling various structural and functional purposes [7]. In the present review I we summarize our studied on changes in PS distribution and shedding during maturation and ageing of erythroid cells.

2. Methodologies

For these studies we have employed two analytical methodologies, Nuclear Magnetic Resonance (NMR) spectroscopy [4] and flow cytometry [8]. Using ^{1}H- and ^{31}P-NMR procedures, we measured absolute concentrations of metabolites in aqueous and organic extracts of the cells [9-12].

Flow cytometry was employed to measure various parameters of cellular oxidative stress: generation of reactive oxygen species (ROS) and membrane lipid peroxides, the intracellular content of reduced glutathione [13], as well as the contents of the labile iron [14] and calcium (Ca). These measurements are based on changes in the fluorescence intensities of specific probes.

To measure the cellular distribution of PS and its shedding from erythroid cells, we developed a two-step fluorescence inhibition assay [8]. PS is usually estimated by staining cells with annexin V which specifically binds to PS. Fluorochrome-conjugated annexin V is used to determine the percentage of PS-carrying cells by flow cytometry [15, 16]. This method is applicable to populations containing a significant fraction of positive cells, for example, following exposure to an apoptosis-inducing agent. However, in vivo, at a given time, only a small fraction of any cell population is apoptotic, making their determination statistically unreliable. In addition, this procedure does not yield information regarding the inner PS, which is not exposed on the outer surface of the cells, nor on the PS shed into the surrounding medium. Moreover, the method refers usually only to strongly positive cells, giving the impression that the process occurs in an "all or none" fashion, neglecting cells with less than maximal amount of bound annexin V. Most importantly, the procedure provides relative comparison rather than absolute quantitative values.

To overcome these limitations, we developed a novel flow cytometry methodology that provides a quantitative measurement of the external PS as well as the intracellular and shed PS. The procedure entails two steps: In the first step, the outer PS of intact cells or the total PS of cell lysates and supernatants, or human serum is bound to excess amount of fluorescent-annexin V. In the second step, the residual, non-bound fluorescent-annexin V is quantified by binding to PS exposed on apoptotic cells (e.g., 6-day old HL-60 cells) which serve as an indicator reagent. The fluorescence of these indicator cells is reciprocally proportional to the amount of PS on the measured cells in the first step [8].

3. PS exposure and shedding during the lifespan of RBCs in the circulation

During their life in the circulation, RBCs are exposed to several stress situations, which are (i) physical, occurring when they squeeze through small capillaries, (ii) hyperosmotic, when they travel through the kidney medulla, and (iii) oxidative, when they pass the oxygenated lung. These stress conditions affect the RBC composition and properties, leading to their senescence and eventually to their elimination from the circulation.

One of the signals of senescence is PS externalization. PS-carrying RBCs undergo phagocytosis (erythrophagocytosis) by macrophages in the reticulo-endothelial system (extravascular hemolysis) [5]. Under normal conditions this occurs in humans after 120 days, but under pathological conditions this process is accelerated, thereby shortening the life-span of RBCs, causing hemolytic anemia. These hemolytic anemias are hereditary, such as the hemoglobinopathies, thalassemia and sickle cell disease, or acquired, such as the myelodysplastic syndromes.

Using the methodologies described above, we studied the externalization and shedding of PS in RBCs during their senescence and compared RBCs derived from the peripheral blood of normal donors and patients with hemolytic anemias. ^{31}P-NMR analysis indicated that compared to normal RBCs, thalassemic RBCs have lower concentrations of total cellular PS which was associated with increased PS shedding [4]. Flow cytometry measurements, using fluorescent annexin V as a probe, confirmed these results and further demonstrated that despite of the decreased total cellular PS, in thalassemic RBCs, the PS exposed on their outer membrane was significantly increased. This was reflected not only by moderate increase in the percentage of annexin V positive cells as measured by the direct method, but also by a significant increase in exposed PS on the entire population as measured by the indirect method. The increased PS exposure reflected the balance between the decrease in the inner membrane PS and the increase in the shedding of PS into the extracellular milieu. The increased PS shedding by thalassemic RBCs was also reflected in the higher PS concentration in sera of thalassemic patients compared with normal donors. It should be mentioned that while shedding is often described in the context of microparticles, i.e., membrane-bound vesicles [3], we have shown that the majority of the shed PS is membrane-free [8].

PS shedding has a profound effect on the membrane composition and functionality. The PLs and cholesterol are the major lipid membrane components. Using a ^{1}H-NMR, we determined their ratio in normal and thalassemic RBC membranes and in supernatants following in vitro incubation [6]. The results indicated a significant decrease in PLs in the membranes and an increase in the supernatants, while cholesterol was only slightly decreased in the membrane and was minimal in the supernatants. These changes resulted in an increased cholesterol/PL ratio in the RBC membranes. Thalassemic RBCs demonstrated a higher basal cholesterol/PL ratio than normal RBCs. These findings suggest that shedding is a selective process involving mainly PLs and leading to relative accumulation of cholesterol in the membrane.

PS shedding and the consequential changes in the membrane composition and properties affect its functionality. It increased its osmotic resistance and the susceptibility of RBCs to undergo erythrophagocytosis. Using cultured macrophages, we have shown that while PS externalization increased phagocytosis, the shed PS prevented it, probably by competitive binding to PS receptors on the macrophages [6].

PS shedding may play a role in the functioning and fate of mature RBCs in the circulation:

a. Shedding of PS-enriched membranes [3, 4] might cause size reduction which characterizes RBC senescence as well as microcytic anemias. Shedding might serve mainly to rejuvenate the plasma membrane of the RBCs by removing its damaged components [17].

b. The cholesterol content of the RBC plasma membrane was reported to affect its mechanical properties (fluidity) [18, 19]. During physiological aging, senescent RBCs showed an increased cholesterol/PL ratio followed by greater membrane strength [20]. We have shown that in RBCs PS shedding and relative accumulation of cholesterol are associated with a greater osmotic resistance [6].

c. PS externalization has been suggested as one of the mechanisms of senescent RBC clearance from the circulation by PS receptor carrying reticuloendothelial system macrophages [5]. We have shown that whereas PS externalization increases phagocytosis, PS shedding decreases it [4]. The latter effect may be attributed to a decrease in the exposed PS, as well as competition by the shed PS for the macrophage PS receptors. Thus, the balance between PS externalization and shedding may play a role in controlling the fate/lifespan of the RBCs in the circulation under both physiological and pathological conditions, e.g., in thalassemia where RBCs were shown to have increased PS shedding [4, 8].

d. Finally, it is worth mentioning that PS has procoagulant properties [21]. Exposed and shed PS could be involved in normal and pathological homeostasis [1]. Thus, thalassemic patients with increased exposed and shed PS are prone to thromboembolic complications [22, 23].

4. PS shedding during development of erythroid cells

RBCs are produced in the bone marrow by a well regulated process (erythropoiesis) that involves proliferation and maturation. PS externalization and shedding have important roles in this process [7]. We studied normal human bone marrow cells as well as two in vitro models of erythropoiesis, primary cultures of human erythroid precursors and a murine erythroleukemia cell line. The human erythroid precursors are derived from progenitors present in the peripheral blood of normal donors. They are stimulated by the physiological inducer erythropoietin to proliferate and mature into hemoglobin-containing nucleated orthochromatophilic normoblasts. This system provides a reliable *in vitro* model that recapitulates many aspects of erythroid maturation [24]. The murine cells, derived originally from the spleen of viral induced leukemia, were stimulated to undergo erythroid maturation by hexamethylene bis acetamide [25] [26]. In all these systems, both PS exposure and shedding were found to be high in early precursors, and to be reduced during maturation.

Several suggestions might be raised regarding the role of PS shedding in the maturation of erythroid cells:

a. Size reduction characterizes not only RBC senescence in the circulation, but also erythroid maturation in the bone marrow. During their maturation erythroid precursors undergo a gradual and continuous, but a significant, reduction in size [27, 28]. This is an important functional adaptation generating mature RBCs small enough to pass through narrow capillaries. It also generates a high surface to volume ratio that promotes gas exchange between the RBCs and tissue cells during this passage. Shedding of PS-enriched membranes [3, 4] during maturation might be the cause or the outcome of the size reduction process. We have shown that inhibition of PS externalization/shedding prevented size reduction in differentiating erythroid cells [7], favoring the first possibility.

b. Apoptosis of nuclear cells involves PS externalization [29]. RBC production is regulated by apoptosis of erythroid precursors, which is controlled by erythropoietin, serving as an anti-apoptotic agent [30]. We found that depletion of erythropoietin during maturation of cultured erythroid precursors results in PS externalization, suggesting that this process is involved in the apoptosis of erythroid precursors as part of normal or pathological (ineffective) erythropoiesis (e.g., in the myelodysplastic syndrome or thalassemia), while PS shedding may have an opposite effect.

c. During their early development in the bone marrow, erythroid precursors are found in erythroblast islands, where they surround a central macrophage [31]. A diverse array of adhesion proteins expressed on the erythroblast surface mediate its interaction with both stromal cells and the extracellular matrix [32, 33]. It is possible that the outer PS on these precursors may assist in their attachment to macrophages carrying PS receptors, thus forming the erythroblast islands. Outer PS shedding (in addition to PS internalization) may lessen this adhesion and facilitate the release of erythroid precursors from the island as they mature. This possibility awaits experimental confirmation.

d. During maturation, erythroid precursors expel their cellular organelles, including the nucleus, mitochondria and ribosomes, by exocytosis through membrane-bound vesicles [34, 35]. Recent results indicated that enucleation is caused by the coalescence of vesicles at the nuclear-cytoplasmic junction, whereas, mitochondria are eliminated through selective autophagy [36]. Plasma membrane remodeling by PS redistribution might also be part of this process. Yoshida et al. have shown that "the nuclei are engulfed by macrophages only after they are disconnected from reticulocytes, and that phosphatidylserine, which is often used as an 'eat me' signal for apoptotic cells, is also used for the engulfment of nuclei expelled from erythroblasts" [37].

5. Mechanisms involved in PS shedding

We studied several mechanisms in relation to the above described changes in PS distribution: the oxidative status of the cells, changes in Ca-flux and microtubule (MT) polymerization.

6. Oxidative stress

The oxidative status of cells depends on the balance between oxidants (such as ROS) and antioxidants. Under pathological conditions, the balance leans towards generation of excess oxidants, which is accompanied by reduced content of antioxidants, resulting in oxidative stress. Although free radicals have important roles in normal physiology, such as in signal transduction, in excess they interact with and damage various components of the cells (e.g., proteins, lipids and nucleic acids). Many diseases are associated with oxidative stress, including hemolytic anemias. Although these anemias vary as to their etiology, in all cases the damage to erythroid cells is mediated by oxidative stress [38]. Using flow cytometry, we have demonstrated oxidative stress in normal mature RBCs treated with various oxidants: increased generation of ROS and membrane lipid peroxides and decreased content of reduced glutathione - the main cellular antioxidant. Similar results were obtained in RBCs derived from patients with thalassemia, sickle cell disease, myelodysplastic syndromes (MDS), paroxysmal nocturnal hemoglobinuria, spherocytosis and other hemolytic anemias. 1H-NMR analysis demonstrated oxidative stress in such RBCs by a high lactate/pyruvate ratio [4].

Oxidative stress reduces the activity of the enzyme translocase [39], causing the equilibrium that exists between the PS on the inner and the outer membrane leaflets to lean towards externalization. We have found that oxidatively stressed RBCs (old vs. young RBCs, thalassemic vs. normal RBCs, oxidant treated vs. non treated normal RBCs) have less total cellular PS but more exposed and shed PS [6]. Ameliorating the oxidative stress, e.g., by treating thalassemic cells with an antioxidant (e.g., vitamin C or N-acetyl cysteine) resulted in opposite results [8].

As mentioned above, in RBCs, exposed PS is one of the signals of senescence [5] and that it induces erythrophagocytosis. This process is accelerated in hemolytic anemias resulting in short survival of RBCs in the circulation. Although in patients with hemolytic anemia the proliferation of erythroid precursors in the bone marrow is increased (by stimulating the production of erythropoietin in the kidneys), when the condition is chronic the production of mature RBCs is futile due to increased premature death (by apoptosis) and lack of maturation of the erythroid precursors (ineffective erythropoiesis) [40]. The supply of mature, functional, RBCs is thus insufficient.

The main cause of oxidative stress in hemolytic anemias is iron overload due to increased iron absorption and repeated blood transfusions. When the iron content in the serum exceeds the binding capacity of transferrin, the iron-transport protein, surplus iron appears as "non-transferrin bound iron", which is taken up by cells, including RBCs, by mechanisms that are transferrin receptor-independent [41]. The incoming iron accumulates intra-cellularly as "labile iron pool" [42, 43], which is of redox potential due to its participation in chemical (Haber-Weiss and Fenton) reactions that generate ROS.

The oxidative status affects PS externalization/shedding also in developing erythroid cells. It is modulated throughout maturation; from being very high in early erythroid precursors it is reduced considerably as the cells mature. This change is most probably related to the decrease in the metabolic rate. Most of the ROS produced by cells are originated in the mitochondria in the process of oxidative energy production [38]. Erythroid maturation involves a loss of mitochondria and a decrease in energy production which results in lower generation of ROS and consequently, in lower PS externalization and shedding.

7. Ca-flux

Increase in the intracellular Ca concentration is a well-known mechanism of PS [44]. We studied the relationship between the oxidative state, changes in Ca-flux and PS shedding [6]. It was found that the oxidatively stressed thalassemic RBCs with their increased PS shedding have high Ca content which could be corrected by treatment with antioxidants. The low Ca content and PS-shedding of normal RBCs could be increased by treatment with oxidants. Modulating the Ca content of normal RBCs by treatment with the Ca ionophore A23187 or by varying the Ca concentration in the medium confirmed that increasing the inward Ca flux induced PS externalization and shedding.

8. Microtubule (MT) polymerization

Several lines of evidence suggest an interaction between the plasma membrane PLs and cytoskeleton components [45, 46], including the MTs [47,48] - the key components of the cytoskeleton [49]. MTs are made up of αβ-tubulin heterodimers [49], and they readily polymerize and depolymerize in cells. MTs are involved in a variety of cellular processes such as cell division, maintenance of cell shape, cell signaling and migration, and cellular transport [50] as well as maturation and stress. During erythroid maturation, MTs undergo dramatic changes in distribution to become absent in mature mammalian RBCs [51]. It has been shown that at early stages of maturation of murine erythroid precursors MTs are radially arranged just under the plasma membrane. Addition of the MT depolymerization promoters, colchicine or vinblastine, caused MTs to disappear completely. This, however, did not affect enucleation [51]. Addition of paclitaxel (Taxol), which enhances MT polymerization and stabilization, to these cells caused the resulting pre-mature RBCs (reticulocytes) to contain abnormally high numbers of polymerized MTs [51]. Treatment of patients with Taxol caused PS externalization and short survival of their RBCs [52].

We investigated the effect of MT depolymerization in developing erythroid cells on their membrane PS distribution and shedding using cultured human and murine erythroid precursors. Cells were treated with the MT depolymerization enhancer - colchicine and inhibitor - Taxol. The effect of these modulators was studied on the constitutive shedding as well as shedding induced by the Ca-ionophore A23187 [53]. We found that treatment with colchicine and Taxol markedly increased both the constitutive and the induced PS externalization. PS shedding, however, was increased by colchicine, but was inhibited by Taxol.

As discussed above, PS shedding is one of the mechanisms of membrane remodeling [54], including changes in the membrane cholesterol/PL ratio [4, 8]. Using ^{1}H-NMR, we showed that colchicine, by enhancing shedding, increased the cholesterol/PL ratio, whereas Taxol, by inhibiting shedding, decreased this ratio.

Many compounds that alter the polymerization dynamics of MTs block mitosis, and consequently, induce cell death by apoptosis [55]. One of these compounds, Taxol, a promoter of MT polymerization and stabilization, is being used for treatment of patients with various malignancies such as breast cancer [56] or ovarian cancer [57]. A significant side effect of this treatment is severe anemia which was related to the effect of Taxol on PS externalization of mature RBC [52]. In line with the importance of PS shedding in erythroid development, the present finding that Taxol affects PS shedding may suggest that anemia in patients treated with Taxol might be also due to its effect on erythropoiesis in the bone marrow.

9. Summary

PS externalization and shedding undergo a bi-phasic modulation in erythroid cells: both are decreased during maturation but increased during aging. This redistribution of PS is the outcome of multiple factors and mechanisms, including changes in the cellular oxidative status, Ca concentration and MT polymerization which affect the inward and outward PS flow and PS shedding. These dynamic processes are ongoing continuously and simultaneously, and may have opposite effects. For example, PS exposure on thalassemic RBCs, induced by their high intracellular oxidative status and Ca concentration, is blunted by increased PS shedding. Only when PS externalization overcomes the ability to remove it by shedding are thalassemic RBCs removed by erythrophagocytosis. Further study on the roles played by PS shedding in the production and clearance of RBCs is crucial for understanding its effect on the pathological consequences of hemolytic anemias and for the planning of novel therapeutic modalities to overcome them.

10. References

[1] R.F. Zwaal, P. Comfurius, E.M. Bevers, Surface exposure of phosphatidylserine in pathological cells, Cell Mol Life Sci 62 (2005) 971-988.
[2] J.A. Op den Kamp, Lipid asymmetry in membranes, Annu Rev Biochem 48 (1979) 47-71.
[3] K. Pattanapanyasat, E. Noulsri, S. Fucharoen, S. Lerdwana, P. Lamchiagdhase, N. Siritanaratkul, H.K. Webster, Flow cytometric quantitation of red blood cell vesicles in thalassemia, Cytometry B Clin Cytom 57 (2004) 23-31.
[4] I. Freikman, J. Amer, J.S. Cohen, I. Ringel, E. Fibach, Oxidative stress causes membrane phospholipid rearrangement and shedding from RBC membranes--an NMR study, Biochim Biophys Acta 1778 (2008) 2388-2394.
[5] M. Foller, S.M. Huber, F. Lang, Erythrocyte programmed cell death, IUBMB Life 60 (2008) 661-668.
[6] I. Freikman, I. Ringel, E. Fibach, Oxidative Stress-Induced Membrane Shedding from RBCs is Ca Flux-Mediated and Affects Membrane Lipid Composition, J Membr Biol 240 (2011) 73-82.
[7] I. Freikman, E. Fibach, Distribution and shedding of the membrane phosphatidylserine during maturation and aging of erythroid cells, Biochim Biophys Acta 1808 (2011) 2773-280.
[8] I. Freikman, J. Amer, I. Ringel, E. Fibach, A flow cytometry approach for quantitative analysis of cellular phosphatidylserine distribution and shedding, Anal Biochem 393 (2009) 111-116.

[9] J. Schiller, K. Arnold, Application of high resolution 31P NMR spectroscopy to the characterization of the phospholipid composition of tissues and body fluids - a methodological review, Med Sci Monit 8 (2002) MT205-222.

[10] D.J. Philp, W.A. Bubb, P.W. Kuchel, Chemical shift and magnetic susceptibility contributions to the separation of intracellular and supernatant resonances in variable angle spinning NMR spectra of erythrocyte suspensions, Magn Reson Med 51 (2004) 441-444.

[11] I. Spasojevic, V. Maksimovic, J. Zakrzewska, G. Bacic, Effects of 5-fluorouracil on erythrocytes in relation to its cardiotoxicity: membrane structure and functioning, J Chem Inf Model 45 (2005) 1680-1685.

[12] J.E. Raftos, S. Whillier, B.E. Chapman, P.W. Kuchel, Kinetics of uptake and deacetylation of N-acetylcysteine by human erythrocytes, Int J Biochem Cell Biol 39 (2007) 1698-1706.

[13] J. Amer, E. Fibach, Oxidative status of platelets in normal and thalassemic blood, Thromb Haemost 92 (2004) 1052-1059.

[14] E. Prus, E. Fibach, Flow cytometry measurement of the labile iron pool in human hematopoietic cells, Cytometry A 73 (2008) 22-27.

[15] J. Amer, O. Zelig, E. Fibach, Oxidative status of red blood cells, neutrophils, and platelets in paroxysmal nocturnal hemoglobinuria, Exp Hematol 36 (2008) 369-377.

[16] F.A. Kuypers, R.A. Lewis, M. Hua, M.A. Schott, D. Discher, J.D. Ernst, B.H. Lubin, Detection of altered membrane phospholipid asymmetry in subpopulations of human red blood cells using fluorescently labeled annexin V, Blood 87 (1996) 1179-1187.

[17] F.L. Willekens, J.M. Werre, Y.A. Groenen-Dopp, B. Roerdinkholder-Stoelwinder, B. de Pauw, G.J. Bosman, Erythrocyte vesiculation: a self-protective mechanism?, Br J Haematol 141 (2008) 549-556.

[18] H.A. Wilson-Ashworth, Q. Bahm, J. Erickson, A. Shinkle, M.P. Vu, D. Woodbury, J.D. Bell, Differential detection of phospholipid fluidity, order, and spacing by fluorescence spectroscopy of bis-pyrene, prodan, nystatin, and merocyanine 540, Biophys J 91 (2006) 4091-4101.

[19] L.J. Gonzalez, E. Gibbons, R.W. Bailey, J. Fairbourn, T. Nguyen, S.K. Smith, K.B. Best, J. Nelson, A.M. Judd, J.D. Bell, The influence of membrane physical properties on microvesicle release in human erythrocytes, PMC Biophys 2 (2009) 7.

[20] P. Caprari, A. Scuteri, A.M. Salvati, C. Bauco, A. Cantafora, R. Masella, D. Modesti, A. Tarzia, V. Marigliano, Aging and red blood cell membrane: a study of centenarians, Exp Gerontol 34 (1999) 47-57.

[21] M.S. Tallman, D. Hakimian, H.C. Kwaan, F.R. Rickles, New insights into the pathogenesis of coagulation dysfunction in acute promyelocytic leukemia, Leuk Lymphoma 11 (1993) 27-36.

[22] A. Eldor, E.A. Rachmilewitz, The hypercoagulable state in thalassemia, Blood 99 (2002) 36-43.

[23] A. Ruf, M. Pick, V. Deutsch, H. Patscheke, A. Goldfarb, E.A. Rachmilewitz, M.C. Guillin, A. Eldor, In-vivo platelet activation correlates with red cell anionic phospholipid exposure in patients with beta-thalassaemia major, Br J Haematol 98 (1997) 51-56.

[24] E. Fibach, D. Manor, A. Oppenheim, E.A. Rachmilewitz, Proliferation and maturation of human erythroid progenitors in liquid culture, Blood 73 (1989) 100-103.

[25] R.C. Reuben, R.L. Wife, R. Breslow, R.A. Rifkind, P.A. Marks, A new group of potent inducers of differentiation in murine erythroleukemia cells, Proc Natl Acad Sci U S A 73 (1976) 862-866.

[26] E. Fibach, R.C. Reuben, R.A. Rifkind, P.A. Marks, Effect of hexamethylene bisacetamide on the commitment to differentiation of murine erythroleukemia cells, Cancer Res 37 (1977) 440-444.

[27] A. Cueff, R. Seear, A. Dyrda, G. Bouyer, S. Egee, A. Esposito, J. Skepper, T. Tiffert, V.L. Lew, S.L. Thomas, Effects of elevated intracellular calcium on the osmotic fragility of human red blood cells, Cell Calcium 47 (2010) 29-36.

[28] J. Jandl, Blood - Textbook of Hematology, Little, Brown and Co., Boston, 1996.

[29] P.A. Leventis, S. Grinstein, The distribution and function of phosphatidylserine in cellular membranes, Annu Rev Biophys 39 (2010) 407-427.

[30] U. Testa, Apoptotic mechanisms in the control of erythropoiesis, Leukemia 18 (2004) 1176-1199.

[31] M.C. Bessis, J. Breton-Gorius, Iron metabolism in the bone marrow as seen by electron microscopy: a critical review, Blood 19 (1962) 635-663.

[32] J.A. Chasis, N. Mohandas, Erythroblastic islands: niches for erythropoiesis, Blood 112 (2008) 470-478.

[33] S. Soni, S. Bala, M. Hanspal, Requirement for erythroblast-macrophage protein (Emp) in definitive erythropoiesis, Blood Cells Mol Dis 41 (2008) 141-147.

[34] S.C. Gifford, J. Derganc, S.S. Shevkoplyas, T. Yoshida, M.W. Bitensky, A detailed study of time-dependent changes in human red blood cells: from reticulocyte maturation to erythrocyte senescence, Br J Haematol 135 (2006) 395-404.

[35] J. Liu, X. Guo, N. Mohandas, J.A. Chasis, X. An, Membrane remodeling during reticulocyte maturation, Blood 115 (2010) 2021-2027.

[36] P.A. Ney, Normal and disordered reticulocyte maturation, Curr Opin Hematol 18 (2011) 152-157.

[37] H. Yoshida, K. Kawane, M. Koike, Y. Mori, Y. Uchiyama, S. Nagata, Phosphatidylserine-dependent engulfment by macrophages of nuclei from erythroid precursor cells, Nature 437 (2005) 754-758.

[38] E. Fibach, E. Rachmilewitz, The role of oxidative stress in hemolytic anemia, Curr Mol Med 8 (2008) 609-619.

[39] A. Lopez-Revuelta, J.I. Sanchez-Gallego, A.C. Garcia-Montero, A. Hernandez-Hernandez, J. Sanchez-Yague, M. Llanillo, Membrane cholesterol in the regulation of aminophospholipid asymmetry and phagocytosis in oxidized erythrocytes, Free Radic Biol Med 42 (2007) 1106-1118.

[40] S. Rivella, Ineffective erythropoiesis and thalassemias, Curr Opin Hematol 16 (2009) 187-194.

[41] E. Prus, E. Fibach, Uptake of non-transferrin iron by erythroid cells, Anemia 2011 (2011) 945289.

[42] W. Breuer, M. Shvartsman, Z.I. Cabantchik, Intracellular labile iron, Int J Biochem Cell Biol 40 (2008) 350-354.

[43] E. Prus, E. Fibach, The labile iron pool in human erythroid cells, Br J Haematol 142 (2008) 301-307.

[44] F. Lang, K.S. Lang, P.A. Lang, S.M. Huber, T. Wieder, Mechanisms and significance of eryptosis, Antioxid Redox Signal 8 (2006) 1183-1192.

[45] G.R. Chichili, W. Rodgers, Cytoskeleton-membrane interactions in membrane raft structure, Cell Mol Life Sci 66 (2009) 2319-2328.

[46] K.F. Meiri, Membrane/cytoskeleton communication, Subcell Biochem 37 (2004) 247-282.

[47] E. Reaven, S. Azhar, Effect of various hepatic membrane fractions on microtubule assembly-with special emphasis on the role of membrane phospholipids, J Cell Biol 89 (1981) 300-308.

[48] J.M. Caron, R.D. Berlin, Interaction of microtubule proteins with phospholipid vesicles, J Cell Biol 81 (1979) 665-671.

[49] B. van der Vaart, A. Akhmanova, A. Straube, Regulation of microtubule dynamic instability, Biochem Soc Trans 37 (2009) 1007-1013.

[50] B. Bhattacharyya, D. Panda, S. Gupta, M. Banerjee, Anti-mitotic activity of colchicine and the structural basis for its interaction with tubulin, Med Res Rev 28 (2008) 155-183.

[51] S.T. Koury, M.J. Koury, M.C. Bondurant, Cytoskeletal distribution and function during the maturation and enucleation of mammalian erythroblasts, J Cell Biol 109 (1989) 3005-3013.

[52] P.A. Lang, J. Huober, C. Bachmann, D.S. Kempe, M. Sobiesiak, A. Akel, O.M. Niemoeller, P. Dreischer, K. Eisele, B.A. Klarl, E. Gulbins, F. Lang, T. Wieder, Stimulation of erythrocyte phosphatidylserine exposure by paclitaxel, Cell Physiol Biochem 18 (2006) 151-164.

[53] E.N. Dedkova, A.A. Sigova, V.P. Zinchenko, Mechanism of action of calcium ionophores on intact cells: ionophore-resistant cells, Membr Cell Biol 13 (2000) 357-368.

[54] T.J. Greenwalt, The how and why of exocytic vesicles, Transfusion 46 (2006) 143-152.

[55] M.A. Jordan, Mechanism of action of antitumor drugs that interact with microtubules and tubulin, Curr Med Chem Anticancer Agents 2 (2002) 1-17.

[56] J.C. Chang, E.C. Wooten, A. Tsimelzon, S.G. Hilsenbeck, M.C. Gutierrez, Y.L. Tham, M. Kalidas, R. Elledge, S. Mohsin, C.K. Osborne, G.C. Chamness, D.C. Allred, M.T. Lewis, H. Wong, P. O'Connell, Patterns of resistance and incomplete response to docetaxel by gene expression profiling in breast cancer patients, J Clin Oncol 23 (2005) 1169-1177.

[57] W.P. McGuire, W.J. Hoskins, M.F. Brady, P.R. Kucera, E.E. Partridge, K.Y. Look, D.L. Clarke-Pearson, M. Davidson, Cyclophosphamide and cisplatin compared with paclitaxel and cisplatin in patients with stage III and stage IV ovarian cancer, N Engl J Med 334 (1996) 1-6.

7

Anaemia in Developing Countries: Burden and Prospects of Prevention and Control

Kayode O. Osungbade[1,2,*] and Adeolu O. Oladunjoye[1,2]
¹Department of Health Policy and Management
Faculty of Public Health
College of Medicine and University College Hospital
University of Ibadan and
²Department of Community Medicine
University College Hospital, Ibadan
Nigeria

1. Introduction

Anaemia constitutes a public health problem in developing countries. Worldwide, about 2 billion people are estimated to suffer from anaemia and it is reported to account for three-quarters of 1 million deaths a year in Africa and South-East Asia. The underlying causes of anaemia are many, varied and largely preventable; these include nutritional deficiencies, infections and haemoglobin disorders.

Cost-effective interventions against anaemia are well documented in the literature. However, there are constraints to diagnosis, treatment and prevention in resource-poor settings of developing countries. Effective management of anaemia includes treatment of the underlying cause, restoration of the haemoglobin concentration to normal levels, and prevention and treatment of complications, among others. Suggested strategies aimed at preventing anaemia focused on the major underlying causes in developing countries.

2. Background

Anaemia is the reduction in the haemoglobin concentration of the peripheral blood below the normal range expected for age and sex of an individual.(1) The World Health Organisation (WHO) defines anaemia as a hemoglobin value below 13 g/dl in men over 15 years of age, below 12 g/dl in non pregnant women over 15 years, and below 11 g/dl in pregnant women.(2) It is a condition in which the number of red blood cells or their oxygen carrying capacity is insufficient to meet physiologic needs and this varies for age, sex, altitude and pregnancy status.(3) However, the determination of hemoglobin concentration should always take the state of hydration and altitude of residence of an individual into consideration.(1)

Anaemia is a global health problem in both developing and developed countries with major consequences on human health as well as social and economic development.(4) Anaemia is

---

*Correspondence Author

the world's second leading cause of disability.(3) Worldwide, the World Health Organisation (WHO) estimated the number of anaemic persons to be about 2 billion and approximately 50% of all cases can be attributed to iron deficiency.(5) Anaemia is responsible for about 1 million death a year, out of which three-quarters occur in Africa and South-East Asia.(6) Anaemia affects over half of preschool age children and pregnant women in developing countries, and at least 30-40% in industrialized countries.(3) Nevertheless, it is apparent that the prevalence of anaemia in developing countries is about four times more than developed countries.(7) In view of the above, this chapter highlights the burden of anaemia in the population and discusses its causes in developing countries. Furthermore, the chapter reviews the prospects and challenges of diagnosis of underlying causes, treatment and prevention in the developing countries.

3. Methods

We reviewed literature using key words of the thrust of the paper; hence, search terms such as prevalence, burden, causes, treatment and prevention of anaemia in developing countries were used. Cross sectional, observational and randomized control trials' literature on the subject published between 2000 and 2010 served as the main sources of information. Commonly used medical databases such as PubMed (Medline), AJOL and Google Scholar were searched as appropriate; in addition, Cochrane Library was used to source for systematic reviews on the subject matter.

4. Results

4.1 Burden of anaemia in developing countries

The most vulnerable groups in the population are children and pregnant women, while others such as the non pregnant women and the elderly are next affected. An estimated 10-20% of preschool age children in developed countries and 30-80% in developing countries are anaemic at 1 year of age.(8) The consequences of anaemia in children are inimical as it affects their cognitive performance, behaviour and physical growth. Children who suffer from anaemia have delayed psychomotor development and impaired performance of tests; in addition, they experience impaired coordination of language and motor skills, equivalent to a 5 to 10 points deficit in intelligent quotient (IQ).(5)

The World Health Organisation (WHO) estimated that 56% of all pregnant women in developing countries are anaemic.(9) In Southern Asia, the prevalence of anaemia in pregnancy is about 75% in contrast to what obtains in North America and Europe with about 17% prevalence. Furthermore, 5% of pregnant women suffer from severe anaemia in the worst affected parts of the world.(9)

The consequences of anemia in women are enormous as the condition adversely affects both their productive and reproductive capabilities. First, anaemia reduces their energy and capacity for work (10), and can therefore threaten household food security and income. Second, severe anaemia in pregnancy impairs oxygen delivery to the fetus and interferes with normal intra-uterine growth, thereby resulting in intrauterine growth retardation, still birth, low birth weight and neonatal deaths.(10-11) Therefore, anaemia is highly contributory to poor pregnancy and birth outcomes in developing countries as it predisposes to premature delivery, increased perinatal mortality and increased risk of death during delivery and postpartum (10).

Worldwide, it is estimated that about 20% of maternal deaths are caused by anaemia; in addition, anaemia contributes partly to 50% of all maternal deaths.(12) Similar situation is found in sub-Saharan Africa where anaemia is reportedly accounted for about 20% of all maternal deaths brought about through three main mechanisms.(13) First, anaemia resulting from blood loss during or after childbirth makes women more susceptible to deaths by lowering their haematological reserve. Second, severe anaemia is associated with increased susceptibility to infection due to lowered resistance to disease; and third, haemoglobin (Hb) level of less than 4 g/dl is associated with high risk of cardiac failure and death particularly during delivery or soon after, if prompt intervention is not instituted.(14-15)

In terms of lost years of healthy life, iron deficiency anemia causes 25 million cases of Disability Adjusted Life Years (DALYs); this accounts for 2.4% of the total global DALYs.(3) Physical and cognitive losses due to iron deficiency anaemia cost developing countries up to 4.05% losses in gross domestic product per annum(16), thereby stalling social and economic development. In the World Health Organisation (WHO)/World Bank rankings, Iron Deficiency Anaemia (IDA) is the third leading cause of disability-adjusted life years lost for females' aged 15–44 years.(17-18)

4.2 Common causes of anaemia in developing countries

Most often, anaemia co-exists with an underlying disease and rarely occurs on its own. The commonest causes of anaemia in developing countries, particularly among the most vulnerable groups (pregnant women and preschool age children) are nutritional disorders and infections.

4.2.1 Iron deficiency

Iron Deficiency Anaemia (IDA) is an underlying risk factor for maternal and perinatal mortality and morbidity; it is estimated to be associated with 115,000 of the 510,000 maternal deaths (i.e. 22%) and 591,000 of the 2,464,000 perinatal deaths (i.e. 24%) occurring annually around the world.(19) Iron is an essential component of haemoglobin (Hb), which is required for basic cellular function in all human tissues, particularly muscle, brain and red blood cells.(20) Therefore, deficiency of iron in the body can lead to anaemia in any age group. Iron deficiency anaemia (IDA) occurs when iron deficiency is sufficiently severe enough to diminish erythropoiesis, thereby leading to a decrease in the number of red cells in the blood and resulting in the development of anaemia.(21) However, mild-to-moderate forms of iron deficiency can occur in which the affected person is yet to become anaemic, but tissues are functionally iron deficient.(5) It is generally assumed that 50% of cases of anaemia are due to iron deficiency(5), but this may vary within population groups or environment.

The risk factors for IDA include a low intake of iron, poor absorption of iron from diets high in phytate or phenolic compounds, and early period of life when iron requirements are expectedly high. (4) Similarly, iron requirements are highest for pregnant women - 1.9 mg/1,000 kcal of dietary energy in the second trimester and 2.7 mg/1,000 kcal in the third trimester. These are followed by iron requirements in infants (1.0 mg), adolescent girls (0.8 mg), adolescent boys (0.6 mg), non pregnant women (0.6 mg), preschool and school age children (0.4mg), and adult men (0.3mg).(22)

Sources of dietary iron include meat, fish and poultry; other sources, though in less quantity, are cereals, dairy products, fruits and vegetables. About 40% of iron content of meat, fish and poultry is in the haem form, out of which about 25% is absorbed;(7) whereas only about 2 - 5% of total iron is absorbed from cereals and legumes. Therefore, these foods have a major influence on iron status.(23) Unfortunately, intakes of these foods especially meat, fish and poultry are low among people of low socio-economic status. Furthermore, some of the foods are avoided or observed as taboos for religious or cultural reasons in certain communities of developing countries.

Inadequate absorption of dietary iron is highly contributory to the high prevalence of anaemia in the developing countries of Asia and other regions, except where it is caused by infections such as hookworm and malaria.(7) Poor absorption of dietary iron can be due to substances which interfere with its absorption such as proton pump inhibitors, calcium supplements and dairy products.(24)

4.2.2 Micronutrient deficiency

Evidence abounds that haemoglobin (Hb) concentration of persons with Vitamin A deficiency (VAD) increases by about 10 g/L when vitamin A supplements are provided.(25) Studies also suggest that vitamin A can improve hematologic indicators and enhance the efficacy of iron supplementation.(26) Thus, it is suggestive that Vitamin A deficiency (VAD) can predispose to anaemia.

It is reported that riboflavin deficiency may be quite common in developing countries where intake of animal products is low, and especially during seasons when there is less intake of vegetables.(7) Vitamin B12 is necessary for the synthesis of red blood cells and its deficiencies have been associated with megaloblastic anemia.(17) Therefore, diets with little or no animal protein, as it is often the case in the developing world, coupled with malabsorption related to parasitic infections of the small intestine, might result in Vitamin B 12 deficiency.(17)

Folic acid is also essential for the formation and maturation of red blood cells and necessary for cell growth and repair. Deficiency of folate reduces the rate of DNA synthesis with consequent impaired cell proliferation and intramedullary death of resulting abnormal cells; this shortens the lifespan of circulating red blood cells and results in anaemia.(27) There is, however, little evidence that folic acid deficiency may be a public health problem in many developing countries.

4.2.3 Infections

4.2.3.1 Malaria

It is now estimated that malaria is responsible for 1.2 million deaths annually and 2.9% of total DALYs in low and middle income countries.(28) About 35% of children with malaria in Africa have anaemia.(29) In sub-Saharan Africa, it is estimated that between 200,000 and 500,000 pregnant women develop severe anemia as a result of malaria.(9) *P. falciparum* malaria in pregnancy is the primary cause of up to 10,000 maternal anaemia related deaths in sub-Saharan Africa annually.(30)

Malaria, especially by the protozoon *Plasmodium falciparum,* causes anaemia by rupturing red blood cells and suppressing production of red blood cells.(31) However, this cannot be explained simply by the direct destruction of parasitized red blood cells at the time of release of meroziotes.(32) Decreased red cell production results from marrow hypoplasia seen in acute infection and dyerythropoiesis.(33) *Plasmodium falciparum* is the primary cause of severe malaria in regions of the world where malaria is endemic, especially sub-Sahara Africa .(7)

4.2.3.2 Parasitic infestation

Helminthes such as flukes, hookworm and whipworm cause chronic blood loss, and consequently iron loss.(34) These parasitic infestations are known to cause chronic haemorrhage and iron deficiency, resulting in the development of anaemia.(35) Blood loss caused by helminthiasis put the mother, fetus and child at risk of iron deficiency, which could lead to anaemia.(36) For example, the trematode, *Schistosomia haematobium* (fluke), predisposes to a significant urinary blood loss in severe infections and infected persons may present with terminal heamaturia, which continues for as long as it is not treated and then results in anaemia. Whereas, *Schistosomia mansoni* eggs can rupture the intestinal lining and result in the leakage of blood, other fluids and nutrients into the lumen.(34)

Hookworm infestation produces a high degree of long-term morbidity by causing iron deficiency anemia.(17) The extent to which this deficiency occurs depends on the host's iron status, the infecting parasites, and the intensity and duration of infection.(36) Blood loss is caused primarily by coagulase released by the parasite and it is responsible for continuous blood loss in the stool.(17) For example, *Ancylostoma duodenale* is estimated to cause up to 0.25 ml of blood loss per worm per day.(30)

A hookworm burden of 40–160 worms (depending on the iron status of the host) is associated with iron deficiency anemia.(37) Several studies in developing countries observed that 51% of anaemic children were iron deficient and if hookworm infection could be reduced by as much as 25%, it would reduce iron deficiency anaemia by 35% and severe anaemia by 73%.(31, 38) The nematode, *Trichuris trichiura* (whipworm) causes anaemia if the worm burden is heavy(31) and colonic lesions are associated with bleeding or there is a chronic reduction in food and micro-nutrient intake caused by anorexia-inducing effects of tumor necrosis factor-α released in response to the infection.(39-40)

4.2.3.3 Human Immuno-deficiency Virus infection (HIV)

Developing countries are the worst hit by the HIV pandemic, which accounts for 22.5 million people (68% of global total) in sub-Saharan Africa and 4.9 million people (15% of global total) in Asia living with HIV/AIDS in 2009.(41) In 2009, 1.3 million Africans died of HIV and this constituted 72% of the global total.(42) Anaemia is a frequent complication among HIV-positive individuals and it has been associated with a rapid HIV disease progression and mortality.(43) The predominant cause of anaemia in the context of HIV is anaemia of inflammation; this is also known as anemia of chronic disease, which is characterized by decreased red blood cell production through a series of mechanisms mediated, in part, by pro-inflammatory cytokines such as tumor necrosis factor-α and interleukin-6.(17)

Studies have also shown that zidovudine (AZT) causes anaemia in pregnant women as early as four weeks of commencing therapy.(44) The cause of anaemia in HIV-positive patients is, therefore, multi-factorial and includes infections, neoplasm, dietary deficiencies, blood loss, medications and antibodies to antiretroviral agents.(45-46) In addition, bone marrow suppression, especially the erythroid lines, by the AIDS virus is also known to cause anaemia in affected persons.(47)

4.3 Sickle cell diseases and thalassemia

About 5% of the world's population carries the genes responsible for haemoglobinopathies.(48) Sickle cell disease is an inherited disorder of hemogblobin and it is among the most common genetic diseases in the world.(17) Each year, about 300,000 infants are born with major haemoglobin disorders – including more than 200,000 cases of sickle-cell anaemia in Africa.(48) It is characterized by lifelong haemolytic anaemia and many other significant morbidities largely related to painful and debilitating vaso-occlusive phenomenon.(49)

Patients present with recurrent anaemia, which sometimes require blood transfusion. *'Sicklers'*, as affected persons are often called, have worsened symptoms of low packed cell volume especially when there is a co-infection or pregnancy. It is a challenge for patients in developing countries, both old and young, in treating their ill conditions as there are usually inadequate supportive measures to restore them back to their stable states.

Thalassemia is the most common single genetic disorder worldwide, resulting from defects in genes producing hemoglobin. (50) It is highly prevalent in many Asian, Mediterranean and Middle Eastern countries.(51) The intermediate clinical forms of thalassemia result in anaemia, with occasional need for transfusions of red blood cells.(17)

5. Prospects and challenges of diagnosis of underlying causes of anaemia

Blood test for serum ferritin seems to be a sensitive and an early indicator of iron deficiency. In most developing countries, it is determined by using an immunoassay kit which is readily available, easily done and relatively inexpensive. (52) However, serum iron concentration, total iron-binding capacity and examination of blood films cannot detect the earliest stages of iron deficiency. (52) On the other hand, bone marrow examination showing absence of stainable iron is the definitive method for diagnosing IDA;(53) however, this is a painful and invasive procedure and it is therefore usually used as a last resort.(54)

The World Health Organisation (WHO) recently recommended prompt parasitologic confirmation by microscopy or alternatively, by rapid diagnostic tests (RDTs) in all patients suspected of malaria before treatment is commenced unless parasitological diagnosis is not accessible; this is with a view to reducing cases of resistance to anti malaria treatment. (55) However, many peripheral health facilities in resource-poor settings of developing countries lack the capacity to conduct quality parasitological diagnosis of malaria by microscopy.(56-57) Nonetheless, rapid diagnostic tests (RDTs) for malaria had recently been shown to offer the potential of extending accurate malaria diagnosis to areas when microscopy services are not available, especially in remote locations of the developing countries.(58-59)

In making a diagnosis of any clinical phase of schistosomiasis, the highly sensitive and specific PCR based assays have been developed for the detection of schistosome DNA in faeces or sera and plasma.(60) However, these tests are either not available or very expensive in many developing countries; thus, clinicians often use clinical acumen to make a diagnosis in majority of cases. Furthermore, fresh water bath is common among children in developing countries; thus, children with pruritic reaction or unexplained febrile illness several weeks after a fresh water bath are suspected to have contracted urinary schistosomiasis.(61) Diagnosis is made by finding parasitic eggs in urine sample, which is best taken at midday after exercise when most eggs are being shed.(61) On the other hand, eggs of hookworm are readily isolated from stool samples in developing countries.

Major challenges facing laboratory systems in HIV testing in resource-poor settings include poor infrastructure, lack of human capacity, lack of laboratory policies, and limited synergies between clinical and research laboratories; these factors compromise the quality of test results and patient management.(62) In addition, HIV stigmatization is a major barrier preventing many people from having voluntary counseling and testing done in developing countries. For instance, in the prevention of maternal to child transmission programme

(PMTCT), challenges of diagnosis in developing countries include HIV-associated stigma. This has been reported to pose a barrier to service utilization, including failure of women to return for HIV test results where rapid testing is not available, low acceptance of short-course preventive ARVs offered to HIV-positive women at antenatal clinics, difficulty in tracking and following up of mothers who deliver their infants at home and complexities of infant feeding for HIV-positive mothers in very low-resource settings.(63)

The major challenge in the diagnosis of haemoglobin disorders is detection of the disease conditions during prenatal period. At this period, laboratory confirmation is critically important to enable a couple at risk in making an informed decision about potential termination of pregnancy.(64) With DNA diagnostics, it has become possible to make definitive diagnoses of different haemoglobin disorders during the first trimester of pregnancy by analyzing foetal DNA obtained from chorionic villous biopsy. There is evidence that neonatal screening for sickle-cell anaemia, when linked to timely diagnostic testing, parental education and comprehensive care, markedly reduces morbidity and mortality from the disease condition in infancy and early childhood.(48, 65).

6. Management of anaemia

The objectives of management of anaemia include(1):

* Treatment of the underlying cause;
* Restoration of the haemoglobin concentration to normal levels; and
* Prevention and treatment of complications.

6.1 Treatment of the underlying cause of anaemia

Iron deficiency anaemia is treated with oral iron supplements as ferrous sulfate, ferrous fumerate or ferrous gluconate given as 200 mg twice or three times daily. Treatment could also be parenteral as iron dextran, especially when there is intolerance to oral iron or anaemia is diagnosed late in pregnancy.

Low birth weight infants are born with low iron stores; therefore, they demand high iron requirements for growth. Furthermore, their iron requirements cannot be readily met from breast milk and it is known that their iron stores are depleted by 2 to 3 months postpartum.(7) The global recommendation is to supply low birth weight infants with supplemental iron drops starting at 2 months of age.(38) A substantial amount of evidence confirms that iron supplementation of anaemic school children improves their school performance, verbal and other skills.(66)

Vitamin A can be given as oral supplementation doses to postpartum mothers irrespective of their breastfeeding options in doses of 200,000 I.U and to less than 5 years of age in doses between 100,000-200,000 I.U. In some countries where vitamin A deficiency is a public health problem, vitamin A supplements in capsule form are administered during National Immunization Days (NIDs) alongside oral polio and measles vaccines.(67) Though, high supplementation dose of vitamin A is of immense benefit to both mother and breast feeding infant, it should be avoided in pregnant women because it can cause miscarriage and birth defects.(68)

Vitamin B 12 is usually given intramuscularly but recent studies have shown that an oral dose is as effective as the injectable administration.(69) The daily requirement of vitamin B_{12} is approximately 2 mcg; the initial oral replacement dosage consists of a single daily dose of 1,000 to 2,000 mcg.

Folic acid supplementation can be given to patients with folate deficiency in doses between 1-5 mg daily. It is routinely given to pregnant women, particularly early in pregnancy, to prevent neural tube defect in the growing foetus in some developing countries. Malaria is treated with a wide range of anti-malaria drugs and most African countries now recommend the Artemisinin-based combination therapy (ACT), which is given to reduce cases of resistance of the parasite to other drugs.

Antihelminthic drugs such as albendazole or mebendale can be given to people infested with hookworm. In addition, iron deficiency aneamia which may co-exist can be treated with iron supplement. Praziquantel is the drug of choice for the treatment of schistosomiasis and it is shown to be effective and safe in pregnancy.(36) Praziquantel can easily be administered according to height using a "dose pole" developed to dispense the drug at 40-60 mg/kg; this is with a view to minimizing under dosage while the "dose pole" helps in identifying five height intervals corresponding to 1½, 2, 2½, 3 and 4 tablets of praziquantel.(70)

The availability of the highly active antiretroviral therapy (HAART) at no cost has been of immense benefits to people living with HIV and AIDS, especially in developing countries where most affected persons cannot afford the drug treatment. Furthermore, WHO introduced revised treatment guidelines in 2010; these guidelines recommended early initiation of antiretroviral therapy, at a CD4 count of < 350 cells/mm3. This has, therefore, increased the total number of people medically eligible for antiretroviral therapy by about 50% i.e. from 10 million to 15 million in 2009 globally.(42) The main aspect of care for persons affected by sickle cell anaemia involves early treatment intervention of preventable health problems such as analgesics, antibiotics, vitamins, folic acid supplementation and high fluid intake are periodically used.

6.2 Restoration of the haemoglobin concentration to normal levels

Generally, blood transfusion is a very important measure in the treatment of anaemia; but it should not be used as a substitute for specific treatment of the underlying cause.(1) Blood can be given as an autologous transfusion, exchange transfusion or direct transfusion with blood products. It is recommended that blood transfusion should be given only if the dangers of failure to transfuse outweigh those of transfusion. (1) In developing countries, problems such as economic constraints may limit blood safety precautions; thus, unsafe blood which ought to have been screed for infections such as HIV, hepatitis B or C and syphilis, is inadvertently transfused.(71)

In addition, many developing countries do not have reliable testing systems because of staff shortage, lack of basic laboratory services, poor quality test kits or their irregular supply.(72) Sometimes, patients receive wrong blood type due to mismatch error and thereafter, develop blood transfusion reaction. These constraints underscore the importance of strengthening blood transfusion services in developing countries; furthermore, the process of obtaining an informed consent from patients, including discussing the risk and benefit of transfusion, except in life-threatening emergencies should be emphasised.(1)

6.3 Prevention and treatment of complications

Complications may arise as a result of the underlying disesase or anaemia itself. The overall goal is to ensure that anaemia does not re-occur or further deteriorates. Once the underlying cause can be treated, the prognosis is good in most cases. Other supportive measures include a balanced diet with adequate protein and vitamins; bed rest can also go a long way to restore blood levels in the body.

7. Strategies to prevent anaemia

Food fortification and dietary diversification with iron are important measures to prevent iron deficiency anaemia(8), especially in the vulnerable groups such as pregnant women and children. A number of strategies are used to deliver additional iron to humans, but food fortification has the greatest potential to improve the iron status of the largest number of people.(7) Ferrous fumarate, ferrous succinate and small particle size iron are suitable iron fortificants for infant cereals.(73) Infant cereals are widely fortified in developed countries and this has resulted in a definite reduction in anaemia. (74) WHO recommends that all pregnant women receive iron supplements of 60 mg daily combined in a pill, which also contains 400 µg folic acid.(75)

In view of the high prevalence of Vitamin A deficiency in developing countries and the potentially high prevalence of deficiencies of other micronutrients required for Hb synthesis and other functions, it is logical to assume that supplementation with multiple micronutrients, rather than just iron or iron plus folate, would be a rational public health strategy.(7) Currently, WHO recommends routine vitamin A supplementation during pregnancy or at any time during lactation in areas with endemic vitamin A deficiency.(76) Vitamin A can be given to children under 5 years of age in doses between 100,000-200,000 I.U as it is practised in some developing countries during national immunization days. Furthermore, absorption of iron from food can be enhanced by increasing intake of vitamin C.

Vector control remains as the most effective measure to prevent transmission of malaria in developing countries; though the methods used may vary considerably in their applicability, cost and sustainability.(77) WHO had recommended a combination of integrated vector management, indoor residual spraying, insecticide treated material and larval control.(78) Insecticide-impregnated bed nets in communities decrease the prevalence of severe anaemia in young children.(7) The home management of malaria (HMM) strategy has been introduced where early recognition, and prompt and appropriate treatment of malaria illness in children under 5 years of age in the home or community can be achieved. If *Plasmodium falciparum* malaria is endemic and transmission of infection is high, women in their first or second pregnancies should be given curative antimalarials at their first prenatal visit followed by locally recommended antimalarial prophylaxis.(7) Malaria control programme is highly necessitated among the highly susceptible group especially in the tropical regions of the world.(7)

In areas endemic with parasitic infections which affect Hb or iron status, the International Nutritional Anemia Consultative Group (INACG), WHO, and United Nations Childrens' Fund (UNICEF) recommended certain complementary control measures.(79) For example, adults and children over 5 years living in hookworm endemic areas (i.e. prevalence of 20-30% and above) are required to be treated with at least an annual dose of albendazole, mebendazole, Levamisole or Pyrantel. These drugs can be given to pregnant and lactating women, but should be avoided in the first trimester of pregnancy.(80)

Other efforts aimed at controlling hookworm infections include sanitary disposal of faeces and educational campaigns on proper use of latrines.(81) Most at risk persons are those who engage in agriculture and fishing, and those who use unsafe water for household chores particularly girls and their mothers.(36) Therefore, primary health care measures such as hand washing and wearing of shoes in hookworm endemic areas can have a major impact on the prevalence of anaemia.(7) All forms of schistosomiasis including intestinal and urinary types can be treated with praziquantel effectively. Prevention is best achieved by eliminating water dwelling snails, which serve as natural reservoirs of the disease.

Effective HIV preventive interventions include condom use, provision of clean injecting equipment, standard precautions, blood safety and post exposure prophylaxis for occupational and non-occupational exposures.(82) Sickle cell anaemia can be prevented if couples at risk of having affected children can be identified by inexpensive and reliable blood test. Periodic prophylaxis against malaria, infections and other factors which may trigger discomfort could improve quality life of affected children.(48)

8. Conclusion and recommendations

In developing countries which are usually characterized by resource-limited settings, slow progress has been made toward reducing the prevalence of anemia; this is largely due to persistent micro-nutrient deficiencies, and high prevalence of parasitic diseases, HIV, sickle cell disease and thalassemia.(17) The best approach to preventing IDA in pregnancy is to ensure adequate maternal iron status early in pregnancy or preferably in the pre-conceptional period.(83) Therefore, micronutrient supplements should be given not only to pregnant women but also to non-pregnant women of reproductive age and adolescent girls; this would reduce the prevalence of anaemia in the community and consequently, improve fertility and maternal health.

The apparent failure to reduce the prevalence of anaemia in developing countries may be partly due to existing interventions, which are usually designed with the assumption that iron deficiency is the main cause.(84) Thus, other important causes of anaemia have been underestimated and neglected, and these have been on the increase. Therefore, adequate attention should be given to the emerging causes of anemia in developing countries such as HIV/AIDS and micronutrient deficiency

The involvement of government of developing countries can effectively combine and balance the needs for programme implementation, monitoring and evaluation, research and community involvement. It is expected that the burden of anaemia will drastically reduce if adequate attention is paid to joint participation of all stakeholders in combating the burden in developing countries. Intervention programmes should address iron deficiency with the focus on both dietary quantity and quality of the micronutrient composition. Strategies which are required to improve nutrition knowledge and awareness of mothers and health workers may also be implemented.

Ultimately, treating the underlying causes of anaemia is critical in eliminating anaemia in all age groups, particularly the vulnerable ones. Therefore, it becomes imperative that all stakeholders harmonize and coordinate their efforts in ensuring that the burden and prevalence of anaemia, and its causes are reduced to the barest minimum in all developing countries.

9. References

[1] Standard treatment guidelines Nigeria. 2008:Pg 12-4.
[2] World Health Organisation. Nutritional anemia: report of a WHO Scientific Group. Geneva, Switzerland: World Health Organisation1968.
[3] World Health Organisation. WHO Vitamin and Mineral Nutrition/ Anaemia 2011.
[4] World Health Organisation. Worldwide prevalence of anaemia 1993-2005: WHO global database on anaemia2005.
[5] WHO/UNICEF/UNU. Iron deficiency anaemia: assessment, prevention, and control. Geneva: World HealthOrganization2001.

[6] World Bank. Public health at a glance. December 2004.

[7] ACC/SCN. What Works? A Review of the Efficacy and Effectiveness of Nutrition Interventions. Geneva in collaboration with the Asian Development Bank, Manila: ACC/SCN2001.

[8] World Health Organization. WHO Global Database on Iron Deficiency and Anaemia, Micronutrient Deficiency Information System. . Geneva: World Health Organisation2005.

[9] World Health Organization. The Prevalence of Anaemia in Women : A Tabulation of Available Information. Geneva: WHO; 1992.

[10] Axemo P, Liljestrand J, Bergstrom S, Gebre-Medhin M. Aetiology of late fetal death in Maputo. Gynaecol Obstet Invest. 1995;39:103-9.

[11] Brabin BJ, Premji Z, Verhoeff F. An analysis of anaemia and child mortality. J Nutr. 2001;132:636S-45S.

[12] Rae Galloway, Erin Dusch, Leslie Elderet. Women's perceptions of iron deficiency and anemia prevention and control in eight developing countries. Science Direct, Social Science & Medicine August 2002;55(4):Pages 529-44.

[13] Buseri FI, Uko EK, Jeremiah ZA, Usanga EA. Prevalence and Risk Factors of Anaemia Among Pregnant women in Nigeria. The Open Hematology Journal. 2008;2:14-9.

[14] Ross J, Thomas EL. Iron Deficiency Anaemia and Maternal Mortality. Washington, D.C: Academy for Educational Development; 1996.

[15] UNICEF State of the World's Population 1994. New York: UNFPA1998.

[16] Horton S, Ross J. The economics of iron deficiency. Food Policy. 2003;28:51-75.

[17] Karine Tolentino, Jennifer F. Friedman. An Update on Anemia in Less Developed Countries. Am J Trop Med Hyg. 2007;77(1):44-51.

[18] Yip R, Ramakrishnan U. Supplement: Forging Effective Strategies to Combat Iron Deficiency Experiences and Challenges in Developing Countries. The American Society for Nutritional Sciences J Nutr. 2002 132:827S-30S.

[19] Stoltzfus, Mullany, Black. Iron Deficiency Anemia, "Comparative quantification of health risks: Global and regional burden of disease attributable to selected major risk factors: WHO2004.

[20] World Health Organization. World Health Report. Reducing Risk, Promoting Healthy Life. Geneva: WHO2002.

[21] Stoltzfus R. Update on Issues Related to Iron Deficiency and Anemia Control. Report of the 2003 International Nutritional Anemia Consultive Group: Integrating Programs to Move Iron Deficiency Anaemia Control Forward Symposium. . Marrakech, Morocco: International Life Sciences Institute2003.

[22] Gillespie SR. Major Issues in the Control of Iron Deficiency. Ottawa: The Micronutrient Initiative/UNICEF.1998.

[23] Allen LH, Ahluwalia N. Improving Iron Status through Diet. The Application of Knowledge Concerning Dietary Iron Bioavailability in Human Populations. In: Arlington VA, editor. Management of Social Transformation Programme1997.

[24] Iron Disorders Institute. Iron Disorders. Taylor: Iron Deficiency Anemia; 2009 [cited 2011 24-07].

[25] Sommer A, West KP. Vitamin A Deficiency: Health, Survival and Vision. New York: Oxford University Press.; 1996.

[26] Fishman SM, Christian P, West KP. The role of vitamins in the prevention and control of anaemia. Public Health Nutr. 2000;3:125-50.

[27] Tolentino K, Friedman JF. An Update on Anemia in Less Developed Countries. The American Society of Tropical Medicine. 2007.

[28] Lopez AD, Mathers CD, Ezzati M, Jamison DT, Murray CJ. Global and regional burden of disease and risk factors, 2001: systematic analysis of population health data. Lancet. 2006;367:1747-57.

[29] United Nations Development Programme, World Bank, World health Organisation. The prevention and management of severe anaemia in children in malaria-endemic regions of Africa: A review of research2001.

[30] Steketee RW, Nahlen BL, Parise ME, Menendez C. The burden of malaria in pregnancy in malaria endemic areas. Am J Trop Med Hyg. 2001;64:28-35.

[31] Onyemaobi GA, Onimawo IA. Risk Factors for Iron Deficiency Anaemia in Under-five Children in Imo State, Nigeria. Journal of Applied Sciences Research. 2011;7(1):63-7.

[32] Menendez C, Fleming AF, Alonso PL. Malaria-related Anaemia. Parasitol Today. 2000;16(11):469-76.

[33] Phillips RE, Pasvol G. Anaemia of Plasmodium falciparum malaria. Epidemiology of Haematological Disease: Part II. 1992;5(2):315-30.

[34] Latham MC. Human Nutrition in the Developing World. Rome: FAO1997.

[35] Chitsulo L, Engels D, Montresor A, Savioli L. The global status of schistosomiasis and its control. Acta Trop. 2000;77:41-51.

[36] Hoque M, Hoque E, Kader SB. Risk factors for anaemia in pregnancy in rural KwaZulu-Natal, South Africa: Implication for health education and health promotion. SA Fam Pract. 2009;51(1):68-72.

[37] Hotez PJ, Brooker S, Bethony JM, Bottazzi ME, Loukas A, Xiao S. Hookworm infection. New England Journal of Medicine. 2004;351(8):799-841.

[38] Stoltzfus RJ, Albonico M, Chwaya HM, Tielsch JM, Schulze KJ, Savioli L. Effects of the Zanzibar school-based deworming program on iron status of children. American Journal of Clinical Nutrition 1998;68(1):179-86.

[39] Stephenson LS, Holland CV, Cooper ES. The public health significance of Trichuris trichiura. Parasitology. 2000;121(Suppl):S73-S95.

[40] Duff EM, Anderson NM, Cooper ES. Plasma insulin-like growth factor-1, type 1 procollagen, and serum tumor necrosis factor alpha in children recovering from Trichuris dysentery syndrome. Pediatrics 1999;103:e69.

[41] WHO. Global Health Observatory (GHO)/HIV2011.

[42] Joint United Nations Programme on HIV/AIDS. Overview of the global AIDS epidemic". UN report on the global AIDS epidemic 20102010.

[43] Johannessen A, Naman E, Ngowi BJ, Sandvik L, Matee MI, Aglen HE, et al. Predictors of mortality in HIV-infected patients starting antiretroviral therapy in a rural hospital in Tanzania. BMC Infectious Diseases. 2008;8:52.

[44] Areechokchai D, Bowonwatanuwong C, Phonrat B, Pitisuttithum P, Maek-a-Nantawat W. Pregnancy outcomes among HIV-infected women undergoing antiretroviral therapy. The Open AIDS Journal. 2009;3:8-13.

[45] Moyle G. Anaemia in persons with HIV infection: prognostic marker and contributor to morbidity. AIDS Reviews. 2002;4:13-8.

[46] Omoregie R, Egbeobauwaye A, Ogefere H, Omokaro EU, Ehen CC. Prevalence of antibodies to HAART agents among HIV patient in Benin City, Nigeria. African Journal Biomedical Research. 2008;11:33-7.

[47] Odunukwe N, Idigbe O, Kanki P, Adewale T, Onwujekwe D, Audu R, et al. Haematological and biochemical response to treatment of HIV-1 infection with a combination of nevirapine stavudine + lamivudine in Lagos Nigeria. Turkish Journal of Haematology. 2005;22:125-31.

[48] World Health Organisation. Sickle Cell anaemia. Geneva: Fifty Ninth World Health Assembly, WHO2006.

[49] Mentzer WC, Kan YW. Prospects for research in hematologic disorders: sickle cell disease and thalassemia. JAMA. 2001;285:640-2.

[50] Olivieri NF. The beta-thalassemias. N Engl J Med. 1999;341:99-109.

[51] Greenberg PL, Gordeuk V, Issaragrisil S, Siritanaratkul N, Fucharoen S, Ribeiro RC. Major hematologic diseases in the developing world- new aspects of diagnosis and management of thalassemia, malarial anemia, and acute leukemia. Hematology (Am Soc Hematol Educ Program). 2001:479-98.

[52] Hamedani P, Raza R, Bachand R, Manji M, Hashml K. Laboratory diagnosis of iron deficiency in a developing country, Pakistan. J Int Med Res. 1991;19(1):19-23.

[53] Trost LB, Bergfeld WF, Calogeras E. The diagnosis and treatment of iron deficiency and its potential relationship to hair loss. J Am Acad Dermatol. 2006;54(5):824-44.

[54] Punnonen K, Irjala K, Rajamaki A. Serum transferrin receptor and its ratio to serum ferritin in the diagnosis of iron deficiency. Blood. 1997;89:1052-7.

[55] WHO. Home management of malaria. 2011 [cited 2011 24-07].

[56] Moerman F, Lengeler C, Chimumbwa J, Talisuna A, Erhart A, Coosemans MT. The contribution of the health-care service to a sound and sustainable malaria-control policy. Lancet Infect Dis. 2003;3:99-102.

[57] Bloland P, Kachur S, Williams H. Trends in antimalarial drug deployment in sub-Saharan Africa. J Rxp Biol. 2003;206(3761-3769).

[58] Wongsrichanalai C, Barcus M, Muth S, Sutamihardja A, Wernsdorfer W. A review of malaria diagnostic tools: microscopy and rapid diagnostic test (RDT). Am J Trop Med Hyg. 2007;77:119-27.

[59] Shillcutt S, Morel C, Goodman C, Coleman P, Bell D, Whitty CJ. Bulletin of the World Health OrganizationFeb 2008.

[60] Gray DJ, Ross AG, Li Y-S. Clinical Review: Diagnosis and management of schistosomiasis. British Medical Journal. 2011;342:d2651.

[61] Paul JF, Verma S, Berry K. Urinary schistosomiasis. Emerg Med J. 2002;19:483-4.

[62] Birx D, de Souza M, Nkengasong J. Laboratory challenges in the scaling up of HIV, TB, and malaria programs: The interaction of health and laboratory systems, clinical research, and service delivery. Am J Clin Pathol. 2009;131(6):849-51.

[63] The United States President's emergency plan for AIDS relief. The challenges of HIV/AIDS and children. PEPFAR; 2004 [cited 2011 02-08].

[64] Frenette PS, Atweh GF. Sickle cell disease: old discoveries, new concepts, and future promise. Journal of Clinical Investigation. 2007;117(4):850-8.

[65] WHO. Sickle Cell anaemia 2006.

[66] Draper A. Child Development and Iron Deficiency: the Oxford Brief. Opportunities for Micronutrient Interventions, and Partnership for Child Development. Washington DC: USAID; 1997

[67] WHO. WHO Vitamin A supplementation. 2011 [cited 2011 23-07];
     http://www.who.int/vaccines/en/vitamina].
[68] Stoltzfus RJ, Hakimi M, Miller KW. High dose vitamin A supplementation of breast-feeding Indonesian mothers: effects on the vitamin A status of mother and infant. J Nutr. 1993;123(4):666-75.
[69] Robert C, Brown DL. Vitamin B12 Deficiency. Am Fam Physician. 2003 Mar1;67(5):979-86.
[70] WHO expert committee on the control of Schistosomiasis. Prevention and control of schistosomiasis and soil transmitted helminthiasis: report of a WHO expert committee. Geneva: World health Organisation2001.
[71] Wake DJ, Cutting WA. Blood transfusion in developing countries: problems, priorities and practicalities. Tropical Doctor. 1998 Jan;28(1):4-8.
[72] WHO. Blood safety and availability. November 2009 [cited 2011 24-07].
[73] Hurrell RF, Furniss DE, Burri J, Whittaker P, Lynch SR, Cook JD. Iron fortification of infant cereals: a proposal for the use of ferrous fumarate or ferrous succinate. American Journal of Clinical Nutrition. 1989;49:1274-82.
[74] Rush D, Leighton J, Sloan NL, Alvir JM, Garbowski GC. The National WIC Evaluation: Evaluation of the Special Supplemental Food Program for Women, Infants, and Children. II. Review of past studies of WIC. American Journal of Clinical Nutrition. 1988;48:394- 411.
[75] Branca F, Lopriore C, Briesid A, Golden MH. Multi-micronutrient fortified food reverses growth failure and anaemia in 2 - 5 year-old stunted refugee children. Scandinavian Journal of Nutrition. 1999;43(25):51S.
[76] WHO. Safe Vitamin A Dosage During Pregnancy and Lactation. Recommendations and a Report of a Consultation. Geneva: WHO1998.
[77] WHO. Vector control of malaria. 2011 [cited 2011 24-07]; Available from:
     www.who.int/malaria/vector_control/en.
[78] WHO. Regional Framework for an Integrated Vector Management Strategy for the South-East Asia Region. New Delhi: World Health Organization Regional Office for South-East AsiaJune 2005.
[79] Stoltzfus RJ, Dreyfuss ML. Guidelines for the Use of Iron Supplements to Prevent and Treat Iron Deficiency Anemia. Geneva: International Nutritional Anemia Consultative Group/ UNICEF/WHO1998.
[80] WHO. Report of the WHO informal consultation on hookworm infection and anaemia in girls and women. Geneva: WHO1996 Contract No.: document WHO/CTD/SIP/96.1.
[81] WHO. Initiative for Vaccine Research: Parasitic disease. 2011 [cited 2011 24-07]; Available from: www.who.int/vaccine_research/disease/soa_parasitic/en.
[82] WHO. HIV/AIDS: Prevention in the health sector. 2011 [cited 2011 24-07]; Available from: www.who.int/hiv/topics/prevention/en.
[83] Okwu GN, Ukoha AI. Studies on the Predisposing Factors of Iron Deficiency Anaemia among Pregnant Women in a Nigeria Community. Pakistan Journal of Nutrition. 2008;7(1):151-6.
[84] Joint World Health Organization/Centers for Disease Control and Prevention. Assessing the iron status of populations : including literature reviews : report of a Joint World Health Organization/Centers for Disease Control and Prevention Technical Consultation on the Assessment of Iron Status at the Population Level. Geneva, Switzerland2004 6-8 April 2004.

8

How Can Cancer-Associated Anemia Be Moderated with Nutritional Factors and How Do *Beta Vulgaris* L. Ssp. *Esculenta Var. Rubra* Modify the Transmethylation Reaction in Erythrocytes in Cancerous Patients?

Anna Blázovics[1] et al.[*]
[1]Department of Pharmacognosy, and II. Department of Medicine, Semmelweis University, Budapest Hungary

1. Introduction

Genetic predisposition, unhealthy dietary or life habits and heavy social circumstances could result in the changes of redox homeostasis, which is very important for the equilibrium between tissue regeneration and apoptosis. When the balance is disturbed, cancer and/or necrosis may develop (Powis et al., 1997). Moderate dietary habits with natural bioactive agents, antioxidants, methyl donor molecules and metal elements can help restore the normal function of the organism, although the immoderate consumption of nutritive components is contraindicated. Long term antioxidant and/or antioxidant-related treatments as well as metal element owerflow can modify redox-homeostasis because these alimentary components effect signal transduction routes and compensatory effects of altered tissues can be observed (Vanherweghem et al., 1993, Blázovics et al., 2007a,b, Blázovics et al., 2008).

Epidemiological, experimental and clinical investigations have shown that food supplements are not effective in cancer therapy because of inappropriate usage in cases of people suffering from cancers with low vitamin and trace element levels. Significant changes of total scavenger capacity, metal element concentrations, bounded HCHO and

*Péter Nyirády[2], Imre Romics[2], Miklós Szűcs[2], András Horváth[2], Ágnes Szilvás[3], Edit Székely[1], Klára Szentmihályi[4], Gabriella Bekő[5] and Éva Sárdi[6]
[1]Department of Pharmacognosy, and II. Department of Medicine, Semmelweis University, Budapest,
[2]Department of Urology, Semmelweis University,
[3]Saint John Hospital, Budapest,
[4]Institute of Materials and Environmental Chemistry, CRC, Hungarian Academy of Sciences, Budapest,
[5]Central Laboratory Pest, Semmelweis University,
[6]Corvinus University, Budapest

protoporphyrin as well as Zn-protoporphyrin concentrations in erythrocytes can be observed in cancerous processes, which are very important in cancer-associated anemia (Blázovics et al., 2008).

Red blood cells do not get enough oxygen to all parts of the body especially in cancer-related anemia, such as cancer in bone marrow directly or in metastasis, as well as in cisplatin or carboplatin chemotherapy, which lower the erythropoietin production in the kidneys and in radiation therapy caused anemia. It is especially significant if the level of the transmethylation ability is too low in the organism. Alterations in DNA methylation play an important role in neoplasia (Baylin, et al. 1997, Calvisi et al., 2007). DNA hypomethylation leads to elevated mutation rates. (Chen et al. 1998). The most studied mechanisms by epigenetics are DNA and histone methylation and the stable and reversible alterations in the genome that affect gene expression and genome function. The nature and role of the mechanisms of promoter hypermethylation during carcinogenesis were studied worldwide, however the mechanism behind one of the earliest epigenetic observations in cancer nowadays, genome-wide hypomethylation, still remains unclear (Wild, and Flanagan 2010)

Tumor hypermethylation predicts a poor prognosis in patients with earlier stages of prostate cancer, and is commonly found in the plasma DNA of patients with castration-resistant prostate cancer (Rosenbaum et al., 2005, Bastian et al. 2009). Low transmethylation ability can be observed in the erythrocyte in different tumors and in different stages (Blázovics et al., 2008, Nyirády et al., 2010). Hypomethylation seems to be a condition of the system, which can be improved with methyl donating molecules from food ingredients, such as different N-, S- and O- methylated compounds.

2. Natural therapy and cancer-related anemia

In spite of an enormous effort and many new excellent experimental data, which come to light in cancer research, cancer therapy is not solved satisfactorily. Several target points are for inhibiting cancerous processes and molecules are developed to modify signal transduction pathways aimed for a better way of using tailored cancer treatment, although the chance of definitive recovery is very different in the various tumors and only half of circa 200 tumor types can be cured nowadays (Blázovics 2011). Therefore new therapeutic solutions are necessary as well as looking for new food ingredients to moderate several problems, such as cancer-related anemia, which improves the erythrocyte function of bone metastatic prostate cancer cases.

It is an endeavor to show attempts of natural therapy with small molecules for inhibiting cancer growth and spreading on the basis of researches. The effectiveness of medicinal therapy can be increased if the therapy is planned for each patient therefore this chapter wants to deal with the importance of the role of transmethylation ability and the question of modification of redox-homeostasis by alimentary supporting therapy.

2.1 Transmethylation processes
Bioactive molecule, the small genotoxic and carcinogen formaldehyde is in connection with the redox homeostasis. This molecule plays an important role with free radicals in the biological system (Lichszteld and Kruk 1977, Nieva and Wentworth 2004). Since

endogenous transmethylation processes occur via HCHO, this molecule can be considered as an ancient and basic compound of life systems. HCHO can be found in animal tissues in specially-bounded, mainly hydroxymethyl forms. Endogenous HCHO is produced partly by the enzymatic demethylation of different N-, S-, and O- methylated compounds (Huszti et al., 1986, Sárdi et al., 2005, Kovács-Nagy et al., 2009). S-adenosylmethionine is an important methyl donor in several biological transmethylation reactions such as in the duplication of virus. The product S-adenosylhomocysteine inhibits the transmethylation process because this molecule is hydrolysed to adenosine and L-homocysteine by the action of S-adenosylhomocysteine hydrolase. The accumulation of homocysteine leads to increased cellular oxidative stress (Gersbeck et al., 1989, Stead et al., 2006).

DNA methylation typically occurs at cytosine–phosphate–guanine site. In this process, methylation results in the conversion of the cytosine to 5-methylcytosine. This reaction is catalysed by DNA methyltransferase. The methylation stage of this region can have a major impact on gene (Watson et al., 2003).

Some quaternary ammonium compounds, such as N^ε–trimethyl-L-lysine, choline and betaine, are potential HCHO generators as well. Data show the important role of HCHO in proliferative as well as in apoptotic processes. Transmethylation ability is lowered in tumorous processes (Blázovics et al., 2008, Nyirády et al., 2010).

It is also verified, that the arginine (38), methionine (65) and the lysine (72) near the methionine (80) are methylated and coordinated towards the central iron of heme (Stryeer 1988). During moderate transmethylation ability, free protoporphyrin can be found near the Zn-protoporphyrin in the erythrocyte in different cancers and it has pro- and antioxidant forms depending on concentrations. Protoporphyrin concentration is low in cancerous patients, but in metastasis its concentration is significantly high. Oxidized hemoglobin, HbA1c correlates significantly with free radical reactions and with decreased antioxidant status of erythrocytes (Blázovics et al., 2008).

In earlier study, significant changes could be observed in erythrocyte function in patients suffering from colon cancer as well as in metastatic prostate cancer. The erythrocyte mobilized formaldehyde was significantly lower in adult colectomysed patients with no metastasis than in controls. Simultaneously protoporphyrin concentration was low in patients without metastasis, when the diagnosis was Dukes C before operation. HbA1c level correlated significantly with the induced free radical level and decreased antioxidant status of erythrocytes (Blázovics et al., 2008, 2011).

2.2 Redox homeostasis

Redox homeostasis can be considered as the cumulative action of free radicals and antioxidant defenses, providing a suitable condition for life. Oxidative stress is a key modulator, which modifies the ligand-receptor interactions extracellularly and intracellularly, and influences gene expression. Free radicals can act as secondary messengers in several transduction pathways, and take part in the activation of chemotactic cytokines and surface adhesion molecules etc. (Abate et al., 1990, Meyer et al., 1993, Polya et al., 2002).

Oxidative stress can induce stress response genes, and moderate oxidative stress by down regulating the gene expression of several genes. DNA synthesis, selective gene expression, enzyme activation and modification of cell proliferation are involved in redoxy signal mechanisms. Moderate free radical production can modify the function of kinases or directly activate the transcription factors, thereby also influencing the gene regulation in the nucleus (Delerive et al., 2000, Kong et al., 2000).

The "antioxidant" concept has meaning only in defense against free radicals for a long period. Its importance is not doubtful in the therapy of diseases in which free radicals are also involved.

Antioxidant consumption is sine qua non for a healthy way of life, but the concentration range is large and dependent on an individual genetic background. Moderate nutritional customs with natural scavengers or antioxidants can help to restore the normal function of tissues and organs, but the immoderate consumption of vitamins and other bioactive agents is contraindicated. The balance between oxidative stress and antioxidant defense is overturned in diseases (Blázovics et al., 1999, Szilvási et al., 1999, Hagymási et al., 2001). Moderate oxidative stress is important in signal transduction pathways and essential for proliferation and apoptosis. The antioxidant overflow as well as oxidative stress mean serious problems. "Janus face" antioxidants can stop protein phosphorylation and the inhibition of activation of transcription factors. They can also therefore stop cell proliferation and injure the adaptation mechanisms against oxidative stress. The direct roles of these antioxidants in original forms are doubtful in transduction therapy (Azzi et al., 2004, Griffiths and Lunec 2001).

Several food-related bioactive agents are important in cancer prevention as well. Metals are also important both in free radical formation and in antioxidant defense in signal transduction.

Four simple redox measurements, H-donating ability, reducing-power property, free SH-group and stimulated chemiluminescent intensity of plasma and erythrocytes can be applied to evaluate the redox homeostasis in several diseases and different treatments compared to the control values. The calculation of total scavenger capacity can be necessary to measure the tissue relative chemiluminescent light. Normal range of healthy peoples is no more 70 RLU%, 80±10% RLU% is the chemiluminescent intensity of erythrocytes in different diseases, e.g. in the severe IBD, where the range is 100±10%, and the range between 100 and 150 RLU% means increased risk for tumors (precancerous stadium and after tumor resection) and >150 RLU% marks the non treated tumors. Very low chemiluminescent intensity - significantly lower than that of healthy control patients - could be observed in metastatic cancerous patients, some weeks before death because of extra high protoporphyrin concentration in the erythrocyte.

Chemiluminescence methods are suitable to differentiate the grade of diseases (Blázovics et al., 1999.) and difference between genders e.g in alcoholic liver diseases (Hagymási et al., 2001), but in both type of IBD and colon cancer gender difference was not observed (Szilvás et al., 1999).

The measured data are in significant correlation with each other and the changes of activity of erythrocyte superoxide dismutase and glutathione peroxidase as well as concentrations of plasma reducing power and H-donating ability. Consequently, erythrocyte total scavenger capacity (inverse of chemiluminescent intensity) is a good predictive factor for neoplasia in early stage (Blázovics et al., 2008). (Figure 1.)

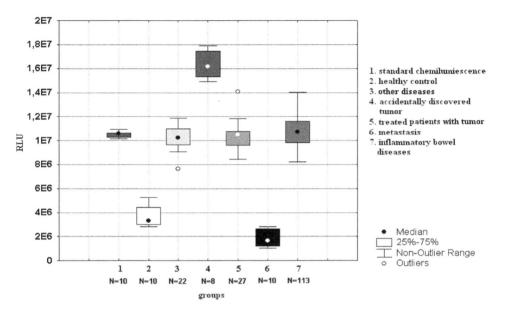

Fig. 1. Chemiluminescent intensity in early state of tumor and metastasis

A significantly higher chemiluminescent intensity of erythrocytes was detected in newly observed tumors. When the patients were operated and treated with chemotherapy and/or irradiation therapy, the erythrocyte chemiluminescence was not altered from that of IBD patients. In severe metastatic stages, before death, the chemiluminescence of erythrocytes was very low, significantly lower than in healthy controls. Plasma chemiluminescence studies rather show only momentary improvement in the course of the therapy of IBD or tumors (Blázovics 2006).

2.3 Nutritional factors in tumor

Besides, genetical disposition it was above mentioned, that lifestyle and nutrition with vitamins, polyphenols, flavonoids and quaterner ammonium derivatives play a decisive role in human health care and inhibit the occurrence of many diseases. It is a proven fact that antioxidants have an important role in preventing cancer and improve redox homeostasis (Lugasi and Hóvári 2002, Polya et al., 2002).

Lack of alimentary factors such as iron, vitamin B12, and folic acid, the formation and function of red blood cells is inhibited. These components are available naturally in several vegetables and food items, therefore eating foods with high iron content, such as red meats, dried beans or fruits, almonds, broccoli, and enriched breads and cereals or high folic acid, such as cereals, green leafy vegetables, asparagus, broccoli, spinach, and lima beans can help (Kuramoto et al., 1996).

Bioactive agent as well as metal element-rich vegetables are important in the food chain and play a decisive role in human health care. Table beet is a particularly important vegetable from this supporting alimentary point of view. Table beet is a vegetable that is rich in content of folic acid, iron, betaine, natural coloring agents, polyphenols, metal elements, etc. (Takács-Hájos 1999, Blázovics et al ., 2007, Sárdi et al., 2009).

A healthy system needs antioxidant and metal element supplementation and can tolerate occasional overflow between wide boundaries. Besides this, redox homeostasis and element homeostasis do not change. However, the reactions of sick organisms - e.g. the Fe accumulating porphyria cutanea tarda and haemochromatosis or Cu accumulating Wilson disease as well as the iron-deficiency anemia and the malnutrition of inflammatory bowel diseases - can be different and that is why everybody must be cautious when recommending table beet root supplements. It can be supposed, that the extreme consumption of table beet root can cause several disturbances among others not only in healthy people but in patients suffering from metal accumulating diseases, although moderate consumption may be beneficial in metal-deficiency diseases (Blázovics et al., 2007b).

2.4 Table beet

Beta vulgaris L. ssp. *esculenta* Gurke var. *rubra* belongs to the *Chenopodiaceae* family and it is in relationship with *Beta vulgaris* L. provar. *altissima*, *Beta vulgaris* L. convar. *crassa* provar. *crassa* and *Beta vulgaris* L. convar. *cicla*. An ancient form of these species is the wild form of *Beta vulgaris* L. var. *maritime* (Takács-Hájos 1999).

The root of the plant *Beta vulgaris* L. ssp. *esculenta* var. *rubra* is commonly called table beet and has been used for centuries as a traditional and popular food in many national cuisines. The Greek Hypocrates, the Roman, but Greek-born Galenus, the Arabian Avicenna, and the Swiss Paracelsus applied table beet in several gastrointestinal diseases, fevers, anemia, wound-healing etc. Nowadays table beet is also an important component of popular medicine (Frank et al., 2005, Pedreno and Escribano 2000).

The applying of table beet in several diseases can be bordered because the natural colored pigment contents of this vegetable are important food coloring matters, which substitute E123 coloring matter in different creams, substituting soya foods, sweets, gelatin deserts, yogurts, ice- creams, dressings and meats etc. (Takács-Hájos 1999).

Beneficial medical effects are due to bioactive components, such as betaine, betanins, betaxanthins, vulgaxanthine, flavonoids, polyphenols, vitamins (thiamine, riboflavine, piridoxine, ascorbic acid, biotin and folic acid) as well as soluble fibre, pectin and different metal elements (e.g. Al, B, Ba, Ca, Cu, Fe, K, Mg, Mn, Na, Zn), which act on various physiological routes (Wang and Goldman 1996, Rice-Evans et al., 1997, Bobek et al., 2000, Kanner et al., 2001).

The coloring matters in table beet are betalains, as red betacyanins and yellow betaxanthins, and they can be used for human nutrition and prevention of numerous diseases, for example skin and lung cancers (Stintzing and Carle 2004, Schwartz et al., 1983, Frank et al., 2005, Boyd et al., 1982, Kapadia et al., 1996, Kapadia et al. 2003).

According to newer researches, these colored pigments have antioxidant activity and play an important role in the development of antioxidant status in the human organism (Cai et al., 2001, Kanner et al., 2001, Pedreno and Escribano 2000., Wettasinghe et al., 2002, Zakharova and Petrova 1998).

Table beets are mainly characterized by the non high-concentration of sucrose. Glucose and fructose can also be found in the samples but their concentrations are significantly low. With regard to glucose quantity, 51% of the varieties were below 0.2 mg/g, 30% of them belong to the 0.2-0.4 mg/g domain and 19% were characterized by a glucose content above 0.4 mg/g. 52.7% of the varieties were in the 10-15 mg/g domain, 33% were between 15-20 mg/g, while 14.3% contained more that 21 mg/g sucrose.

Among the quarternary ammonium compounds, which have human health significance due to their biological activity, a high concentration of betaine can be found.

In earlier examinations, among the quaternary ammonium compounds, in the table beet samples betaine was found in the highest concentration, carnitine was also detectable but in low concentration (the value was not measurable) and other quaternary ammonium compounds were not detectable. 28.5% of the varieties fall under the 0.6 mg/g level, another 28.5% are above the 0.8 mg/g level and 43% can be characterized by a betaine concentration of 0.6-0.8 mg/g per fresh mass. Betaine was found in significantly higher concentration in the lyophilized samples. Fresh samples contained betaine in a concentration of 0.35-1.3 mg/g, while the concentration of lyophilized ones was between 10.3-18.0 mg/g of dry mass. On the basis of the total phenol concentration of table beet squeezed juice, 23.8% of the compared varieties are under the level of 0.6-0.8 mg/ml in the fresh samples, one-third are 0.80-1.0 mg/ml, another one-third are 1.0-1.20 mg/ml and the phenol concentration of 9.5% of the varieties is between 1.20-2.0 mg/ml (Sárdi et al., 2009). On the basis of the comparison of studied variants, those with a higher concentration of betanine contained a higher amount of phenol as well. The value of betanine is 0.40-1.1 mg/g, total phenol shows significant differences between 0.60-1.90 mg/ml, correlation. Betaine concentrations were different in varieties. Where betaine was higher, betanine and polyphenol were also higher along with antioxidant capacity (Hájos et al., 2004). Between red coloring matter and total polyphenol concentration, significant correlation was calculated (r=0,7577) (Sárdi et al., 2009).

Schiebler already discovered betaine in *Beta vulgaris* in 1869 and since then betaine was observed in several living organisms (Blunden and Gordon 1986, Hougaard et al., 1994) and human cells as well (Lever et al., 1994).

In modern medicine, betaine is an important natural molecule for treating homocysteinuria, alcoholic steatosis, chemically induced liver, lung and skin cancers (Wilcken et al., 1983, Barak et al., 1996, Eikelboom et al., Murakami et al., 1998). This molecule helps to create choline, can help synthesize of carnitine and helps to convert homocysteine into methionine and it takes part in biologic methylation (Finkenstein and Martin 1984, Slow et al., 2004, Awad et al., 1983, Skiba et al., 1982, Evans et al., 2002, Millan and Garrow 1998).

2.5 Metal elements in tumor

Metal elements are important in nutrition and prevention of diseases, as anemia could be treated with supplementation of Fe. Concentration of essential metal elements is rigorously regulated in the metabolic pathways in contrary to toxic elements in healthy organisms. Concentration changes of some transition metal elements Cu, Fe, Mn, Zn and non-metal elements S, Se, P can significantly modify the signal transduction. Therefore, their optimal tissue concentrations are not doubtful and daily intake of these elements from natural sources is very important (Szentmihályi et al., 2000a,b, Máday et al., 2000). These elements are ubiquitous in biological systems and play a key role in the catalysis of redox processes. Heavy metals in higher concentrations may inhibit enzyme activities and influence the acute phase protein synthesis and gene expression, as well as the pro-oxidant and antioxidant forms of scavenger molecules. Mainly the free Fe(II) and Cu(I) and Cu(II) redox active metal ions catalyze the formation of reactive oxygen radicals, but they occur in the body in a small amount (Kasprzak et al., 1987). CuZnSOD in the cytoplasm and the nucleus, MnSOD in the mitochondrial matrix, catalase in peroxisomes or in the cytoplasm and glutathione peroxidase in the cytoplasm are known metalloproteins, which take part in the defense mechanism against toxic concentration of free radicals (Yuregir et al., 1994, Schroeder and Cousins 1990, Dinkova-Kostova et al., 2005). Cu occurs in the ceruloplasmin, and it has an oxidase function. It is able to oxidize biogen amines and its phenoxidase activity is also proved (Floris et. al., 2000, Pena, et al., 1999). Zn is a key element in antioxidant superoxide dismutase enzyme as well as Zn-metallothionein, which has hydroxyl scavenging ability (Brando-Neto et al., 1994). Mn also takes part in the enzymatic antioxidant defense system, since the superoxide dismutase enzyme scavenges superoxide anions. In blood, Mn(II) ions take on the forms of free aqua-complexes or are bounded to albumin, α macroglobulin and other glycoproteins (Critchfield and Keen 1992). Mn(II) is an antioxidant, since in fast reaction it exterminates the alkyl peroxyl radicals formed by the peroxidation of fatty acids, while Fe(II) ions generate alkoxy and hydroxyl radicals by splitting the ROOH bond and continue the chain reaction (Siegel and Sigel 1999). Mn(II) ions, similarly to Zn ions, are able to decrease the formation of superoxide radicals by forming Mn_2(NADPH) complexes (Schramm 1986). Metal ions are important for the activation of NF-kappaB, AP-1 and in the cases of NF-kappaB proteasome degradation as well as the regulation of IkappaB kinases and other redoxy sytems. The joining of the NF-kappa B to the DNA is the function of the redoxi state of apo 62 cystein in p50 subunit in the DNA bond domain. This connection is injured by the effect of heavy metals such as As, Cd, Co, Cr, Ni and Pb (Kudrin 2000). The risk of tumor formation is increased in the presence of Ni, Cr and As ions, because DNA repair systems are very sensitive targets of these elements (Hartwig 1998). Divalent cations, such as Zn, Cu, Cd, Mn and Ni can modulate the function of tumor suppressor protein p53 in vitro (Maehle et al., 1992). The excess of Zn and Cd cause inhibition of the apoptosis (Chukhlovin et al., 2001).

In several biochemical pathways Ni, Cr and As toxic metal elements compete with Mg ions. Competition between Ni(II) and Mg(II) may provide an important mechanism for interfering with DNA-protein interactions involved in the repair process, because the inhibition of DNA repair is partly reversible by the addition of Mg(II) (Kasprzak et al., 1987, Hartwig et al., 1994). Presumable Ni(II), Co(II) and As(II) ions displace Zn ion in the zinc-finger structure of DNA repair enzymes (Hartwig 1998). Ni, Cr and As elements are established carcinogens in humans. These heavy metals can induce adhesion molecules and cytokines (Hayat 1996).

Magnesium deficiency alters calcium homeostasis via Ca^{2+}/Mg^{2+} antagonism, leading to transient increase in the concentration of intracellular calcium. Magnesium may act as a physiological „antioxidant", e.g. against lipoprotein oxidation. The transient increase in the intracellular calcium level induced by magnesium deficiency, enhances the production of pro-oxidant cytokines (IL-1, IL-6, IL-8, TNF-α, -β), different growth factors (EGF-α, TGF-β, NFGF, FGF, PDGF), and interferons (IFN-α, -γ) by activation of phosphoinositol diphosphate (PIP_2) and MAP kinases (Dolmetsch et al. 1997, Caddell 2000).

The enhanced synthesis of cytokines induces gene expressions of enzymes of reactive oxygen species including NADPH oxidase, xanthine-oxidase/dehydrogenase, cyclooxygenase, lipoxygenase, cytochrome P450, NO synthase, proteins containing iron, and superoxide dismutase, copper zinc and manganase enzymes that are regulated at transcripitional level by phosphorylation of transcription factors. On the contrary, the increase in the intracellular magnesium level inhibits the production of pro-oxidant cytokines via the activation of corresponding protein phosphatases, therefore the generation of reactive oxygen species can be attenuated. Therefore the intake of the right amount of magnesium and magnesium-calcium rations is essential.

2.6 Clinical investigation of table beet supplementation
Adenocarcinoma of the prostate is still one of the major reasons of cancer-related mortality in populations of Western countries, but the current understanding of its etiology and pathogenesis is still lacking (Jemal et al., 2008).

Although, prostate cancer is silent and creates no early warning symptoms, after the extensive use of serum prostate specific antigen (PSA) testing, it has increasingly been reported at earlier stages. In case of localized prostate cancer, for a man in good condition, radical prostatectomy is the preferred treatment with more than 10 years life expectancy. Furthermore, radical surgery might provide a therapy for well-selected locally advanced prostate cancer. However, it is still not possible to distinguish who is at a high risk of tumor recurrence after primary local therapy, so will not benefit from surgery. In addition it can not be predicted who will benefit from hormonal therapy and who will become soon hormone resistant in cases of advanced prostate cancer. Nowadays, although using more promising indicators to distinguish between surgically curable and oncologically treatable prostate cancer, there has not still been an optimal factor found which would tell us the prognosis (Barqawi et al., 2004, Nyirády and Romics 2009a,b).

Several papers report effect of table beet supplements in the improvement of quality of life of different diseases, although their physiological investigation is poor. Table beet affects numerous biochemical reaction ways, enzymes and metabolic-synthesis occurring in vivo (Kuramoto et al., 1996, Váli et al., 2007, Blázovics et al., 2007b). In this clinical study 10g natural table beet lyophilized product was given twice daily for 1 month for 24 patients (mean age 68±8 years) with hormone-resistant and metastatic prostate cancer treated with taxan chemotherapy, who reported their complaints themselves first, mean 3.6±2.8 years before. 18 men's data were amenable after treatment for evaluation. (Permission number of clinical study: Semmelweis University 127/2006.) The lyophilized product was purchased from commercial service (Permission number: 1361/004/2003 BFAEE) GPS Powder Kft. Budapest, Hungary) (Nyirády et al., 2010).

In addition to routine laboratory examination values of HbA1c, 9 cytokines and levels of 3 growth factors, the global parameters of redox-homeostasis, few elements, Zn- and level of free protoporphyrin, trans-methylation processes were determined before and one month after treatment.

Results showed that in most of the patients the favorable impact of beet was enforced and significantly high levels of Zn- and free protoporphyrin decreased; furthermore trans-methylation processes fastened which all characterize patients with tumor (Nyirády et al., 2010). Table1. shows the element concentrations of lyophilized table beet powder applied in human study.

The calculated metal element intake concentration, on the basis of daily dose of lyophilized table beet powder, is very low. The essential element concentrations compared to the

elements	lyophilized table beet powder (µg/g)	daily intake (µg)	percentage of daily needs *, and percentage of average daily intake **
Al	21.62 ± 4.60	432.4	13.1**
B	8.56 ± 4.91	171.2	7.4*
Ba	3.79 ± 0.16	75.8	5.1**
Ca	701.0 ± 15.6	14020	1.4*
Co	0.146 ± 0.003	2.92	0.5**
Cr	0.311 ± 0.037	6.22	17.8*
Cu	3.13 ± 0.59	62.6	6.9*
Fe	17.68 ± 0.03	353.6	4.4*
K	8057 ± 512	161140	3.4*
Li	< 0.1		
Mg	829.9 ± 9.7	16598	4.0*
Mn	9.99 ± 0.11	199.8	9.1*
Mo	0.205 ± 0.059	4.1	9.1*
Na	661.4± 30.9	13228	0.9*
Ni	0.469 ± 0.125	9.38	9.4**
P	1545 ±83	30900	4.4*
Se	0.142 ± 0.011	2.84	5.2*
Si	53.96 ± 1.48	1079.2	5.4**
Sr	3.89 ± 0.05	77.8	1.7**
Zn	6.09 ± 0.21	121.8	1.1*

Table 1. Element concentration of lyophilized table beet powder (dose 20g/day) ; (mean±SD).

proposed daily intake (RDA, DRI) and non-essential or toxic element concentrations compared to average daily intake, can be seen in Table 1. The important intake (>15%) can be considered in the case of Cr.

Alteration of metal element homeostasis may elevate the risk of prostate diseases, e.g. intake of high amount of Fe or Zn deficiency may increase the oxidative processes in which NF-kappaB, IL-6 and IL-8 etc. are activated and the incidence of prostate cancer elevates as well as toxic metal elements (Salnikow et al., 2008). Zn depletion in the prostate's peripheral zone is found to correlate with the Gleason score.

Erythrocyte element status of patients with prostate cancer significantly changed versus controls in cases of Al (1.90±1.67 vs 0.537±0.260), Ni (0.722±0.565 vs 0.265±0.195) and Pb (0.309±0.301 vs 0.094±0.053), and these ion concentrations were significantly high in prostate cancer patients with PSA>9 (Nyirády et al., 2009b).

Toxic metal elements and free radicals influence the function of several receptors and genes such as tyrosine kinases, epidermal growth factor (EGF), platelet-derived growth factor (PDGF), vascular endothelial growth factor (VEGF); src and ras genes and signal proteins, nuclear factors - kappaB (NF-kappaB), activated protein–1 (AP-1), p53, nuclear factor of activated cells family (NFAT), hypoxia induced factor (HIF-1) (Suzuki 1997, Atmane 2003).

The plasma concentrations of Ca-, Cu- and Mg in patients did not change significantly during the treatment and they were between the normal range in all cases. Nevertheless, the Fe concentration decreased significantly by the effect of table beet supplementation and moved toward the normal value range. The Se level increased by the effect of treatment, although it reached the normal value only in some cases. The Zn concentration decreased significantly, the mean value was in the normal range. These data show that the metal ion homeostasis begins to restore, the metal ions stay in cells compartments by the effect of table beet consumption (Table 2.).

groups	Ca normal value:98	Cu normal value:1.2	Fe* normal value:1.1	Mg normal value:22	Zn* normal value:1.4	Se* normal value:0.08
	(mg/kg)					
control (N=9)	61.38±22.85	0.79±0.25	4.37±1.47	32.09±10.80	7.22±3.22	0.080±0.026
metastatic postate tumor (N=18)	77.82±11.03	1.25±0.28	12.52±9.63	21.47±3.51	1.46±0.60	0.011±0.006
metastatic postate tumor + table beet (N=18)	77.02±16.44	1.17±0.37	5.49±3.83	20.95±4.93	1.03±0.44	0.050±0.061

significance (p<0.05)* ; (mean±SD).

Table 2. Effect of table beet treatment on the plasma element concentrations of metastatic prostate cancer patients with taxan chemotherapy.

IFN-α, β, γ, IL-1α, β, IL-6, IL-10, IL-12, TNF-α, β, MIF and chemokines inflammatory cytokines, which initiate the activation of specific immune cells and regulate their differentiations (Haddad 2002). Chemokines affect the increasing of cell adhesion and chemotaxis, as well as activation of effector leucocytes are increased by them. During leucocyte activation, free radicals and lipid derivatives are liberated (Malaguarnera 2001).

Special components (betaine, folic acid, Fe, flavonoids and vitamins) of table beet could modify the erythrocyte total scavenger capacity and element concentrations as well as improve the transmethylation ability.

The levels of proinflammatory cytokines shown of a declining tendency, but these changes were not significant (IL1a P=0.084; IL6 P=0.154; IL8 P=0.578). The effect was beneficial. Measured parameters of anti-inflammatory cytokines also decreased (IL2 P=0.255; P=0.38; P=0.204). At the same time VEGF was not changed, although EGF was higher (p=0.003), and PSA (P=0.441) was elevated non significantly after supplementation. The levels of IL-6, CRP, IFNG and MCP1 were decreased in small amounts in the sera; these were disadvantageous results (Nyirády et al., 2010).

Consumption of beetroot decreased the proinflammatory cytokines and in some patients (44%) increased the level of IL2. In other patients (52%) we measured lower level of PSA. There were hopeful results, but increased EGF levels draw attention to the fact, that further investigations and correlation analysis must be performed, in which beneficial effects on patients can be observed. Data can be seen in Table 3.

parameters	patient groups			
	healthy controls (N=26)	early stage (N=28)	metastatic (N=18)	metastatic+ table beet (N= 8)
IL-1 alpha (pg/ml)	0.64±0.50	0.10±0.30	0.54±0.42	0.35±0.17
IL-1 beta (pg/ml)	1.57±1.3	0.80±2.20	1.18±1.60	0.42±0.50
IL-2 (pg/ml)	4.18±2.80	4.70±5.60	7.80±4.4	5.5±7.2
IL-4 (pg/ml)	4.56±1.84	2.30±5.40	4.70±2.05	4.0±2.01
IL-6 (pg/ml)	1.51±1.34	1.20±2.30	14.2±24.20	5.6±6.5
IL-8 (pg/ml)	25.21±16.16	9.10±16.30	31.20±87.00	25.3±29.6
IL-10 (pg/ml)	1.08±0.69	0.20±0.50	1.54±1.91	0.88±0.99
TNF-alpha (pg/ml)	7.45±4.23	3.00±3.60	3.41±1.65	3.50±0.98
VEGF (pg/ml)	190±150	183±94	272±116	282±160
IFNG (pg/ml)	1.78±1.41	0.8±1.50	4.28±4.21	2.21±1.97
MCP1 (pg/ml)	346±158	306±93	347±171	323±157
EGF (pg/ml)	212±81	66.8±58.3*	59.3±40.4*	110±58.8**
CRP (mg/l)	<5	5.6±12.8	14.4±24.9	5.9±4.9
PSA (pg/ml)	<2	10.66±7.79*	93±120**	133.5±182.5**

significance (p<0.05): control vs *; * vs **; (mean±SD).

Table 3. Immune parameters of prostate cancerous patients with and without table beet treatment in different stages and PSA levels.

Table 4. summarizes the redox parameters of patient groups. Table beet consumption moderated the erythrocyte free radical level in tendency and significant difference was observed in plasma in treated group compared to control. The large SD means that metastatic processes are different in time. There were no differences between HbA1c values.

groups	plasma (RLU%)	erythrocyte (RLU%)	HbA1c (%)
Control (N=11)	4.51±1.25	73.19±12.09	<6.1
postate tumor (metastatic) (N=18)	3,25±4,93	71,78±60,07	6,1±0,7
postate tumor (metastatic) + table beet (N=18)	1,69±1,39*	54,71±43,81	6,1±0,9

significance (p<0.05) control vs*; (mean±SD).

Table 4. Effect of table beet treatment on the redox parameters of prostate cancer patients with taxan chemotherapy.

On the basis of linear regression between chemiluminescent intensity (RLU%) and free protoporphyrin/Zn-protoporphyrin ratio, where y = -237.49x + 156.08 and R^2 = 0.6177 were calculated, significance could be observed. If the free protoporphyrin and HCHO ration was analyzed, the linear regression was better: y = -272.77x + 1024.6 and R^2 = 0.8331 (Nyirády et al., 2009).

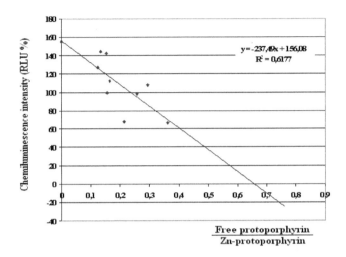

Fig. 2. Correlation between free protoporphyrin/Zn-protoporphyrin and chemiluminescent intensity (RLU%) in erythrocyte of cancerous patients.

Free protoporphyrin is accumulated generally in more cancerous cells than in healthy ones and autofluorescence lifetime is extended in cancer tissues (Chang et al., 2005). The results showed that in cancerous patients protoporphyrin – according to concentration – induces free radicals in small concentration and scavenges in higher concentration.

Accumulation of toxic metal elements and high protoporphyrin and Zn-protoporphyrin concentrations and low bond HCHO in erythrocyte with high PSA level mean wrong diagnosis.

According to the findings it seems that moderate and permanent consumption of table beet product affect favorably the life expectancy of patients, improves the erythrocyte function by the increasing methyl groups and diminishes the Zn-protoporphyrin and free protophorphyrin concentrations, but because of the increasing values of EGF and PSA in 44% of patients with bone metastasis, carefulness is needed. Further examinations are needed in this field.

Table 5. shows the erythrocyte Zn-protoporhyrin-, free- protoporhyrin-, erythrocyte formaldehyde – concentrations and PSA levels of cancerous patients with and without table beet treatment in different stages.

Before the table beet treatment, the HCHO concentration was 1.02 x 10^{-3} ± 2,73 x 10^{-4} μmol/mg erythrocyte, and after treatment the HCHO concentration was 3.72 x 10^{-3} ± 1,08 x 10^{-3} μmol/mg erythrocyte. Consequently, the HCHO concentration was elevated and therefore the function of erythrocyte was improved.

patients	Zn-protoporhyrin (nmol/l ery)	free-protoporhyrin (nmol/l ery)	erythrocyte formaldehyde (μmol/ml)	PSA (ng/ml)
healthy control (N=14)	nd	nd	1.52×10^{-2} ± 1.25×10^{-3}	nv
prostate tumor (histology -) (N=10)	1282 ± 513*	325 ± 50*	1.06×10^{-2}* ± 1.44×10^{-3}	9.66 ± 5.28*
prostate tumor (histology +) (N=30)	1043 ± 372*	582 ± 782*	7.830×10^{-3}** ± 2.56×10^{-3}	13.68 ± 21.91*
prostate tumor (metastatic) (N=18)	1470±768*	334±420*	1.02×10^{-3}*** ± 2.73×10^{-4}	93 ± 120**
prostate tumor (metastatic) + table beet (N=18)	857±308*	301±276*	3.72×10^{-3} ± *****1.08×10^{-3}	133.5±182.5**

nd non detected; nv value is in normal range (normal value of PSA is 0.01-4.00 ng/ml); (mean±SD) significance: control vs *,**,***; * vs **; **vs***, ****.

Table 5. Erythrocyte parameters of cancerous patients with and without table beet treatment in different stages.

3. Conclusion

HCHO and protoporphyrin concentrations and the induced free radical level of erythrocytes are very important indexes in cancer. The changes of their concentrations mean changes in tumor stages.

Generally the valuation of beneficial effects of nutrition supplements on patient life quality in tumor is empirical, and clinical studies are very rare. *Beta vulgaris* L. ssp. *esculenta* var. *rubra* is rich in bioactive compounds therefore it affects numerous biochemical reactions, enzyme activities and metabolic pathways. Homeostasis depends on table beet metal ion concentrations. This vegetable can be considered as a functional food, because among others, table beet is a good alimentary factor in cases of fatty liver, it has beneficial lipid lowering effects in obesity. Dietary betaine may need to be factored into the dietary sources of labile methyl groups and increase the methyl-pool. Treatment of betaine lowered plasma homocysteine concentration in homocystinuric patients.

The favorable impact of *Beta vulgaris* is enforced because significantly high levels of Zn- and free protoporphyrin decrease and furthermore trans-methylation processes fasten in cancerous patients. These results clearly verify that iron, folic acid and betaine components as well as colorful compounds with antioxidant activity of table beet extract demand more attention as a preventive therapy in chemotherapy induced anemia. Table beet will have a great impact and application in human cancer, but because of the increasing values of EGF close medical control is necessary for patients especially during chemotherapy.

4. Acknowledgements

This study was supported by the Health Sciences Scientific Committee ETT 354/2006, ETT 012/02, ETT 02/02.
Authors express their thanks to Mrs. Sarolta Bárkovits, Mrs. Edina Pintér and Mrs. Judit Sablyán for their excellent technical assistance.

5. Abbreviations

CRP = C reactive protein
DNA = deoxy-ribonucleic acid
EGF = epidermal growth factor
HbA1c = glycated hemoglobin
HCHO = formaldehyde
IBD = inflammatory bowel diseases
IFNG = interferon-gamma
IL-1 alpha/beta, IL-2, IL-4, IL-6, IL-8, IL-10, = interleukins
MCP-1 = monocyte chemoattractant protein-1
PSA = prostate-specific antigen
RLU = relative light unit
TNF-α = tumor necrosis factor-alpha

6. References

Abate, C., Patel, L., Rauscher, I.F.J., Curran, T. (1990). Redox regulation of Fos and Jun DNA: binding activity in vitro. *Science,* Vol.249, No. 4973, (Sept 1990), pp. 1157–1161, ISSN: 0036-8075

Atmane, N., Dairou, J., Paul, A., Dupret, J.M., Rodrigues-Lima, F. (2003). Redox regulation of the human xenobiotic metabolizing enzyme arylamine N-acetyltransferase 1 (NAT1). Reversible inactivation by hydrogen peroxide. *Journal of Biological Chemistry,* Vol. 278, No. 37, (Jun 2003), pp. 35086-35092, ISSN: 0021-9258

Awad, W.M.J., Whitney, P.L., Skiba, W.E., Mangum, J.H., Wells, M.S. (1983). Evidence for direct methyl transfer in betaine:homocysteine S-methyl-transfrease. *Journal of Biological Chemistry,* Vol. 258, No.258, (1983 Nov 10), pp. 12790-12792, ISSN: 0021-9258

Azzi, A., Gysin, R., Kempná, P., Munteanu, A., Villacorta, L., Visarius, T., Zingg, J,M. (2004). Regulation of gene expression by alpha-tocopherol.. *Biological Chemistry,* Vol.385, No 7, (Jul 2004), pp. 585-591, ISSN: 0021-9258

Barak, A.J., Beckenhauer, H.C., Tuma, D.J. (1996). Betaine, ethanol and the liver: a review. *Alcohol,* Vol.13, No.4, (Jul-Aug 1996), pp. 395-398, ISSN: 0741-8329

Barqawi, A., Thompson, I.M., Crawford, E.D. (2004). Prostate cancer chemoprevention, an overview of United States trials, *Journal of Urology,* Vol.171, No.2, (Febr 2004), pp. S5-8, ISSN: 0022-5347

Baylin, S.B., Herman, J.G., Graff, J.R., Vertino, P.M., Issa, J.P. (1997). Alterations in DNA methylation: a fundamental aspect of neoplasia. *Advances in Cancer Resesearch,* Vol. 72, No.72, pp. 141-196, ISSN: 0065-230X

Bastian, P.J., Palapattu, G.S., Yegnasubramanian, S., et al. (2008). CpG island hypermethylation profile in the serum of men with clinically localized and hormone refractory metastatic prostate cancer. *Journal of Urology*, Vol. 179, No.2, (Febr 2008), pp. 529–534, ISSN: 0022-5347

Blázovics, A. (2011). Small molecules in cancer therapy: cytotoxics and molecularly targeted agents. *Current Signal Transduction Therapy*, Vol.6, No.1, (Jan 2011), pp. 2-19, ISSN: 1574-3624

Blázovics, A., Kovács, Á., Lugasi, A. (2007a). The effect of short and long term antioxidant treatments on redox homeostasis in experimental and clinical studies. In: *Nutritional Research Advances*, (Ed.) Sarah V. Watkins, Nova Science Publisher, ISBN: 978-1-60021-516-2, Chapter 4, pp. 1-34, USA

Blázovics, A., Kovács, Á., Szilvás, Á. (2009). Redox homeostasis in gastrointestinal diseases. Acta Biologica. Szegediensis Vol. 53, Suppl. 1, 3-6, pp. 41-45, ISSN: 1588-4082

Blázovics, A., Kovács, Á., Lugasi, A., Hagymási, K., Bíró, L., Fehér, J. (1999). Antioxidant defence in erythrocytes and plasma of patients with active and quiescent Crohn's disease and ulcerative colitis: A chemiluminescence study. *Clinical Chemistry*, Vol.6, No.45, pp. 895-896, ISSN: 0009-9147

Blázovics, A., Nyirády, P., Bekő, G., Székely, E., Szilvás, Á., Kovács-Nagy, E., Horváth, A., Szűcs, M., Romics, I., Sárdi, É. (2011). Changes in erythrocyte transmethylation ability are predictive factors for tumor prognosis in prostate cancer, *Croatica Chemica Acta*, Vol. 84, No.3. pp. 127-131, ISSN: 001-1643

Blázovics, A., Sárdi, E., Szentmihályi, K., Váli, L., Takács-Hájos, M., Stefanovits-Bányai, E. (2007b). Extreme consumption of Beta vulgaris var. rubra can cause metal ion accumulation in the liver. Acta Biologica Hungarica. Vol.58, No.3. pp. 281-286, ISSN: 0236-5383

Blázovics, A., Szilvás, Á., Székely, Gy., Tordai, E., Székely, E., Czabai, G., Pallai, Zs., Sárdi É. (2008). Important bioactive molecules of erythrocytes in colorectal cancer patients after colectomy. *The Open Medicinal Chemistry Journal*, No.2, (Febr 2008), pp. 6-10, ISSN: 1874-1045

Blunden, G., Gordon, S.M. (1986). Betaines and their sulphonio analogues in marine algae. *Progress in Phycological Research*, Vol.4, pp. 41-80, ISSN: 0167-8574

Bobek, P., Galbavy, S., Mariássyová M. (2000). The effect of red beet (Beta vulgaris var. rubra) fiber on alimentary hypercholesterolemia and chemically induced colon carcinogenesis in rats. *Nahrung*, Vol.44, No.3 S. (Jul 2000), pp. 184-187, ISSN: 0027-769X

Boyd, J.N., Babish, J.G., Stoewsand, G.S. (1982). Modification by beet and cabbage diets of aflatoxin B_1-induced rat plasma α-foetoprotein elevation, hepatic tumorigenesis, and mutagenicity of urine. *Food and Chemical Toxicology*, Vol.20, No.1, (Feb 1982), pp. 47-52, ISSN: 0278-6915

Brando-Neto, J., Stefan, V., Mendoca, B.B. et al. (1995). The essential role of zink in growth, *Nutrition Research*, Vol. 15, No.3, (Marc 1995), pp. 335-338, ISSN: 0271-5317

Caddell, J.L. (2000). Geriatric cachexia: a role for magnesium deficiency as well as for cytokines? *American Society for Clinical Nutrition*, Vol. 71 No.3, (Marc 2000), pp. 851-852, ISSN: 0212-1611

Cai, Y., Sun, M., Corke, H. (2001). Antioxidant activity of betalains from plants the Amaranthaceae. *Journal of Agricultural and Food Chemistry*, Vol.51, No.49, (Apr 2003), pp. 2288-2294, ISSN: 1579-4377

Calvisi, D.F., Ladu, S., Gorden, A., Farina, M., Lee, J.S., Conner, E.A., Schroeder, I., Factor, V.M., Thorgeirsson, S.S. (2007). Mechanistic and prognostic significance of aberrant methylation in the molecular pathogenesis of human hepatocellular carcinoma, *Journal of Clinical Investigation*, Vol. 117, No.9, (Sept 2007), pp. 2713-2722, ISSN: 0895-4356

Chang, C.L., You, C., Chen, H.M., Chiang, C.P., Chen, C.T., Wang, C.Y. (2004). Autofluorescence lifetime measurement on oral carcinogenesis. Conference Publications - IEEE Engineering in Medicine and Biology Society, Vol. 4, pp. 2349-2351. **ISSN:** 1557-170X.

Chen, R.Z., Pettersson, U., Beard, C., Jackson–Grusby, L., Jaenisch, R. (1998). DNA hypomethylation leads to elevated mutation rates. *Nature*. Vol.395, No.6697, (Sept 1989), pp. 89-93, ISSN: 0028-0836

Chukhlovin, A.B., Tokalov, S.V., Yagunov, A.S., Westendorf, J., Reincke, H., Karbe, L. (2001). In vitro suppression of thymocyte apoptosis by metal-rich complex environmental mixtures: potential role of zinc and cadmium excess. *The Science of The Total Environment*, Vol.281, No.1-3, (Dec 2001), pp. 153-163, ISSN: 0048-9697

Critchfield, J.W., Keen, C.L. (1992). Manganese^{+2} exhibits dynamic binding to multiple ligands in human plazma. *Metabolism: Clinical and Experimental*, Vol.41, No10,(Oct 1992), pp. 1087-1092 ISSN: 0026-0495.

Delerive, P., Furman, C., Teissier, E., Fruchart, J., Duriez, P., Staels, B. (2000). Oxidized phospholipids activate PPARα in a phospholipase A2-dependent manner. *FEBS Letters*, Vol. 471, No.1, (Apr 2000), pp. 34-38, ISSN: 0014-5793

Dinkova-Kostova, AT, Holtzclaw, W.D., Wakabayashi, N. (2005). Keap1, the sensor for electrophiles and oxidants that regulates the phase 2 response, is a zinc metalloprotein. *Biochemistry*. Vol.10, No.44, (May 2005), pp. 6889-6899, ISSN: 0001527X

Dolmetsch, R.E., Lewis, R.S., Goodnow, C.C., Healy, J.I. (1997). Differential activation of transcription factors induced by Ca2+ response amplitude and duration. *Nature*, No.386, (Apr 1997), pp. 855-858, ISSN: 0028-0836

Eikelboom, J.W., Lonn, E., Yusuf, S. (1999). Homocysteine and cardiovascular disease: a critical review of the epidemiologic evidence. *Annals of Internal Medicine*, Vol.131, No. 7, (Sept 1999), pp. 363-375, ISSN: 0003-4819

Evans, J.C., Huddler, D.P., Jiracek, J., Castro, C., Millian, N.S., Garrow, T.A., Ludwig, M.L. (2002). Betaine-homocysteine methyltransferase zinc in distorted barrel. *Structure*, Vol.10, No.9, (Sept 2002), pp. 1159-1171, ISSN:0022-2860

Finkenstein, J.D., Martin, J.J. (1984). Inactivation of betaine-homocysteine methyltransferase by adenosylmethionine and adenosylethionine. *Biochemical and Biophysical Research Communication*, Vol.118, No.118, (Jan 1984), pp. 14-19, ISSN: 0006-291X

Floris, G., Medda, R., Padiglia, A., et al., (2000). The physiological significance of ceruloplasmin. A possible therapeutical approach. *Biochemical Pharmacology*, Vol 60, No.12, (Dec 2000), pp. 1735-1741, ISSN: 0006-2952

Frank, T., Stintzing, F.G., Carle, R., Bitsch, I., Quaas, D., Strass, G., Bitsch, R., Netzel, Z. (2005). Urinary pharmacokinetics of betalains following consumption of red beet juice in healthy humans. *Pharmacological Research,* Vol.52 No.4, (Oct 2005), pp. 290-297, ISSN: 1043-6618

Gersbeck, N., Schönbeck, F., Tyihák, E. (1989). Measurement of formaldehyde and its main generators in *Erysiphe graminis* infected barley plants by planar chromatographic techniques. *Journal of Planar Chromatography,* Vol. 2, No.1, pp. 86-89, ISSN:1789-0993

Griffiths, H.R., Lunec, J. (2001). Ascorbic acid in the 21st century: more than a simple antioxidant. *Environmental Toxicology and Pharmacology,* .Vol. 10, No.4, (Sept 2001), pp. 173-182, ISSN: 1382-6689

Haddad, J.J. (2002). Oxygen-sensitive pro-iflammatory cytokines, apoptosis signaling and redox-responsive transcription factors in development and pathophysiology. *Cytokines Cellular and Molecular Therapy,* Vol. 7, No.1, (Marc 2002, pp. 1-14, ISSN: 1368-4736

Hájos, M.T., Varga, I.Sz., Lugasi, A., Fehér, M., Bányai, É.S. (2004): Correlation between pigment contents and FRAP values in beet root (Beta vulgaris ssp. esculenta var. rubra). *International Journal of Horticultural Science,* Vol.10, No.4, pp. 85-89, ISSN: 1585-0404

Hagymási, K., Blázovics, A., Lengyel, G., Kocsis, I., Fehér, J. (2001). Oxidative damage in alcoholic liver disease. *European Journal of Gastroenterology and Hepatology,* Vol.13, No.1, (Jan 2001), pp. 49-53, ISSN: 0954-691X

Hartwig, A. (1998). Carcinogenicity of metal compounds: Possible role of DNA repair inhibition. *Toxicology Letters,* Vol.102-103, (Dec 1998), pp. 235-239 ISSN: 0378-4274

Hartwig, A., Mullenders, L.H.F., Schlepegrell, R., Kasten, U., Beyersmann, D. (1994). Nickel(II) interferes with the incision step in nucleotide excision repair in mammalian cells. *Cancer Research,* Vol. 54, No.15, (Aug 1994), pp. 4045-4051, ISSN. 0008-5472

Hayat, L.(1996). Cations in malignant and benign brain tumors. *Journal. Environmental Science and Health. Part. A* Vol. 31, No.8,(Aug 1996), pp. 1831-1840.ISSN: 1093-4529

Hougaard, L., Anthoni, U., Christophersen, C., Larsen, C., Lever, C., Lever, P.H.N. (1991). Characterization and quantitative estimation of quaternary ammonium compounds in marine demosponges. *Comparative Biochemistry and Physiology Part B: Biochemistry and Molecular Biology,* Vol.99, No.2, (2, 1991), pp. 469-472, ISSN: 1096-4959

Huszti, Z., Tyihák, E. (1986). Formation of formaldehyde from S-adenosyl-L-(mehyl-3H) methionine during enzymatic transmethylation of histamine. *FEBS Letters.* Vol.209, No.2, (Dec 1986), pp. 362-366, ISSN: 0014-5793

Jemal, A., Siegel, R., Ward, E., Hao, Y., Xu, J., Murray, T., Thun, M. (2008). Cancer statistics, *CA: a Cancer Journal for Clinicians,* Vol.58, No.2, pp. 71–96, ISSN:0007-9235

Kanner, J., Harel., S., Granit, R. (2001). Betalains-A New class of Dietary cationized antioxidants. *Journal of Agriculture and Food Chemistry,* Vol. 49, No.11, (2001 Nov), pp. 5178-5185, ISSN: 0021-8561

Kapadia, G.J., Azuine, M.A., Sridhar, R., Okuda, Y., Tsuruta, A., Ichiishi, E., Mukainake, T., Takasaki, M., Konoshima, T., Nishino, H., Tokuda, H. (2003). Chemoprevention of DMBA-induced UV-B promoted, NOR-1-induced TPA promoted skin carcinogenesis, and DEN-induced phenobarbital promoted liver tumors in mice by extract of beetroot. *Pharmacological Research,* Vol.47, No.2, (2003 Feb), pp. 141-148, ISSN: 1043-6618

Kasprzak, K.S., Waalkes, M.P., Poirier, L.A. (1987). Effect of essential divalent metals on carcinogenicity and metabolism of nickel and cadmium. *Biological Trace Element Research*, No.13, (Aug 1987), pp. 253-273, ISSN: 0163-4984

Kapadia, G.J., Tokuda, H., Konoshima, T., Nishino, H. (1996). Chemoprevention of lung and skin cancer by *Beta vulgaris* (beet) root extract. *Cancer Letters*, Vol.100, No.1-2, (Febr 1996), pp. 211-214, ISSN: 0304-3835

Kong, A.N., Yu, R., Chen, C., Mandlekar, S., Primiano, T. (2000). Signal transduction events elicited by natural products: role of MAPK and caspase pathways in homeostatic response and induction of apoptosis. *Archives Pharmacological Research*, Vol.23, No.1, (Febr 2000), pp. 1-16, ISSN:0253-6269

Kovács-Nagy, E., Blázovics, A., Fébel, H., Szentmihályi, K., Sárdi, É. (2009). Chromatographic analytical opportunities on a thin film of mobilizable methylgroups of different biological objects under the influence of exogenic treatment. *Acta Biologica Szegediensis*, Vol.53, Suppl. 1, pp. 54. ISSN: 1588-385X

Kuramoto, Y., Yamada, K., Tsuruta, O,, Sugano, M. (1996). Effect of natural food colorings on immunoglobulin production in vitro by rat spleen lymphocytes. *Bioscience Biotechnology and Biochemistry*, Vol.60, No.10, (Oct 1996), pp. 1712-1713, ISSN: 0916-8451

Lever, M., Sizeland, P.C., Bason, L.M., Hayman, C.M., Chambers, S.T. (1994). Glycine betaine and proline betaine in human blood and urine. *Biochim Biophys Acta*, Vol. 1200, No.3, (Aug 1994), pp. 259-264, ISSN: 0304-4165

Lichszteld, K., Kruk, L. (1977). Singlet molecular oxygen in formaldehyde oxidation. *Zeitschrift für Physicalische Chemie. (N F)* Vol.108, pp. 167-172, ISBN: 0044-3336

Lugasi, A., Hóvári J. (2002). Flavonoid aglycons in food of plant origin II. Fresh and dried fruits. Acta Alimentaria, Vol. 31, No.1, (Feb 2002), pp. 63-71. ISSN: 0139-3006

Máday, E., Szentmihályi, K., Then, M., Szőke, É. 2000. Mineral element content of chamomile. *Acta Alimentaria*, Vol. 29, No.1, (Febr 2000), pp. 51-57, ISSN:0139-3006

Maehle, L., Metcalf, R.A., Ryberg, D., Bennett, W.P., Harris, C.C., Haugen, A. (1992). Altered p53 gene structure and expression in human epithelial cells after exposure to nickel. Cancer Research, Vol.52, No.1,(Jan 1992), pp. 218-221, ISSN: 0008-5472

Malaguarnera, L., Ferlito, L., Imbesi, R.M, Gulizia, G.S., Di Mauro, S., Maugeri, D., Malaguarnera, M., Messina, S.S. (2001). Immunosenescence: a review. *Archives of Gerontology and Geriatritcs,*. Vol. 32, No.1, (Febr 2001), pp. 1-4, ISSN: 0167-4943

Meyer, M., Schreck, R., Baeuerle, P.A. (1993), H_2O_2 and antioxidants have opposite effects on activation of NF-kappa B and AP-1 in intact cells: AP-1 as secondary antioxidant-responsive factor. *EMBO Journal*, Vol.12, No.5, (May 1993), pp. 2005-2015, ISSN: 0261-4189

Millan, N.S., Garrow, T.A. (1998). Human betaine-homocysteine methyltransferase is a zinc metalloenzyme. *Archives of Biochemistry and Biophysics*, Vol.356, No.1 (Aug 1998), pp. 93-98, ISSN: 0003-9861

Murakami, T., Magamura,Y., Hirano, K., (1998). The recovering effect of betaine on carbon tetrachloide indiced liver injury. *Journal of Nutritional Science and Vitamology, (Tokyo), Vol.*44, No.2, (Apr 1998), pp. 249-255, ISSN:0301-4800

Nieva, J., Wentworth, P.Jr. (2004). The antibody-catalyzed water oxidation pathway - a new chemical arm to immune defence? *Trends in Biocheical Science*, Vol.29, No.5, (May 2004), pp. 274-278, ISSN: 0968-0004

Nyirády, P., Blázovics, A., Romics, I., May, Z., Székely, E., Bekő, G., 1 Szentmihályi, K. (2009a). Microelement concentration differences between patients with and without prostate adenocarcinoma. Vol. 3. Deficiency or excess of trace elements in the environment as a risk of health, Eds. Szilágyi M. and Szentmihályi K. Hungarian Academy of Sciences, pp. 26-30. TEFC. Budapest, ISBN:

Nyirády, P., Romics, I. (2009b). Textbook of Urology 2009. Semmelweis Kiadó és Multimédia Stúdió, ISBN: 9789639879232

Nyirády, P., Sárdi, É., Bekő, G., Szűcs, M., Horváth, A., Székely, E., Szentmihályi, K., Romics, I., Blázovics, A. (2010). Effect of bioactive molecules of Beta vulgaris L. ssp. Esculenta var. rubra on metastatic prostate cancer. *Orvosi. Hetilap*, Vol.151, No. 37, (Sept 2010), pp. 1495-1503, ISSN: 0030-6002

Pedreno, M.A., Escribano, J. (2000). Studying the oxidation and the antiradical activity of betalain from beet root. *Journal of Biological Education*, Vol.35, No.1, (Jan 2000), pp. 49-51, ISSN: 0021-9266

Pena, M.M., Lee, J., Thiele D.J. (1999). A delicate balance: homeostatic contol of copper uptake and distribution, *Journal of Nutrition*, Vol.129, No.7, (Jul 1999), pp. 1251-1260, ISSN: 0022-3166

Polya, G.M., Polya, Z., Kweifio-Okai, G. (2002). Biochemical pharmacology of anti-inflammatory plant secondary metabolites. In Recent Progress in Medicinal Plants Vol.8, (Ed) E. Sighn, J.N. Govil, V.K. Sighn, SCI TECH Publishing, Houston, Texas, USA., pp. 1-22. ISBN: 1930813139

Powis, G., Gasdanska, J.R., Baker, A. (1997). Redox signaling and the control of cell growth and death. *Advances in Pharmacology*, Vol.38, pp. 329-358, ISSN: 0009-9236

Rice-Evans, C.A., Miller, N.J., Paganga, G. (1999). Antioxidant properties of phenolic compounds. *Trends Plant Science*. Vol.2, No.4, (April 1997), pp. 152-159, ISSN: 1360-1385

Rosenbaum, E., Hoque, M.O., Cohen, Y., Zahurak, M., Eisenberger, M.A., Epstein, J.I., Partin, A.W., Sidransky, D. (2005). Promoter hypermethylation as an independent prognostic factor for relapse in patients with prostate cancer following radical prostatectomy. *Clinical Cancer Research*, Vol.11, No.23, (Dec 2005), pp. 8321-8525, ISSN: 1078-0432

Salnikow, K., Zhitkovich, A. (2008). Genetic and epigenetic mechanisms in metal carcinogenesis and cocarcinogenesis: nickel, arsenic, and chromium, *Chemical Research in Toxicology,*. Vol.21, No.1, (Jan 2008), pp. 28-44, ISSN: 0893-228X

Sárdi, É., Stefanovits-Bányai, É., Kocsis, I., Takács-Hájos, M., Fébel, H., Blázovics, A. (2009). Effect of bioactive compounds of table beet cultivars on alimenary induced fatty livers of rats. *Acta Alimimentaria,* Vol.38, No.3, (Sept 2009), pp. 267-280, ISSN: 0139-3006

Sárdi, É., Tordai E. (2005). Determination of fully N-methylated compounds in different cabbage and beetroot varieties. *Acta Biologica Szegediensis*, Vol.49. No.1-2, pp. 43-45, ISSN: 1588-385X

Schroeder, J.J., Cousins, R.J. (1990). Interleukin 6 regulates metallothionein gene expression and zinc metabolism in hepatocyte monolayer cultures. *Proceedings of the National Academic of Science U S A*. Vol.87, No.8, (Apr 1990), pp. 3137-3141. ISSN: 0027-8424

Schwartz, S.J., von Elbe, J.H., Pariza, M.W., Goldsworthy, T., Pitot, H.C. (1983). Inability of red beet betalain pigments to initiate or promote hepatocarcinogenesis. *Food and Chemical Toxicology*, Vol.21, No.5, pp. (Oct 1983), 531-535, ISSN: 0278-6915

Sigel, A., Sigel, H. (1999). Interactions between Free Radicals and Metal Ions in Life Processes. Metal Ions in Biological Systems, Marcel Dekker Inc., New York, Vol. No.36, pp. 1-797.

Skiba, W.E., Taylor, M.S., Wells, M.S., Mangum, J.H., Awad, W.M.J. (1982). Human hepatic methionine biosynthesis. Purification and characterization of betaine:homocysteine S/methyltransferase. *Journal of Biological Chemistry*, Vol.257, No.24, (Dec 1982). pp. 14944-14948, ISSN: 0021-9258

Slow, S., Lever, M., Lee, M.B., George, P.M., Chambers, S.T., (2004). Betaine analogues alter homocysteine metabolism in rats. *The International Journal of Biochemistry and Cell Biology*, Vol.36, No.5, (May 2004), pp. 870-880, ISSN: 1357-2725

Stead, L.M., Brosman, J.T., Brosman M.E., Vance D.E., Jacobs, R.L. (2006). Is it time to reevaluate methyl balance in humans? *The American Journal of Clinical Nutrition*, Vol.83, No.1, (Jan 2006), pp. 5–10. ISSN: 0002-9165

Stintzing, F.G., Carle, R. (2004). Functional properties of anthocyanins and betalains in plants food and in human nutrition. *Trends Food Science and Techology*, Vol.15, No.1, (Jan 2004), pp. 19-38, ISSN: 0924-2244

Stryeer, L. Biochemistry 3rd (1988). ed. V.H. Freeman and Co., New York, ISBN: 0716719207

Suzuki, Y.J., Forman, H.J., Sevanian, A. (1997). Oxidants as stimulators of signal transduction. *Free Radical Biology and Medicine*, Vol.22, No.1-2, pp. 269-285, ISSN: 0891-5849

Szentmihályi, K., Blázovics, A., Lugasi, A., Kéry, Á., Lakatos, B., Vinkler, P. (2000a). Effect of natural polyphenol-type antioxidants (Sempervivum tectorum and Raphanus sativus L. var. niger extracts) on metal ion concentrations in rat bile fluid. *Current Topics Biophysics*, Vol. No.24, pp. 203-07, ISSN:

Szentmihályi, K., Csiktusnádi-Kiss, G.A., Keszler, Á., Kótai L., Candeaias, M., Bronze, M.R., Boas, L.V., Spauger, I., Forgács, E. (2000b). Method development for measurement of elements in Hungarian red wines by inductively coupled plasma optical emission spectrmetry (ICP-OES). *Acta Alimentary*, Vol,29, pp. 105-121, ISSN: 0139-3006

Szilvás, Á., Blázovics, A., Székely, Gy., Fehér, J. (1999). Free radical status and tumor markers in gastrointestinal tumors, European Congress, I.H.P.B.A. Budapest, (Ed) L. Flautner, P.K. Kupcsulik, I. Rózsa, Monduzzi Editore. International Proceeding Divison, pp. 409-412, ISSN: 2039-4632

Takács-Hájos, M. (1999). Color components of different table beet root varieties. *International Journal of Horticulture Science*, Vol. 5, pp. 3-4, ISSN: 1585-04040

Váli, L., Stefanovits-Bányai, E., Szentmihályi, K., Fébel, H., Sárdi, E., Lugasi, A., Kocsis, I., Blázovics, A. (2007). Liver-protecting effects of table beet (Beta vulgaris var. rubra) during ischemia-reperfusion. *Nutrition*, Vol.23, No2, (Feb 2007), pp. 172-178, ISSN: 0899-9007

Wang, M., Goldman, I.L. (1996). Phenotypic variation free folic acid content among F1 hybrids and open-pollinated cultivars of red beet. *Journal of the Amarican Society for Horticultural Science*. Vol.121, No.6, (Nov 1996), pp. 1040-1042, ISSN: 0003-1062

Vanherweghem, J.L., Depierreux, M., Tielemans, C., Abramowicz, D., Dratwa, M., Jadoul, M,, Richard, C., Vandervelde, D., Verbeelen, D., Vanhaelen-Fastre, R, et al. (1993). Rapidly progressive interstitial renal fibrosis in young women: association with slimming regimen including Chinese herbs. *Lancet*, Vol.13, No.341, (Feb 1993), pp. 387-391, ISSN: 0140-6736

Watson, R.E., Curtin, G.M., Doolittle, D.J., Goodman, J.I. (2003). Progressive alterations in global and GC rich DNA methylation during tumorigenesis, *Toxicological Sciences*, Vol.75, No.2, (Oct 2003), pp. 289-299, ISSN: 1096-6080

Wettasinghe, M., Bolling, B., Plhak, L., Xiao, H., Parkin, K. (2002). Phase II enzyme-inducing and antioxidant activities of beetroot (*Beta vulgaris* L.) extracts from phenotypes of different pigmentation. *Journal of Agricultural and Food Chemistry*, Vol.50, No.23, (Nov 2002), pp. 6704-6707, ISSN: 0021-8561

Wilchen, B., Dudman, N., Tyrrell, P.A. (1983). Homocystinuria-the effects of betaine. *New England Journal of Medicine*, Vol. 309, No.8, (Aug 1983), pp. 448-453, ISSN: 0028-4793

Wild, L., Flanagan, J.M. (2010). Genome-wide hypomethylation in cancer may be a passive consequence of transformation. *Biochimica et Biophysica Acta*, Vol.1806, No.1, (Aug 2010), pp. 50-57, ISSN: 0304-419X

Yuregir, G.T., Kayrin, L., Curuk, M.A., Acarturk, E., Unlukurt, I. (1994/1995). Correlation between trace elements and lipid profiles. *Journal of Trace Elements in Experimental Medicine, Vol.7, pp. 113-118, ISSN: 0896-548X*

Zakharova, N.S., Petrova, T.A. (1998). Relationship between the structure and antioxidant activity of various betalains. *Prikladnaya Biocimimija i Mikrobiologiya*, Vol.34, No.2, (March April 1998), pp. 199-202, ISSN: 0555-1099

9

Nutritional Anaemia

Alhossain A. Khallafallah[1,2,*] and Muhajir Mohamed[1]
[1]Launceston General Hospital, Launceston, Tasmania
[2]School of Human Life Sciences, University of Tasmania
Australia

1. Introduction

Data available in Australia regarding the prevalence of iron deficiency anaemia (IDA) in pregnant women show that about 17.4% of pregnant women suffer from IDA, while the World Health Organization (WHO) global database on anaemia has suggested a prevalence of 14% based on a regression-based analysis.

There is a suggested association between IDA and the following maternal risks: increased fatigue antenatally and postnatally, poor exercise tolerance, impaired thermoregulation, decreased resistance to infection, reduced tolerance of bleeding or surgical intervention at delivery, delayed instigation of lactation and increased risk of postnatal depression. IDA is also a risk factor for preterm delivery and subsequent low birth weight and may be associated with inferior neonatal health. Infants born to women with IDA are more likely to become anaemic themselves which, in turn, is known to have a detrimental effect on an infant's mental and motor development. Although iron supplementation during pregnancy is one of the most widely practiced public health measures, there remain many controversial issues with this practice.

Oral iron supplementation has long been a standard treatment for IDA worldwide. However, patients do not always respond adequately to oral iron therapy due to difficulties associated with ingestion of the tablets and their side effects, which can play a significant role in rates of compliance. The side effects include gastrointestinal disturbances characterized by colicky pain, nausea, vomiting, diarrhoea, and or constipation, and occur in large cohort of patients taking iron preparations. In addition, the presence of bowel disease can affect the absorption of iron and thereby minimize the benefit received from oral iron therapy.

In the past, intravenous iron had been associated with undesirable and sometimes serious side-effects and was therefore limited in use. In recent years, the new type II and III iron complexes have been developed which are better tolerated and can be used for a rapid reversal of iron deficiency anaemia. Despite increasing evidence of the safety of the newer preparations, intravenous iron continues to be underutilized.

1.1 Iron deficiency anaemia in the general population

Anaemia occurs in different age groups in a number of clinical situations associated with iron deficiency, iron deficiency anaemia and blood loss. Usually in the presence of intact

*Correspondence Author

erythropoiesis iron therapy is very effective in restoring the depleted iron stores and accordingly improving the haemoglobin.   Other treatment strategies that stimulate erythropoiesis such as erythropoietin will also require the presence of iron in order to be an effective treatment.   Intravenous iron offers a rapid repletion of iron and is superior to oral iron as proven in many clinical trials.

In this regard, we will describe different clinical scenarios for iron deficiency anaemia in different cohorts of patients and numerate the available management options in the literature.

1.2 Other causes for nutritional anaemia

In this part, we are discussing other common nutritional deficiencies apart from iron that result in anaemia such as vitamin B12 and folate deficiencies. Furthermore, we discuss rare nutritional anaemia due to copper and selenium deficiencies and highlighting the most appropriate management approaches and treatment strategies.

2. Iron deficiency

Nutritional iron deficiency is the most common deficiency disorder in the world, affecting more than two billion people worldwide, with pregnant women at particular risk.[1-3] World Health Organization (WHO) data show that iron deficiency anaemia (IDA) in pregnancy is a significant problem throughout the world with a prevalence ranging from about 15% of pregnant women in industrialized countries to an average of 56% in developing countries (range 35-75%).[2,3]

Furthermore, IDA is affecting a large number of children and women not only in the developing world, but is also considered the only nutrient deficiency that is significantly prevalent in the developed world too. The numbers of patients with ID and IDA are overwhelming as more than 2 billion people, over 30% of the world's population, are iron deficient with variable prevalence, distribution and contributing factors in different parts of the world.[1-3]

Iron deficiency affects more people than any other condition, constituting an epidemic public health crisis. It is usually present with subtle manifestations and sometimes considered as a chronic slowly progressing disease that is often underestimated and untreated worldwide despite several warnings and awareness efforts of the World Health Organisation.[1-3]

It is worth noting that IDA has a debilitating effect as it reduces the work capacity of individuals and perhaps entire populations, with resultant serious economic consequences and obstacles to national development.[1,4-6]

The high prevalence of IDA has substantial health consequences with subsequent socio-economic hazards, including poor pregnancy outcome, impaired educational performance, and decreased work capacity and productivity.[1,6]

Targeted iron supplementation, iron rich diet, or both, can improve iron deficiency. However, variability of bioavailable iron compounds limit its value against nutritional iron deficiency. Therefore, laboratory measures of iron stores should be utilised to determine iron deficiency and monitor the therapy.[3,4,6]

Iron deficiency anaemia is quite often underestimated despite the high prevalence of iron deficiency. Blood loss is a major cause of anaemia in the general population.[5,6] This review highlights the importance of early diagnosis of IDA and hence offers the most appropriate treatment in order to avoid serious complications of anaemia.

2.1 Causes of iron deficiency anaemia

Nutritional iron deficiency generally arises when physiological requirements cannot be met by daily dietary iron ingestion as well as iron absorption. Religious beliefs in some countries and the dietary attitude of individuals may contribute to lack of iron supply when certain populations consume monotonous plant-based diets and hence reduces dietary iron bioavailability.

Women are at particular risk for developing IDA especially in their childbearing period as they have greater iron requirement because of menstrual blood loss and also during the pregnancy and lactation period when they have increased iron demands.[2]

Iron deficiency can also be caused by other types of chronic blood loss including gastro-intestinal blood loss from gastritis, peptic ulcers, inflammatory bowel disease, parasitic infestations (such as *hookworms*, *Ancylostoma*) as well as haemorrhoids.[7]

The recommended dietary daily iron for men over the age of puberty and women over the age of menopause are 8 mg per day, while for women in the child bearing period the recommended daily dietary iron dose is 18 mg per day.[8] In the typical diet, major sources of iron are meat, poultry, nuts and seeds, legumes and bean products, green leafy vegetables, raisins, whole grains and fortified cereals.[8]

2.2 Symptoms of iron deficiency

The presenting symptoms of IDA are variable and usually are the general symptoms of anaemia, including lethargy; unusual fatigue after exertion; signs of iron deficiency including paleness of the skin or eyes, intestinal problems, cognitive problems such as impaired learning ability, spoon nails, easy brittle and fragile nails, leg cramps especially in night time (restless leg syndrome) and sometimes hair loss.[6,7]

2.3 Diagnosis of Iron deficiency

Although a study of bone marrow iron stores is an accurate tool for assessing the body stored iron, it remains an impractical, invasive procedure to apply for most patients.

Measurement of both soluble transferrin receptor and serum ferritin provide a tool for accurate diagnosis of IDA. However, transferrin receptor is not a well-standardized test that can be reliably reproduced with high precision in most of laboratories worldwide.

In the meantime, ferritin estimation is an easy automated test to perform in most laboratories in the world; however its use is limited in case of inflammation or infection as it is considered as an acute phase reactant that is affected by many conditions including inflammation or infection and hence negatively influences its value.

Therefore, new technology such as hypochromic reticulocytes and reticulocyte haemoglobin testing, reportedly have higher sensitivity, specificity, reproducibility and cost effectiveness as a screening tool for iron deficiency.[9,10] This may offer a reliable screening test for iron deficiency in the future.

2.4 Iron metabolism

The main source of iron in humans comes from the destruction of erythrocytes by macrophages of the reticuloendothelial system including the spleen (recycled internal iron supply), while the daily requirement of external iron remains as little as between 1 to 8 mg daily. However, more external iron is required in case of increased demand for iron such as physiological requirements during growth, pregnancy or in a pathological condition such as bleeding (increase iron loss).[3,4,6,8] Recent studies have shown how the human body up- and down-regulate iron absorption in response to changing iron status via intestinal and hepatic proteins.[6,10]

Transferrin is an important protein synthesized by the liver that provides both a high affinity and high avidity mechanism to increase iron yield required for active erythropoiesis.[11]

Hepcidin is a peptide hormone that is also synthesized by liver that regulates iron and plays a significant role in iron metabolism.[12-15] Hepcidin was first described in January 1998 by Tomas Ganz and colleagues,[12] who sequenced this peptide and found that it contained 25 amino acids and 4 disulfide bonds. This peptide circulates in the plasma and responds to various stimuli that regulate iron stores and serum iron and is usually renally excreted.[13]

Ferroportins are considered as hepcidin receptor/iron exporter in the regulation of iron absorption, recycling, and tissue distribution. Ferroportin 1A (FPN1A) works as an element for translational repression in iron-deficient cells, while FPN1B is expressed in duodenal enterocytes, enabling them to export iron.[12]

Hepcidin, controls ferroportin and hence, the inflows of iron into plasma from main sources; duodenal enterocytes absorbing iron intake and from macrophages involved in the recycling of iron as well as from hepatocytes involved in iron storage.[12-15]

During pregnancy, fetal hepcidin controls the placental transfer of iron from maternal plasma to the fetal circulation. When hepcidin concentrations are low, iron enters blood plasma at a high rate. When hepcidin concentrations are high, ferroportin is internalized, and iron is trapped in enterocytes, macrophages, and hepatocytes [14,15]

Plasma iron concentrations and transferrin saturation are usually reflecting the difference between the hepcidin and ferroportin-regulated transfer of iron to plasma and iron consumption by the erythropoietic bone marrow tissue and, to a lesser extent, other tissues. Although, plasma transferrin compartment is considered relatively small, its iron content turns over every few hours, allowing iron concentrations to respond rapidly to changes in hepcidin concentrations.[12-15]

The role of hepcidin is mainly to regulate the absorption of dietary haeme, which is the main form of absorbable iron in human. Usually haeme is metabolized to ferrous iron by the enterocytes, however, its transfer to plasma will require ferroportin and hence is subjected to hepcidin-regulation.[12-15]

2.5 Treatment of iron deficiency anaemia

Although oral iron therapy is the most widely practiced treatment for iron deficiency anaemia, there are many issues that limit oral iron success in the management of IDA.

For instance, many patients do not respond adequately to oral iron therapy due to difficulties associated with ingestion of the tablets and their side effects, which can play a significant role in rates of compliance.[16-17]

The side effects of oral iron therapy include gastrointestinal disturbances characterized by colicky pain, nausea, vomiting, diarrhoea and or constipation, and occur in about 50% of patients taking iron preparations.[6]

Furthermore, the most widely prescribed oral iron is mainly composed of ferrous salts.[18,19] Ferrous salt is characterized by low and variable absorption rates and also its absorption can be limited in conjunction with ingestion of certain foods as well as mucosal luminal damage.[18-21] Therefore, ferric compounds were introduced to avoid such obstacles. However, these compounds are generally less soluble and have poor bioavailability.[21]

The usual recommended oral iron sulphate dose for the treatment of iron deficiency should be at least 80 mg daily of elemental iron, which is equivalent to 250 mg of oral iron sulphate tablets (Abbott, Australasia Pty Ltd).

In addition to oral iron side effects, patients with chronic bowel disease do not absorb oral iron readily and thereby minimise the benefit received from oral iron treatment.[21]

Although it is debatable whether intravenous iron should be administered or would oral iron have the same effect, many queries remain and are required to be addressed in further research and randomised trials.

The major challenges in the management of IDA are related to the tolerability and side effects of iron therapy in its different forms. Therefore, it is crucial to determine the most appropriate form and dose of iron as well as duration of treatment in order to successfully replenish the iron stores. Traditionally, the oral iron was widely used worldwide, however the effectiveness of oral formulations, due to the several facts mentioned before, is compromised by lack of absorption, poor compliance, adverse effects (up to 56%) and discontinuation of treatment (up to 20%).[6,18,21]

On the other hand, parenteral iron seems to be an attractive alternative to oral iron and is likely to be more popular option due to the introduction of new intravenous iron preparations, which allow high doses of iron to be administered rapidly in a single treatment.

In the past, intravenous iron had been associated with undesirable and sometimes serious side-effects and was therefore limited in use.[22-23] However, in recent years, the new type II and III iron complexes have been developed which are better tolerated and can be used for rapid repletion of iron stores.[24,25] Despite increasing evidence of the safety of the newer preparations, both in pregnant and general populations, intravenous iron continues to be underutilised because of previous concerns with tolerability of older intravenous iron preparations.[26]

Review of infusions of iron dextran among 481 patients revealed that about 25% of patients had mild side effects that have been self-limited. However about 2% experienced severe allergic reactions and about 0.6% were considered as anaphylactic reactions. Most of these reactions occurred immediately during the infusion of the test dose.[27]

On the other hand, iron gluconate is considered to have a lower reaction rate and therefore a test dose is not recommended. During the 1990s, only 3.3 allergic events per million doses per year with iron gluconate were reported.[28] During mid 1970s to mid 1990s There were no life-threatening reactions recorded as a result of iron gluconate infusion.

In contrast, during the same period, there were 31 fatalities among 196 allergic/anaphylactic reactions were reported for iron dextran, with about 16% of case fatality rate.[28]

The high incidence of adverse reactions of iron dextarn including serious adverse events have limited its application in practice.[29-31] Nonetheless, the application of iron gluconate is considered safe, it remains impractical in theory as it requires multiple infusions with huge implications on the often-limited health system resources as well as on patients' compliance.

There are new forms of intravenous iron that have recently been developed and are available in some countries that permit treating physicians to administer safely relatively high doses of iron in a single dose treatment. Furthermore, relatively older and established iron preparation such as intravenous iron polymaltose (Ferrosig, Sigma Pharmaceuticals,

Australia) demonstrated a high safety profile in treatment of IDA in both obstetric and general populations without a maximum dose-limit for treatment of IDA.[26] The total dose of IV iron polymaltose is calculated according to the patient's body weight and entry Hb level according to the product guidelines as following; iron dose in mg (50 mg per 1 ml) = body weight (maximum 90 kg) in kg x (target Hb (120 g/L) - actual Hb in g/L) x constant factor (0.24) + iron depot (500).[26] Recent reports demonstrate the feasibility of rapid infusion over 2 hours.[26,32,33] However, a test-dose of iron polymaltose (100 mg) should be first administered over 30 minutes and premedication is recommended prior to iron treatment for better toleration (antihistamine and or low dose steroids).[26,32,33]

Furthermore, in 2009, the United States Food and Drug Administration (FDA) approved ferumoxytol (AMAG Pharmaceuticals, Inc., USA)[34] for the treatment of iron-deficiency anaemia in adult patients with chronic kidney disease (CKD).[34] However, the maximum dose allow only 510 mg of ferumoxytol in a single administration and is limited to use initially in CKD, although with the expected expansion of its spectrum to include other forms of IDA.[35]   Another form of iron is ferric carboxymaltose (Vifor Pharma, Glattbrugg, Switzerland), which can be rapidly administered in 15 minutes in doses of 15 mg/kg body weight, with a maximum dose of 1000 mg.[36,37] There is no need for a test-dose of ferric carboxymaltose and its use is not restricted as ferumoxytol. More recently, in July 2010 a new intravenous iron isomaltoside (MonoFer, Pharmacosmos A/S, Holbaek, Denmark)[38] is introduced without the requirement of a test dose and it can be administered in 60 minutes at a rate of 20 mg/kg body weight in a single infusion without a maximum dose.[38,39] Iron isomaltoside administration was effective, safe, and was well tolerated when used to replenish iron stores in patients with anaemia of CKD.[39]

Intravenous iron including iron sucrose was employed in randomised controlled trials with improved effectiveness of intravenous iron only or in combination with oral iron compared to oral iron only based on Hb levels.[40,41]

A single IV iron sucrose dose has been reported to produce an increased incidence of thrombosis (9/41; 22%).[42] In contrast, 6 small doses of intravenous iron sucrose were administered over a three-week period without infusion-associated thrombosis as intravenous iron sucrose was administered in 5 daily doses to 45 pregnant women, also well tolerated.[34] In the first study, utilising intravenous iron sucrose, there was no significant difference between intravenous iron sucrose versus oral iron sulphate in the Hb levels at any time as measured at days 8, 15, 21, 30 and at delivery,[42] while in the second trial, with the 6 small doses of iron sucrose, there was a significant difference in Hb levels in favour of the intravenous iron sucrose group as measured at 2 and 4 weeks after administration of IV iron and at delivery.[40]

However, both trials administered IV iron sucrose at the expense of a vastly greater effort from the patients as well as extra demands on hospital resources.[40,41]

Certainly, the new intravenous iron preparations represent a medical revolution in effective, rapid and safe iron repletion in the management of iron deficiency anaemia.[34-39] This will reflect positively in the treatment of IDA in different populations by application of a single high-dose intravenous iron treatment with subsequent repletion of the iron stores effectively and hence, to improve subjective and objective outcomes in IDA.

Although iron deficiency is a precursor of IDA, many clinical studies treat it similarly to IDA. In case of severe IDA, a blood transfusion has been the traditional efficient approach to correct the anaemia, especially if patients did not respond to oral iron therapy or when a rapid correction of anaemia is clinically required.

Currently, the development of new intravenous iron formulations that offer higher doses in a single administration has provided the treating physicians with the opportunity to employ intravenous iron as an effective, rapid and safe treatment for IDA[34-39] avoiding the use of blood transfusion with its known hazards.[43] There are increasing evidence-based research that support the safety and efficacy of IV iron in IDA. There is also increasing evidence for inadequacy of oral iron in terms of adverse effects, lack of compliance as well as lack of absorption and slow and often questionable effect in IDA patients, especially in patients with ongoing blood loss.[44-47]

A common requirement across the range of clinical situations is the need for safe, effective higher, less frequent doses to achieve optimal clinical outcomes. The major goals of such strategy include overall cost reduction, relief to overstretched health system(s), improved patient convenience, improved compliance, preservation of venous access and reduced blood transfusion.[35-41,43,46] This will ultimately reduce the demand for blood transfusions, especially in the case of short supply. Furthermore, some of the new iron preparations such as ferric carboxymaltose and iron isomaltoside, do not require a test dose and therefore, ease the application of intravenous iron in a timely and cost effective fashion. This certainly will enhance the use of intravenous iron in clinical practice.

The WHO identified the problem of IDA as the most debilitating nutritional deficiency worldwide in the twenty first century. Such problem, if left untreated and not addressed properly can have a devastating effect on entire populations with adverse socio-economical consequences. Therefore, the use of intravenous iron should be considered as an effective, rapid and safe treatment option in some clinical scenarios with intravenous iron being employed to avoid or reduce the demand for blood transfusions or when rapid repletion of iron stores are required. Treatment options for IDA should consider the recently developed intravenous iron formulations, which is considered a milestone in the management of IDA.

Overall, the developing world is most vulnerable, especially the poorest and the least educated countries that are disproportionately affected by iron deficiency, and therefore they will gain the most by eradication of IDA. Therefore, awareness of the magnitude and scale of the IDA problem will help in recognising the most appropriate ways of diagnosis and treatment, which is crucial to overcome such devastating health problem. Perhaps consensus guidelines set by world experts in managing IDA incorporating new intravenous iron therapies are warranted.

3. Vitamin B12 deficiency anaemia

Cobalamin (vitamin B12) along with folic acid is normally required for DNA synthesis. Deficiency of one or both can cause defect in DNA synthesis, with lesser defect in RNA and protein synthesis, leading to a state of unbalanced cell growth and impaired cell division. The aberrant DNA synthesis causes arrest in S phase of cell cycle, affecting mitosis and cell division. This results in nucleo-cytoplasmic asynchrony and megaloblastic anaemia. [1]

3.1 Cobalamin

Cobalamin is a complex organo-metallic compound in which the cobalt atom is situated within a corrin ring. The two active coenzyme forms are methylcobalamin and 5-deoxyadenosyl cobalamin[1].

3.2 Main functions of cobalamin[2]
1.   Conversion of methyl malonyl coA to succinyl coA in the mitochondria.
2.   Methylation of homocysteine to methionine in the cytoplasm.

3.3 Effects of cobalamin deficiency
a.   Impairment of DNA synthesis
      Cobalamin deficiency causes reduced methionine, which leads to reduced
      tetrahydrofolate and high methyl tetrahydrofolate in the cells (methyl folate trap
      hypothesis). This in turn causes low dTMP synthesis with high dUMP levels which
      results in impairment of DNA synthesis due to uridine for thymidine substitution in
      base pairing.
b.   Defective myelin synthesis and neurological problems.
      Cobalamin and folate have fundamental roles in CNS function at all ages, especially the
      methionine-synthase mediated conversion of homocysteine to methionine, which is
      essential for nucleotide synthesis and genomic and non-genomic methylation[3].
      Prolonged cobalamin deficiency causes defective conversion of propionate to succinyl
      coA and also causes high serum methyl malonic acid and homocysteine. Both of these
      can cause defective myelin synthesis and neurological dysfunction, since methionine is
      required for synthesis of choline.
c.   Venous and arterial thrombosis.
      Plasma homocysteine levels are increased in both folate and cobalamine, which can
      lead to venous and arterial thrombosis[4].

3.4 Sources of cobalamin and dietary requirements
Cobalamin cannot be synthesized in human beings and needs to be supplied in the diet.
Animal sources like meat, liver, fish, egg, milk and cheese are good sources of cobalamin.
The estimated daily requirement of cobalamin is 1 mcg/day. The recommended daily
allowance is 2.4 mcg/day. The daily requirement is so small relative to stores that deficiency
typically takes years to develop in adults.[5]

3.5 Absorption, transport and cellular uptake
Absorption:
1.   Stomach
      Gastric digestion releases cobalamin from the bound proteins. Gastric R-binder (also
      called haptocorrin) binds with cobalamin forming cobalamin - R binder complex. R-
      binder is also present in saliva, milk, gastric juice, bile, plasma and phagocytes.
2.   Duodenum:
      Cobalamin - R binder complex is digested by pancreatic proteases. Cobalamin binds to
      Intrinsic Factor (IF). IF is produced by gastric parietal cells and is resistant to proteolytic
      digestion. IF has two binding sites, one for cobalamin and another for cubulin in Ileal
      cells.
3.   Distal ileum:
      In the Ileal mucosal cell, IF is bound to cubulin. IF is destroyed and cobalamin binds to
      TCII forming a complex and absorbed into the blood.
4.   Blood:
      Cobalamin – TCII complex in the blood is rapidly taken up by liver, bone marrow and
      other cells. Most cobalamin in the blood is bound to TCI, present in secondary granules
      of neutrophils, a group closely related to R binder. The function of TCI is not known.

5.	Cellular uptake:
	Cobalamin – TCII complex is rapidly taken up by liver, bone marrow and other cells. Cobalamin – TCII is released into lysosomes.	Lysosomal degradation leads to cobalamin release. Most of the cobalamin (~95%) is bound to two intracellular enzymes.
a.	Methyl malonyl coA mutase in the mitochondria catalyses methyl malonyl coA to succinyl coA.
b.	Methionine synthase in the cytosol: Methyl cobalamin acts as coenzyme for methionine synthase allowing transfer of methyl group from homocysteine to methionine. 5 methyl tetrahydrofolate donates methyl group to cobalamin thus regenerating methyl cobalamin.

3.6 Causes of cobalamin deficiency
a.	Nutritional cobalamin deficiency:
Causes: Strict vegans, [6] breast-fed infants of mothers with low cobalamin levels.
b.	Cobalamin malabsorption
1.	Intrinsic Factor deficiency
	Pernicious anaemia
	Total gastrectomy
2.	Food-bound cobalamin malabsorption (FBCM)
Gastritis can cause FBCM. Progression of anaemia is slower than in IF-related malabsorption and may extend beyond a decade. [7]
3.	Disorders causing cobalamin malabsorption in small intestine:
-	Pancreatic insufficiency
-	Blind loop syndrome
-	Fish tape worm (Diphyllobothrium latum)
-	Mucosal damage :
Causes: Tropical sprue, nontropical sprue, Crohn's disease , Small intestinal tumours like lymphoma, granulomatous disease.
4.	Other causes of cobalamin deficiency
	Gastric achlorhydrria
	Partial gastrectomy
-	Drugs: H2 receptor antagonists, proton pump inhibitors, Cholestryamine, Neomycin etc.

3.7 Perinicious Anaemia (PA)
PA is the most common cause of cobalamin deficiency is intrinsic factor deficiency due to atrophic gastritis or autoimmune destruction of parietal cells. The age of onset is usually after 40 years and more common in Northern European descent.
In autoimmune PA, the gastric parietal cells are affected by cytotoxic T cells. There is an increased incidence of circulating antibodies – antiparietal cell antibodies (90%) & anti-intrinsic factor antibodies (60%). PA can be associated with other autoimmune disorders like Grave's disease, Hashimoto's thyroiditis, Addison's disease and hypo-parathyroidisim.
Gastric atrophy affects acid and pepsin areas of the stomach while the antrum is spared. Atrophic gastritis usually precedes the onset of megaloblastic anaemia by many years. All

the cells which have a high proliferation exhibit megaloblastic changes, e.g. epithelial cells lining the gastrointestinal tract (buccal mucosa, tongue and small intestine), cervix, vagina, and uterus. There is a higher risk of gastric cancer and carcinoids in patients with pernicious anaemia.[8]

3.8 Clinical features of cobalamin deficiency
Haematologic: Pancytopenia with megaloblastic anaemia
Cardiopulmonary: Congestive heart failure
Gastro-intestinal: Beefy red tongue (glossitis), broad spectrum malabsorption, diarrhoea
Skin: Melanin pigmentation, premature greying of hair
Genitals: Cervical and uterine dysplasia
Reproductive: Infertility or sterility

3.9 Central nervous system (CNS)
CNS involvement is unique to cobalamin deficiency. Peripheral nerves, posterolateral columns of spinal cord, cerebrum, optic nerve and rarely autonomous nervous system are affected. Pathological changes are demyelination, axonal degeneration and neuronal death. Symptoms are paraesthesia, numbness in extremities, weakness and ataxia. Psychotic changes can occur in cobalamin deficiency, which can vary from mild irritability and forgetfulness to severe dementia or frank psychosis.

3.10 Lab investigation in megaloblastic anaemia
3.10.1 Full blood count & blood film
High MCV usually precedes anaemia. Low red cell count, Hb and reticulocyte counts are common. Low white cell count and low platelet counts can occur in moderate to severe deficiency.
Blood film shows macro-ovalocytes, hypersegmented neutrophils (greater than 5% PMNs with more than five lobes or a single PMN with more than six lobes are pathognomonic). In severe deficiency, leuko-erythroblastic blood picture, tear drop poikilocytes, basophilic stippling, Howell Jolly bodies, nucleated red cells and Cabot's ring can be seen.

3.10.2 Bone marrow analysis
Hypercellularity is prominent in all the three cell lines. Erythroid hyperplasia is more marked than the others. Abnormal erythropoiesis with abnormally large red cell precursors (megaloblasts) with less mature nuclei (nuclear – cytoplasmic asynchrony) is common. Nuclear chromatin is more dispersed with fenestrated pattern, a characteristic feature of megaloblastic anaemia.
In severe megaloblastic anaemia up to 90% of RBC precursors are destroyed before they become mature, when compared to 10 % in normal marrow (ineffective erythropoiesis).
Abnormal leucopoiesis - giant metamyelocytes and band forms are characteristic. Hypersegmented neutrophils are also seen in bone marrow. Abnormal megakaryocytes can be seen (pseudohyperdiploidy).

3.10.3 Serum cobalamin levels[9]
Normal levels : 120 - 680 pmol/L measured using Immunoassay.
The limitations of serum cobalamin levels are

Falsely low levels (in patients with normal cobalamin)
Severe folate deficiency (in 30% of patients)
Low TC- I levels
Physiologically low levels in pregnancy
Intake of large doses of Vitamin C
Falsely normal or high levels (in patients with low cobalamin)
Myeloproliferative disorders (Cobalamin binders like TC-I &TC-II are increased)
Acute liver disease (release of cobalamin from hepatocytes).

3.10.4 Other tests

3.10.4.1 Schilling test

The Schilling test measures cobalamin absorption by assessing increased urine radioactivity after an oral dose of radioactive cobalamin. Malabsorption due to any cause produces low radioactivity in urine. The test is useful in demonstrating that the anaemia is caused by an absence of IF. Schilling test helps to identify abnormal IF-related absorption and also to distinguish between gastric and intestinal defects.

If the Schilling test result is normal, non-malabsorptive disorders and FBCM are considered. A modified absorption test, in which the test dose of cobalamin is bound to food, was created specifically to identify FBCM.[10]

3.10.4.2 Serum homocysteine and methyl malonic acid

Elevated serum methylmalonic acid and homocysteine levels are found in patients with cobalamin deficiency. Clinical deficiency often features serum MMA above 1000 nmol/L and homocysteine above 25 uM. In folate deficiency, serum methylmalonic acid levels are normal and homocysteine levels are high.[11, 12,13]

Patient Condition	Homocysteine	Methylmalonic Acid
Healthy	Normal	Normal
Vitamin B-12 deficiency	Increased	Increased
Folate deficiency	Increased	Normal

Table 1. Serum homocysteine and methylmalonic acid values in healthy persons, cobalamin and folic acid deficiency

The advantage of these tests is they measure tissue vitamin stores and may diagnose the deficiency even when the serum cobalamin and folate levels are borderline or normal.

3.10.4.3 Other tests

1. The indirect bilirubin level may be elevated because pernicious anaemia causes haemolysis associated with increased turnover of bilirubin. The serum lactic dehydrogenase (LDH) concentration usually is markedly increased.
2. Intrinsic Factor (IF) antibodies in serum by Immunoassay.[14]
3. Type 1 (blocking) antibody prevents the attachment of vitamin B12 to intrinsic factor: present in 50-60% of patients with pernicious anaemia. Type 2 (precipitating) antibody

prevents attachment of the vitamin B12-intrinsic factor complex to ileal receptors: present in 30% of patients with pernicious anaemia, and only in those who also have Type 1 antibodies. IF antibody has high specificity for PA (>95%). It is used to help diagnose when pernicious anaemia is suspected. As recent vitamin B12 administration is associated with a high rate of false positive results the sample must be collected prior to commencing therapy or at least one week after vitamin B12 administration. This test shows rarely false positivity in diabetes and thyroid disorders.

4.   Parietal cell antibodies

Parietal cell antibodies can be measured using indirect IF. Antibodies react with sub-units of the gastric parietal cell proton pump. Antibodies are positive in 80% of patients with pernicious anaemia and in 40-50% of patients with other organ specific autoimmune diseases.[15]

4. Treatment

4.1 Cobalamin deficiency
4.1.1 Specific replacement therapy

The 1000-mcg intramuscular dose begins repletion of stores (up to 150 mcg is retained from that injection by most patients).[5] Cyanocobalamin and hydroxocobalamin are commonly available preparations. 8 to 10 injections are given over the first 2 to 3 months followed by monthly injections.[16] Hydroxocobalamin injections can be spaced at twice the interval for cyanocobalamin.[17] The toxicity of cobalamin is minimal with rare allergic reactions which can be anaphylactic.[18]

In a randomized study with cobalamin deficiency, 2 mg of cyanocobalamin administered orally on a daily basis was as effective as 1 mg administered intramuscularly on a monthly basis.[19] For patients who refuse monthly parenteral therapy or prefer daily oral therapy or in those with disorders of haemostasis, cobalamin (1–2 mg/day as tablets) can be recommended for patients with cobalamin malabsorption (where cobalamin is passively absorbed at high doses).[1]

Patients with FBCM may need to take cobalamin supplements on an empty stomach to prevent in vitro binding of cobalamin to food. 1000 mcg oral doses may be necessary in many cases of FBCM, but the undesirable effects of long term high doses, if any, are not known.[20]

4.1.2 Response to treatment

The response to treatment is generally predictable and can be used as a therapeutic trial. Patients have a sense of well-being within 12 to 24 hours, which is an early feature of response. In bone marrow the megaloblastic erythropoiesis starts changing to normoblastic within 12 hours and complete resolution by 48 hours. Brisk reticulocytosis starts at 3 to 4 days and peaks at 5 to 7 days. Hypersegmented neutrophils continue to remain in the blood for 10 to 14 days. Mean corpuscular volume (MCV) will take eight weeks or more to normalize.[1] All these responses will be impaired if there is associated iron deficiency, anaemia of chronic disease or hypothyroidism.

Neurologic improvement also begins within the first week and is typically complete in 6 weeks to 3 months. Its course is not as predictable as a haematologic response. Severe hypokalemia can occur after cobalamin therapy, which requires careful monitoring and management.

4.1.3 Causes of non-responsiveness of megaloblastosis to medication
1. Wrong diagnosis (eg: Myelodysplastic syndrome)
2. Combined cobalamin + Folate deficiency ,medication with one vitamin
3. Drugs eg: Hydroxyurea, azathioprine
4. Factors associated with B12 deficiency causing impaired response
c. Iron deficiency
d. Haemoglobinopathy
e. Hypothyroidism

4.2 Transfusions
Complications can occur during transfusions, particularly congestive heart failure in elderly. Transfusion should be restricted to symptomatic anaemia, rather than by low haemoglobin values. In severe anaemia, exchange transfusion after removing 250- 300ml of anaemic blood and replacing packed red cells may be beneficial.

4.3 Maintenance regimens
High dose cobalamin tablets (1000 mcg) can be used for maintenance therapy. Despite the advantages of ease, cost, and comfort, oral therapy has its own limitations. Oral cobalamin is less effectively absorbed after a meal than when fasted.[21] Monthly parenteral cobalamin injections are a better alternative in patients who are non-compliant with oral therapy.

4.4 Cobalamin prophylaxis in clinical practice
The value of general supplementation or dietary fortification with cobalamin are not proven.[22] In some situations, like strict vegetarians, patients with gastric surgery and in elderly persons, life-long supplementation with cobalamin will be essential.

5. Folate deficiency anaemia

Folic acid is also known as pteroyl-monoglutamic acid. Fruits and vegetables constitute the main dietary source of the vitamin. Dietary folic acid is heat labile and may be destroyed by cooking. The daily requirement is usually about 50 mcg. The requirement may be increased to many folds during pregnancy.

Folates in various foodstuffs are largely conjugated as polyglutamates. Conjugases in the lumen of the gut convert polyglutamates to mono- and diglutamates, which are readily absorbed in the proximal jejunum. Plasma folate is primarily in the form of N5-methyltetrahydrofolate which is a monoglutamate and is transported into cells by a carrier. In the cell, the N5-methyl group is removed and the folate is then converted again to the polyglutamate form. Conjugation to polyglutamate may be useful for retention of folate within the cell.

The normal body store of folic acid is 5 to 20 mg. Nearly 50% of the body stores are present in the liver. Folate deficiency usually occurs within 4 to 5 months with dietary deficiency, in contrast to cobalamin deficiency which takes many years.

5.1 Role of folate in DNA synthesis
Folate serves as an intermediate carrier of 1 carbon fragment and is essential for denovo synthesis of purines, dTMP and methionine. Its active form is tetrahydrofolate, which acquires 1 carbon from serine and converted to glycine.

For purine synthesis, the 1 carbon is oxidised to formic acid, then transferred to substrate. For methionine synthesis, cobalamin is required and 1 carbon fragment is reduced to the level of methyl group, which is then transferred to homocysteine. In these reactions, the cofactor is released as tetrahydrofolate which can immediately participate in another 1-carbon transfer cycle.

Conversion of dUMP to dTMP is catalysed by thymidylate synthase and dihydrofolate is released. To participate in further 1- carbon transfer cycle, the dihydrofolate is catalysed by dihydrofolate reductase to tetrahydrofolate.

5.2 Folate deficiency
5.2.1 Causes
1. Inadequate intake
    Alcoholics, infants, anorexia nervosa, malnutrition, prolonged cooking of vegetables.
2. Increased requirements
    a. Pregnancy and lactation
    b. Infancy and childhood
    c. Haemolytic anaemias
    d. Cancers
    e. Exfoliative dermatitis
3. Malabsorption
    a. Tropical sprue and non-tropical sprue
    b. Partial gastrectomy
    c. Crohn's disease
    d. Intestinal Lymphoma
4. Impaired Metabolism
    a. Alcoholism
    b. Dihydrofolate reductase inhibitors: Methotrexate, pentamidine, trimethoprim
5. Reduced hepatic stores
    a. Alcoholism
    b. Chronic liver disease and cirrhosis
    c. Hepatic malignancy

5.3 Alcoholism
The common cause of Folate deficiency is alcohol intake. Folate deficiency in alcoholics can be attributed to multiple factors.
a. Dietary malabsorption
b. Reduced food intake
c. Depletion of liver stores of folate
d. Impaired intracellular folate utilization
Prolonged and excessive alcohol can lead to megaloblastic changes in the bone marrow.

5.4 Tropical sprue / coeliac disease
In tropical sprue and coeliac disease, low folate levels are caused by folate malabsorption. Steatorrhoea is the major symptom.
In tropical sprue there will be high foecal fat and jejunal biopsy shows subtotal or total villous atrophy. In coeliac disease, d- xylose test is positive.

In coeliac disease, a gluten free diet can correct folate malabsorption.

5.5 Anti convulsant drugs
Drugs like phenytoin and phenobarbitone can cause folate deficiency. This is usually due to inhibition of dietary folate absorption caused by reduced levels of small intestinal conjugases.

5.6 Pregnancy
Since the foetus accumulates folate, the demand is high during pregnancy.

5.7 Haemolytic states
Haemolytic states like hereditary spherocytosis, auto-immune haemolytic anaemia, sickle cell anaemia, thalassaemias and paroxysmal nocturnal haemoglobinuria cause erythroid hyperplasia. Increased erythroid turnover causes an increase in folate demand, thus causing folate deficiency.

5.8 Exfoliative disorders
Patients can lose folate in exfoliated skin. In exfoliative skin disorders, folate deficiency can occur.

5.9 Neoplastic disorders
In acute leukaemias, myeloproliferative disorders, myeloma and metastatic carcinomas, the neoplastic tissue utilize folate more rapidly than the host tissue.

5.10 Clinical features of folate deficiency
Clinical features of folate deficiency are similar to cobalamin deficiency, except that neurological manifestations are not common in folate deficiency.
Haematological – pancytopenia with megaloblastic anaemia
Cardiopulmonary - congestive heart failure
Gastrointestinal – glossitis, broad spectrum malabsorption and diarrhoea
Folate deficiency can also be implicated in:
1.   Increased arteriosclerosis risks due to elevated homocysteine[1]
2.   Foetal neural tube defects[2]
3.   Cancer pathogenesis[3]

5.11 Laboratory investigations
5.11.1 Full blood count & blood film
The features are similar to cobalamin deficiency. Macrocytic anaemia with ovalocytes and tear drop cells are seen in the blood film. Hypersegmented neutrophils are commonly seen. Neutropenia and thrombocytopenia are less common. In rare cases, the absolute neutrophil count can drop below $1.0 \times 10^9/L$ and the platelet count below $50 \times 10^9/L$.

5.11.2 Bone marrow analysis
Bone marrow features are also similar to that seen in cobalamin deficiency. Hypercellularity is prominent in all the three cell lines. Erythroid hyperplasia is more marked than the others.

Abnormal erythropoiesis with abnormally large red cell precursors (megaloblasts) with less mature nuclei (nuclear – cytoplasmic asynchrony) is common.

5.11.3 Serum folate levels
Normal serum folate levels are 7-45 nmol/L measured by immunoassay.
Limitations of serum folate assay:
Levels vary with levels of folate in the recent diet. Falsely high values of serum folate can occur in haemolysis (in vivo and in vitro) and in cobalamin deficiency.

5.11.4 Red cell folate levels
Normal serum folate levels are 360-1400 nmol/L, measured by immunoassa. Red cell folate is a good index of folate stores and not affected by dietary folate intake. Low red cell folate levels are a better predictor for folate deficiency than low serum folate levels.

However, there are few limitations in this assay. Low to subnormal range occurs only after all the stores are depleted. In two-thirds of patients with severe cobalamin deficiency, falsely low red cell folate levels are common. Since reticulocytes have increased folate concentrations, haemolytic states may produce falsely normal or high red cell folate despite folate deficiency.

5.11.5 Serum homocysteine and methyl malonic acid
In folate deficiency, serum methyl malonic acid levels are normal and homocysteine levels are high.[4]

6. Treatment of folate deficiency

The usual treatment dose of folic acid tablets is 1mg/day. Sometimes up to 5mg/day may be required as in haemolytic anaemias. Adequate absorption with such doses usually occurs even in chronic folate malabsorption. Therapy should be continued until complete hematologic recovery. If the underlying cause is not correctable, folate should be continued. Folinic acid (leucovorin) can be used to rescue drugs with antifolate activity e.g. antimetabolites (methotrexate or 5-fluorouracil) or other drugs like sulfamethoxazole- trimethoprim and pentamidine. Haematological response after folate is similar to cobalamin deficiency.

6.1 Prophylaxis
Folic acid prophylaxis is essential in the following situations
a.   Pregnancy and lactation: The dose is usually 400mcg daily.
b.   Mothers at risk of delivery of neural tube defects: The dose of folic acid is 4mg/day during the peri-conception period and throughout the first trimester.
c.   Haemolytic anemias and hyperproliferative haematological states: The dose is usually between 1mg to 5mg daily.
d.   Patients with rheumatoid arthritis or psoriasis on medication with methotrexate.[6]

7. Other rare nutritional deficiencies that can cause anaemia

Deficiencies of trace elements like copper and selenium can cause anaemia.
Copper is present in legumes, meats, and nuts with a very low daily requirement.[1] It is absorbed through the mucosa of the stomach and proximal duodenum.[2]

Copper is an essential trace metal acting as a ligand to many proteins and enzymes.[2] Dopamine ß-hydroxylase is a copper containing enzyme responsible for conversion of dopamine to norepinephrine, which mediates many neurologic functions. Copper also acts as a ligand to ferroxidase II, which oxidizes iron, helping in the mobilization and transport from hepatic stores to the bone marrow for erythropoiesis.[3] Thus, copper deficiency results in excessive iron in the liver but defective transport of iron to the marrow for effective erythropoiesis.[4]

7.1 Causes of copper deficiency
Acquired copper deficiency is rare. The few potential causes are
1. Gastric and bariatric surgery causing malabsorption[5,6]
2. Intravenous hyperalimentation without copper supplementation
3. Hyperzincaemia
4. Menkes disease, an inherited copper deficiency disorder, in which there is a failure of transporting absorbed copper to the rest of the body from mucosal cells.

7.2 Haematological manifestations of copper deficiency
Copper deficiency can cause anaemia and leukopenia. Sideroblastic changes and nuclear maturation defects in erythroid precursors leading to anaemia have been observed in patients with copper deficiency.[1] Peripheral smear often reveals sideroblastic anaemia with hypochromic microcytic red cells. Leucopenia and thrombocytopenia are less common.[7] The MCV is normal or increased in anaemia of copper deficiency.

7.3 Other manifestations
Copper deficiency is known to cause neurologic deficits due to demyelination. Manifestations include myelopathy, polyneuropathy, ataxia and optic neuritis.[8] The combination of myelopathy, polyneuropathy and anaemia in copper deficiency can mimic the deficits seen with vitamin B12 deficiency.

7.4 Treatment
Copper deficiency can be treated with either oral copper supplementation or intravenous copper.[9] If zinc intoxication is present, discontinuation of zinc may be sufficient to restore copper levels back to normal, but this is usually a very slow process.[9] They will also need to take copper supplements in addition to stopping zinc consumption. Haematological manifestations are often quickly restored back to normal.[9] The neurological symptoms will often cease, but the symptoms are not always restored back to normal.

7.5 Selenium
Selenium is a vital trace element for efficient and effective operation of many functions of the human immune system.[10,11] Selenium is a mineral that is required by the body in trace amounts. Daily requirement of selenium is 50 micrograms. It is present in most organs of the body like kidneys, spleen, liver, pancreas. Selenium is a component of glutathione peroxidase and can be used as an antioxidant and also plays a large role in cell metabolism and cancer prevention.

7.5.1 Selenium deficiency

Selenium deficiency is relatively rare in healthy well-nourished individuals.
Causes of selenium deficiency
1.   Eating foods predominantly grown in selenium-deficient soil.
2.   Severely compromised intestinal function
3.   Total parenteral nutrition
4.   Gastrointestinal bypass surgery

Manifestations of a selenium deficiency include cardiovascular disease, nerve degeneration, hypothyroidism, arthritis and anaemia. A selenium deficiency may even increase the chances of developing some forms of cancer.

Selenium deficiency may play a role in causing or aggravating anaemia as glutathione peroxidase protects red blood cells from free radical damage and destruction. In a prevalence study there was low serum selenium found independently associated with anaemia among older men and women.[12] Mean serum selenium among non-anaemic and anaemic adults was 1.60 and 1.51 umol /L (P=0.0003). The prevalence of anaemia among adults in the lowest to highest quartiles of serum selenium was 18.3, 9.5, 9.7 and 6.9%, respectively (P=0.0005).[12]

7.5.2 Supplements

There are many forms of selenium supplements including organic selenium rich yeast, selenium in the form of selenomethionine, and inorganic sodium selenite. Selenium yeast increases the blood selenium levels and sodium selenite helps to increase the activity of glutathione peroxidase. Organic selenium is better absorbed and less toxic than the inorganic forms. People who are at risk of selenium deficiency will benefit from supplements.

8. References

8.1 References part 1 (1-2)

[1] Worldwide prevalence of anaemia 1993-2005 (2008) Editors: Bruno de Benoist, Erin McLean, Ines Egli, Mary Cogswell, 2008. ISBN: 978 92 4 159665 7.

[2] World Health Organization [WHO], Division of Family Health, Maternal Health and Safe Motherhood Programme, Division of Health Protection and Promotion, Nutrition Programme; WHO. The Prevalence of Anaemia in Women: a tabulation of available information. 2nd ed. Geneva, Switzerland, World Health Organization. 1992.

[3] ACC/SCN (United Nations Administrative Committee on Coordination/Standing Committee on Nutrition). 2004. Fifth report on the world nutrition situation: Nutrition for improved development outcomes. Geneva, 2004, available at accscn@who.org.

[4] Maberly GF, Trowbridge FL, Yip R, Sullivan KM, West CE. programs against micronutrient malnutrition: Ending hidden hunger. Annu Rev Public Health 1994; 15:277-301.

[5] Iron deficiency anaemia: assessment, prevention and control. 2001. World Health Organization Publication WHO/NHD/01.3.

[6] Zimmermann MB, Hurrell RF. Nutritional iron deficiency. Lancet 2007; 370, 9586, 511-520. doi:10.1016/S0140-6736.

[7] Looker AC, Dallman PR, Carrol MD, Gunter EW, Johnson CL. Prevalence of Iron Deficiency in the United States. JAMA. 1997;277:973-976.

[8] Institute of Medicine. Dietary Reference Intakes (DRIs) for Vitamin A, Vitamin K, Arsenic, Boron, Chromium, Copper, Iodine, Iron, Manganese, Molybdenum, Nickel, Silicon, Vanadium, and Zinc. Washington, DC: National Academy Press; 2002, 18-19.

[9] Zini G, Di Mario A, Garzia M, Bianchi M, d'Onofrio G.Reticulocyte population data in different erythropoietic states J. Clin. Pathol. 2011 64:159-163.

[10] Goddard AF, James MW, McIntyre AS, Scott BB; on behalf of the British Society of Gastroenterology. Guidelines for the management of iron deficiency anaemia. Gut. 2011 Jun 6. [Epub ahead of print]

[11] Andrews NC. Disorders of iron metabolism. N Engl J Med. 1999;341:1986–1995.

[12] Tomas Ganz. Hepcidin and iron regulation, 10 years later. BLOOD, 2011; 117, 4425-4433.

[13] Park CH, Valore EV, Waring AJ, Ganz T. Hepcidin, a urinary antimicrobial peptide synthesized in the liver. J Biol Chem. 2001;276:7806–7810.

[14] Weinstein DA, Roy CN, Fleming MD, Loda MF, Wolfsdorf JI, Andrews NC. Inappropriate expression of hepcidin is associated with iron refractory anemia: implications for the anemia of chronic disease. Blood. 2002;100:3776–3781.

[15] Nemeth E, Ganz T. The role of hepcidin in iron metabolism. Acta Hematol. 2009; 122: 78-86.

[16] Auerbach M, Ballard H, Glaspy J. Clinical update: intravenous iron for anaemia. Lancet 2007; 369: 1502-4.

[17] Kumar A, Jain S, Singh NP, Singh T. Oral versus high dose parenteral iron supplementation in pregnancy. Int J Gynaecol Obstet 2005; 89:7-13.

[18] Jacobs P, Johnson G, Wood L. Oral iron therapy in human subjects, comparative absorption between ferrous salts and iron polymaltose. J Med. 1984;15:367-377.

[19] Maxton DG, Thompson RP, Hinder RC. Absorption of iron from ferric hydroxypyranone complexes. Br J Nutr. 1994;71:203-207.

[20] Sharma N. Iron absorption: IPC therapy is superior to conventional iron salts. Obstet Gynecol. 2001;515-19.

[21] Geisser P. In vitro studies on interactions of iron salts and complexes with food stuffs and medicaments. Arzneimittelforschung 1990;40:754-760.

[22] Jenkins A. Using iron dextran to treat iron-deficiency anemia. Hospital Pharmacist. 2005; 12: 224-225.

[23] Lawrence R. Development and comparison of iron dextran products. PDA J Pharm Sci Technol. 1998; 52:190-7.

[24] Auerbach M, Goodnough LT, Picard D, Maniatis A. The role of intravenous iron in anemia management and transfusion avoidance. Transfusion 2008; 48:988-1000.

[25] Auerbach M, Rodgers GM. Intravenous iron. N Engl J Med 2007; 357:93-4.

[26] Khalafallah A, Dennis A, Bates J, Bates G, Robertson IK, Smith L, Ball MJ, Seaton D, Brain T, Rasko JE. A prospective randomized, controlled trial of intravenous versus oral iron for moderate iron deficiency anaemia of pregnancy. J Intern Med. 2010; 268:286-95. Epub 2010 May 19.

[27] Hamstra RD, Block MH, Schokert AL. Intravenous iron dextran in clinical medicine. JAMA. 1980; 2;243:1726-31.

[28] Faich G, Strobos J. Sodium ferric gluconate complex in sucrose: safer intravenous iron therapy than iron dextrans. Am J Kidney Dis. 1999;33:464-70.

[29] Burns DL, Pomposelli JJ. Toxicity of parenteral iron dextran therapy. Kidney Int Suppl. 1999; 69:S119-24.

[30] Michael B, Coyne DW, Fishbane S. et al. Sodium ferric gluconate complex in hemodialysis patients: adverse reactions compared to placebo and iron dextran. Kidney Int. 2002; 61:1830-9.

[31] Fishbane S, Kowalski EA. Comparative safety of intravenous iron dextran, iron saccharate and sodium ferric gluconate. Semin Dial. 2000;13:381-4.

[32] Garg M, Morrison G, Friedman A, Lau A, Lau D, Gibson PR. A rapid infusion protocol is safe for total dose iron polymaltose: time for change. Intern Med J. 2011;41:548-54. doi: 10.1111/j.1445-5994.2010.02356.x.

[33] Manoharan A, Ramakrishna R, Pereira B. Delayed adverse reactions to total-dose intravenous iron polymaltose. Intern Med J. 2009;39:857.

[34] Monograph ferumoxytol (Feraheme). (2009) AMAG Pharmaceuticals Inc.

[35] Rosner MH, Auerbach M. Ferumoxytol for the treatment of iron deficiency. Expert Rev Hematol. 2011;4:399-406.

[36] Kulnigg S, Stoinov S, Simanenkov V et al. A novel intravenous iron formulation for treatment of anemia in inflammatory bowel disease: the ferric carboxymaltose (FERINJECT) randomized controlled trial. Am J Gastroenterol. 2008; 103:1182-1192.

[37] Qunibi W, Dinh Q, Benjamin J. Safety and Tolerability Profile of Ferric Carboxymaltose (FCM) a New High Dose Intravenous Iron, across Ten Multi-Center Trials. J Am Soc Nephrol. 2007; 18: SU-PO1029.

[38] Kalra PA. Introducing iron isomaltoside 1000 (Monofer®)-development rationale and clinical experience. NDT Plus; 2011; 4 (s1): doi: 10.1093/ndtplus/sfr042

[39] Jahn MR, Andreasen HB, Fütterer S, Nawroth T, Schünemann V, Kolb U, Hofmeister W, Muñoz M, Bock K, Meldal M, Langguth P. A comparative study of the physicochemical properties of iron isomaltoside 1000 (Monofer®), a new intravenous iron preparation and its clinical implications. Eur J Pharm Biopharm. 2011;78:480-91. Epub 2011 Mar 23.

[40] Al RA, Unlubilgin E, Kandemir O, Yalvac S, Cakir L, Haberal A. intravenous versus oral iron for treatment of anemia in pregnancy: a randomized trial. Obstet Gynecol 2005; 106:1335-40.

[41] Bayoumeu F, Subiran-Buisset C, Baka NE, Legagneur H, Monnier-Barbarino P, Laxenaire MC. Iron therapy in iron deficiency anemia in pregnancy: intravenous route versus oral route. Am J Obstet Gynecol 2002; 186:518-22.

[42] Reveiz L, Gyte GML, Cuervo LG. Treatments for iron-deficiency anaemia in pregnancy. Cochrane Database Syst Rev. 2007; Issue 2. Art. No.: CD003094. DOI: 10.1002/14651858.CD003094.pub2.

[43] Isbister JP, Shander A, Spahn DR, Erhard J, Farmer SL, Hofmann A. Adverse blood transfusion outcomes: establishing causation. Transfus Med Rev. 2011;25:89-101. Epub 2011 Feb 23.

[44] Aickin M, Gensler H. Adjusting for multiple testing when reporting research results: the Bonferroni vs Holm methods. Am J Public Health 1996; 86:726-8.

[45] Reveiz L, Gyte GML, Cuervo LG. Treatments for iron-deficiency anaemia in pregnancy. Cochrane Database Syst Rev. 2007; Issue 2. Art. No.: CD003094. DOI: 10.1002/14651858.CD003094.pub2.

[46] Auerbach M, Goodnough LT, Picard D, Maniatis A. The role of intravenous iron in anemia management and transfusion avoidance. Transfusion 2008; 48:988-1000.

[47] Auerbach M, Rodgers GM. Intravenous iron. N Engl J Med 2007; 357:93-4.

8.2 References part 2 (3-4)

[1] Antony AC: Megaloblastic anemias. In: Hoffman R, Benz Jr EJ, Shattil SJ, et al ed. Hematology: Basic Principles and Practice, 5th ed. Churchill-Livingstone; 2008, chapter 39.

[2] Stover P: Physiology of folate and vitamin B12 in health and disease. Nutr Rev 2004; 62:S3.

[3] Reynolds E, Vitamin B12, folic acid, and the nervous system. Lancet Neurol. 2006 Nov;5(11):949-60. Review.

[4] Remacha AF, Vitamin B12 deficiency, hyperhomocysteinemia and thrombosis: a case and control study, Int J Hematol. 2011 Apr;93(4):458-64. Epub 2011 Apr 8.

[5] Chanarin I. The Megaloblastic Anaemias, 1st ed. Blackwell Scientific; 1979.

[6] Antony AC. Vegetarianism and vitamin B-12 (cobalamin) deficiency. Am J Clin Nutr. 2003;78:3-6.

[7] Carmel R. Malabsorption of food cobalamin. Baillieres Clin Haematol. 1995;8:639-655.

[8] Kokkola A, Sjoblom S-M, Haapiainen R, et al.. The risk of gastric carcinoma and carcinoid tumours in patients with pernicious anaemia. Scand J Gastroenterol. 1998;33:88-92.

[9] Curtis AD et al. Clin Lab Haematol 1986; 8: 135-140.

[10] Doscherholmen A, Swaim WR. Impaired assimilation of egg Co57 vitamin B12 in patients with hypochlorhydria and achlorhydria and after gastric resection. Gastroenterology. 1973;64:913-919.

[11] Savage DG, Lindenbaum J, Stabler SP, Allen RH. Sensitivity of serum methylmalonic acid and total homocysteine determinations for diagnosing cobalamin and folate deficiencies. Am J Med. 1994; 96:239-246.

[12] Allen RH, Stabler SP, Savage DG, Lindenbaum J. Diagnosis of cobalamin deficiency: usefulness of serum methylmalonic acid and total homocysteine concentrations. Am J Hematol. 1990;34:90-98.

[13] Lindenbaum J, Savage DG, Stabler SP, Allen RH. Diagnosis of cobalamin deficiency: II. Relative sensitivities of serum cobalamin, methylmalonic acid, and total homocysteine concentrations. Am J Hematol. 1990;34:99-107.

[14] Yao Y et al. J Fam Pract 1992; 35: 524-528.

[15] Oh R et al. Am Fam Physician 2003; 67(5): 993-994.

[16] Savage D, Lindenbaum J. Relapses after interruption of cyanocobalamin therapy in patients with pernicious anemia. Am J Med. 1983;74:765-772.

[17] Tudhope GR, Swan HT, Spray GH. Patient variation in pernicious anaemia, as shown in a clinical trial of cyanocobalamin, hydroxocobalamin, and cyanocobalamin-zinc tannate. Br J Haematol.1967;13:216-228.

[18] Tordjman R, Genereau T, Guinnepain MT, et al. Reintroduction of vitamin B12 in 2 patients with prior B12-induced anaphylaxis. Eur J Haematol. 1998;60:269-270.

[19] Antoinette M. Kuzminski, et al. Effective treatment of cobalamin deficiency with oral cobalamin. Blood, 1998 92: 1191-1198.

[20] Carmel R: How I treat cobalamin (vitamin B12) deficiency, Blood, 2008, Volume 112,6

[21] Berlin H, Berlin R, Brante G. Oral treatment of pernicious anemia with high doses of vitamin B12 without intrinsic factor. Acta Med Scand. 1968;184:247-258.
[22] Carmel R. Efficacy and safety of fortification and supplementation with vitamin B12: biochemical and physiologic effects. Food Nutr Bull. 2008;29(suppl):S177-S187.

8.3 References part 3(5-6)

[1] Varela-Moreiras G, Murphy MM, Scott JM. Cobalamin, folic acid, and homocysteine. Nutr Rev. May 2009;67 Suppl 1:S69-72.
[2] Wolff T, Witkop CT, Miller T, Syed SB. Folic acid supplementation for the prevention of neural tube defects: an update of the evidence for the U.S. Preventive Services Task Force. Ann Intern Med. May 52009;150(9):632-9.
[3] Blount BC, Mack MM, Wehr CM, et al. Folate deficiency causes uracil misincorporation into human DNA and chromosome breakage: implications for cancer and neuronal damage. Proc Natl Acad Sci U S A. Apr 1 1997;94(7):3290-5
[4] Savage DG, Lindenbaum J, Stabler SP, Allen RH. Sensitivity of serum methylmalonic acid and total homocysteine determinations for diagnosing cobalamin and folate deficiencies. Am J Med. 1994; 96:239-246.
[5] Herbert V. Development of Human Folate Deficiency. In: Picciano MF, Stokstool ELR, Gregory, JF, eds.Folic Acid Metabolism in Health and Disease (Contemporary Issues in Clinical Nutrition). 13. New York,NY: 1990:195-210.
[6] Whittle S, Hughes R: Folate supplementation and methotrexate treatment in rheumatoid arthritis: A review. *Rheumatology* 2004; 43:267.

8.4 References part 4 (7)

[1] Williams DM. Copper deficiency in humans. Semin Hematol 1983; 20: 118-28.
[2] Wu J et al, Copper Deficiency as Cause of Unexplained Hematologic and Neurologic Deficits in Patient with Prior Gastrointestinal Surgery, *JABFM*, 19:191-194 (2006)
[3] Turnlund J. Copper. In: Shils M, Olson J, Shike M, editors. Modern nutrition in health and disease. Philadelphia: Lippincott; 1998. p. 241.
[4] Fields M, Bureau I, Lewis CG. Ferritin is not an indicator of available hepatic iron stores in anemia of copper deficiency in rats. Clin Chem 1997; 43(8 Pt 1): 1457-9.
[5] Kumar N, Ahlskog JE, Gross JB, Jr. Acquired hypocupremia after gastric surgery. Clin Gastroenterol Hepatol 2004; 2: 1074-9.
[6] Thaisetthawatkul P, Collazo-Clavell ML, Sarr MG, Norell JE, Dyck PJ. A controlled study of peripheral neuropathy after bariatric surgery. Neurology 2004; 63: 1462-70.
[7] Hayton BA, Broome HE, Lilenbaum RC. Copper deficiency-induced anemia and neutropenia secondary to intestinal malabsorption. Am J Hematol 1995; 48: 45-7.
[8] Kumar N, Crum B, Petersen RC, Vernino SA, Ahlskog JE. Copper deficiency myelopathy. Arch Neurol 2004; 61: 762-6.
[9] Kumar, N. Copper deficiency myelopathy (human swayback). Mayo Clinic Proceedings. 2006; 81, 1371-1384.
[10] Rayman MP. The importance of selenium to human health. Lancet. 2000;356:233-241.
[11] 14. Arthur JR, McKenzie RC, Beckett GJ. Selenium in the immune system. J Nutr. 2003;133:1457-1459.
[12] Semba RD, Low serum selenium is associated with anemia among older adults in the United States, Eur J Clin Nutr. 2009;63:93-9. Epub 2007 Sep 5.

Nutritional Anemia in Developing Countries

Frank T. Wieringa, Jacques Berger and Marjoleine A. Dijkhuizen

¹NutriPass – UMR204, Institute for Research for Development (IRD),
IRD-UM2-UM1, Montpellier
²Department of Human Nutrition, Copenhagen University
¹France
²Denmark

1. Introduction

As described in earlier chapters, anemia is characterized by an insufficient concentration of the protein hemoglobin in the circulation, causing a lack of oxygen transporting capacity. Hemoglobin is the principal component of red blood cells, erythrocytes, and is synthesised in the bone marrow with iron as the key oxygen binding site. Before discussing causes and consequences of nutritional anemia in developing countries, it is important to consider briefly how anemia is diagnosed.

Anemia can be diagnosed clinically, for example by looking at the paleness of the skin or mucosa or by a history of weakness and dizziness. This clinical assessment is often the only method available in resource-poor settings, but unfortunately has a low sensitivity and specificity (Critchley and Bates 2005). A more direct and thus more sensitive and specific approach is to measure hemoglobin concentrations in the blood, using one of many different techniques in blood samples obtained by either finger prick or vena-puncture. The obtained values are then compared to those from a matching, normal population, using pre-defined cut-offs for anemia. It is important to realize that different cut-off thresholds are used for different situations. For example, there are different cut-off points for young children, pregnant women, non-pregnant women and men, as well as ethnic differences and differences between smokers and non-smokers. Moreover, altitude affects hemoglobin concentrations and hence cut-offs for anemia. Therefore, it is very important to select the correct reference population for the subjects studied. Cut-off thresholds are normally chosen as the point at which 2.5% of the normal population (or 2 standard deviations) has a value that is lower. Hence, in a normal population, 2.5% of the people will be anemic according to this definition. From an epidemiological viewpoint, this means that if a survey finds a prevalence of anemia close to 2.5%, the studied population can be regarded as normal. From an individual viewpoint however, if a subject from that same population was diagnosed with anemia, s/he would not regard this as normal, would like to know the cause, and if indicated, s/he would like to be treated! Moreover, cut-offs are certainly not absolute or unequivocal, rather, they should be regarded as a proposed value that is accepted by consensus, and are sometimes challenged if found insufficiently accurate. For example, there is currently discussion regarding the cut-off for anemia in infants. Domellof et al. have proposed more precise, stratified cut-off thresholds for anemia at hemoglobin concentrations of <105 g/L for infants 4 – 6 months of age and <100 g/L for infants 9 mo of age (Domellof et al. 2002a), but as shown in Table 1, these revised cut-offs have not been implemented by the public health community yet.

Reference group	cut-off (g/L)	Categories of anemia (g/L)		
		Mild	Moderate	Severe
Pregnant women	110	100-110	70-99	<70
Non-pregnant women	120	110-119	80-109	<80
Children 6 – 59 months of age	110	100-109	70-99	<70
Children 5 – 11 years of age	115	110-114	80-1-9	<80
Children 12 – 14 years of age	120	110-119	80-109	<80
Men	130	110-129	80-109	<80

Table 1. Cut-off values used by the World Health Organization to define anemia in different population groups (WHO 2001).

There are many different causes of anemia. Pathophysiologically speaking, anemia occurs either through a) blood loss in quantities higher than the body can replete through synthesis, b) an increased breakdown in the body of erythrocytes or c) a defect in the synthesis of hemoglobin protein or of new erythrocytes. An increased breakdown of erythrocytes occurs for example in sickle cell disease (sickle cell anemia) and in malaria. However, almost all anemias caused by nutritional deficiencies affect the production of new erythrocytes or hemoglobin, thereby causing anemia.

A large part of the human population is affected by anemia, with an estimated 1.6 billion people being anemic. Iron deficiency (ID) is most often, but certainly not the only cause of nutritional anemia. Indeed, many studies have shown that iron deficiency accounts roughly for only half of the anemia cases (Wieringa et al. 2007a), meaning that improving iron status in an anemic population will only reduce the prevalence of anemia to a certain extent. On the other hand, more people have insufficient iron stores than anemia, as anemia only occurs at the end stage, when iron deficiency eventually leads to so-called iron-deficiency anemia (IDA). Indeed, the World Health Organization (WHO) estimates that roughly twice as many people are affected by iron deficiency than by iron deficiency anemia (WHO 2001).

Prevalences of anemia and iron deficiency are much higher in developing countries than in affluent countries. However, large differences in anemia prevalence exist among different continents and among different countries on the same continent. Reasons for these differences are many and include differences in basic health and nutrition characteristics (such as diet, prevalence of nutritional deficiencies, prevalence of anemia-causing illnesses such as intestinal parasites or malaria) and other factors affecting hemoglobin and erythrocyte concentrations such as sickle cell anemia or other hemoglobinopathies and altitude. To appreciate the extent of anemia as a public health problem, one only has to review the data on anemia prevalence around the world.

The highest burden of anemia and ID is found in Africa and South Asia, with many studies showing the significant public health impact of anemia in these populations. In India, the prevalence of anemia is >50% in both pregnant and non-pregnant women (WHO 2008). Low birth weight and perinatal mortality increase two-fold when hemoglobin concentrations are <80 g/L during pregnancy. Not surprisingly, anemia is estimated to be responsible for 40% of maternal deaths in India (Kalaivani 2009). In rural Bangladesh, more than 30% of nulliparous married women were anemic when entering pregnancy, with 15% being iron deficient and 11% having IDA (Khambalia et al. 2009). And already more than 80% had inadequate iron stores, which was defined as <500 mg of iron. In Pakistan, anemia prevalence was even higher: in a large prospective observational study in ~1400 pregnant women, 90.5% were anemic (Hb<110 g/L) (Baig-Ansari et al. 2008). In Africa, the prevalence of anemia in women of reproductive age (WRA) is estimated to be ~47% and in pregnant women ~57% (WHO 2008), although prevalence rates differ widely from country to country (Lartey 2008). In Mali, anemia was present in 47% of pregnant women (Hb<110 g/L), but only 13% of the women had ID (serum ferritin <12 µg/l) (Ayoya et al. 2006). Infectious diseases were a major contributor to anemia in this study. Among pregnant women in northern Nigeria, 30% was classified as anemic (Hb< 105 g/l); Here, the major contributing factor to anemia was ID (ferritin<10 µg/L) (Vanderjagt et al. 2007). Besides ID, vitamin B12 and folic acid deficiencies were probably prevalent also. In Ghana, anemia (Hb < 110 g/L) was observed in 34 % of the pregnant women from urban areas, with 16% of the women having ID (ferritin≤ 16 µg/l) and only 7.5% having IDA (Engmann et al. 2008). Malaria was a greater risk factor than ID for being anemic in this study. Hence, in Sub-Saharan Africa ID is prevalent, but not as strongly related to anemia, as other causes of anemia such as malaria infection are also prevalent in vulnerable groups. Other areas in the world are affected by a high prevalence of anemia also. In Vietnam, more than half of 900 women investigated in a representative community survey in healthy women of reproductive age were anemic (Trinh and Dibley 2007). In contrast, in Thailand in a similar survey only 14.1 % of 590 women was found to be anemic (Hb< 11g/dl), and 6.0% had IDA, according to the WHO criteria (Sukrat et al.). These last figures are more typical for developed countries. IDA was found in 4% of French children <2 yrs (Hercberg et al. 2001), and in the USA iron deficiency was found in 14.4% of children between 1 and 2 yrs, and in 9.2% of women of reproductive age (Cogswell et al. 2009). Worryingly, there appears to be no decrease in the prevalence of iron deficiency in young children over the last decades, with especially overweight children at risk for ID (Cogswell et al. 2009).

From above data, it is clear that anemia is widespread throughout the world, and given the negative effects of anemia on health and development, a world-wide public health concern. Indeed, for decades the urgent need for interventions to reduce the prevalence of anemia has been recognized, but most interventions have had little impact (Stoltzfus 2008; Yip 2002). From the above studies, it is also clear that the distinction between anemia, IDA and ID is important, not only because of differences in prevalence and health effects of these entities, but also because the etiology and underlying determinants are distinct and call for different intervention strategies. Anemia, IDA and ID are of course interrelated and overlapping diagnoses but do not constitute a complete continuum, and specific factors, causes and determinants play a different role in each entity. Furthermore, the above studies also show that prevalence patterns of anemia and iron deficiency indicators can vary widely among populations, depending on baseline health and nutritional determinants. Below, some key aspects of the etiology, the measurement and the public health impact of anemia will be reviewed, before discussing what can be done to reduce the global burden of anemia.

2. Nutritional causes of anemia with special reference to developing countries

For some micronutrients, such as iron and vitamin B_{12}, there is a clear understanding on why deficiency leads to anemia. For others, such as selenium or vitamin A, the underlying mechanisms are less clear. Moreover, it appears that some nutrients act synergistically, where deficiency of one micronutrient might either aggravate or mask the effects of deficiency of another micronutrient, such as is the case for Vitamin B_{12} and folic acid. Furthermore, anemia is the end result of a long process, often with a multi-factorial etiology, with other health determinants often also playing a role. Therefore, anemia has been difficult to address from a public health point of view, and remains present in many populations despite countless intervention efforts.

As the etiology of anemia has been covered extensively in previous chapters and in other books, this chapter will focus mainly on strategies to prevent anemia from nutritional causes and reduce the prevalence in various populations, especially in those vulnerable groups that have the largest burden or the largest health impact of anemia. For more detailed information on the etiology of nutritional anemia, interested readers can freely download the book 'Nutritional Anemia' from the Sight and Life website (Sight_and_Life 2007). However, as some nutritional aspects of the etiology of anemia are important for understanding the ratio behind certain interventions, these are highlighted in this chapter when necessary.

Anemia is often considered a synonym for iron deficiency. However, as described above, anemia and iron deficiency are distinct, albeit overlapping, conditions. Anemia occurs in the later stages of iron deficiency, when iron stores are completely depleted. However, before anemia occurs, iron deficiency is already affecting other functions, such as the immune system and the nervous system, leading to reduced immunocompetence, decreased physical activity and cognitive impairment (Beard 2001). Physiologically, iron deficiency occurs when requirements exceed the amount of iron absorbed from the diet. Requirements are increased by rapid increases in body mass (such as in pregnant women, young children) or by high losses of iron (menstruation, hookworm infection). This explains in part the high prevalence in vulnerable groups such as children and pregnant women, and on the other hand, the association of anemia with poverty and poor health. A special situation is sequestration of iron in the body, making it less available for utilisation for e.g. hemoglobin synthesis, such as happens in (chronic) infection by the acute phase response or in massive erythrocyte breakdown (such as in malaria). Looking at the uptake of iron, it is found that in general iron absorption is low (~5%) from plant-based diets (developing countries) because of iron-uptake inhibiting factors (phytates, polyphenols) and iron absorption is higher (~15%) from diets containing more meat and fish (developed countries) because iron in animal products is often bound in heme protein structures that greatly facilitates absorption. This explains in part the much higher prevalence of ID in developing countries.

Other nutrients in the diet are also important, and deficiencies of other nutrients can directly or indirectly contribute to anemia and sometimes even to ID. The role of vitamin A in iron metabolism was recognized already in the 1980's (Mejia and Chew 1988), when studies showed that the effect of iron supplementation on hemoglobin concentrations could be enhanced by the addition of vitamin A (Suharno et al. 1993). The mechanisms by which vitamin A enhances hemoglobin formation are not completely understood, but vitamin A is thought to play a role in the absorption of iron and/or in the utilization of iron stores for new heme production (Zimmermann et al. 2006). Because interactions are probably on the level of gene expression and protein synthesis, it is an intricate and finely balanced interplay and deficiencies or excess can have indirect and sometimes unanticipated effects. In the latter case, this means that providing vitamin A to subjects with a marginal iron status would make these subjects more iron deficient, as extra iron would be used for the production of hemoglobin, and is no longer available for other tissues such as the brain. Indeed, we showed in a large multi-country trial in SE Asia that vitamin A supplementation in infancy, without interventions to improve iron status, was associated with anemia (Wieringa et al. 2007a). This is an important reminder that understanding of the underlying mechanisms is important, even though the final public health effect is the objective of an intervention.

Nutrient	(proposed) mechanism leading to anemia	Ref
Iron	Essential part of heme. Deficiency: reduced production of hemoglobin	(Bates et al. 1989)
Folic Acid	Deficiency: Impaired DNA synthesis leading to reduced number of erythrocytes	(Koury and Ponka 2004)
Vitamin B_{12} (Cobalamin)	Deficiency: Interference with folic acid metabolism (see above)	(Koury and Ponka 2004)
Vitamin B_2 (Riboflavin)	Likely involved in iron absorption in gut mucosa	(Powers 2003)
Vitamin B_6 (Pyridoxal)	Possibly involved in heme biosynthesis	(Sight_and_Life 2007)
Vitamin A	Possibly involved in heme biosynthesis, perhaps also involved in regulating availability of iron from liver stores	(Roodenburg et al. 1996; Zimmermann et al. 2006)
Vitamin E	Deficiency: Oxidative stress of the erythrocytes leading to increased hemolysis	(Sight and Life 2007)
Vitamin C	Availability in gut enhances conversion $Fe3+$ to $Fe2+$, increasing iron bioavailability.	(Bates et al. 1989)
Selenium	Deficiency: Possibly oxidative stress or increased inflammation	(Van Nhien et al. 2008)
Copper	Deficiency: Interference with red cell maturation and iron absorption	(Sight_and_Life 2007)

Table 2. Nutrients associated with anemia in developing countries.

Other deficiencies clearly related to the development of anemia are vitamin B_{12} and folic acid deficiency. Deficiency will lead to a characteristic megaloblastic anemia, meaning larger than normal erythrocytes, with poorly differentiated nuclei (Sight_and_Life 2007). Neither vitamin B_{12} nor folic acid deficiency is a rare condition in developing countries, and both contribute to the overall high rates of anemia seen in developing countries. Folic acid is also involved in the neural development of the fetus, and deficiency can result in very distinct malformations. Indeed, flour fortification with folic acid in the USA has resulted in a dramatic decrease in neural tube defects (Berry et al. 2010), making it a very cost-effective intervention (Grosse et al. 2005). The role of vitamin E and selenium in the etiology of anemia is less clear. Suggested mechanisms involve increased oxidative stress, leading to earlier breakdown of erythrocytes or increased inflammation.

Inflammation itself is associated with anemia, and this is often referred to as the 'anemia of chronic disease'. Immune activation leads to a decrease in erythropoiesis (synthesis of new erythrocytes), which eventually will lead to lower hemoglobin concentrations and anemia. Immune activation, and especially the so-called acute-phase response, which is the generalized reaction of the body to infection or trauma, also results in a re-distribution of many nutrients in the human body. This re-distribution makes it more difficult for pathogens to replicate, and has been termed 'nutritional immunity' (Weinberg 1975). However, this re-distribution of nutrients such as iron, vitamin A and zinc by the acute phase response also distorts the measurement of micronutrient status by changing the plasma concentration of indicators commonly used to assess status. We and others have been trying to quantify the extent of this distortion by the acute phase response on several indicators (Wieringa et al. 2002), and have proposed factors (Table 3) to correct for the effects of inflammation (Thurnham et al. 2010; Thurnham et al. 2003). This is important for the estimation of the prevalence of micronutrient deficiencies in populations. If inflammation prevalence is high, e.g. in areas with endemic malaria, the perceived prevalence of vitamin A and zinc deficiencies will be significantly higher, as plasma retinol and zinc concentrations are reduced by inflammation. On the other hand, the perceived prevalence of ID and IDA will be significantly lower, as ferritin concentrations are increased in inflammation. Hence, the acute phase response should be taken into account when using indicators of micronutrient status sensitive to it by concomitantly measuring concentrations of acute phase proteins such as C-reactive protein (CRP) and α1-acid glycoprotein (AGP).

	Incubation phase (only CRP elevated)	Early convalescence phase (CRP and AGP raised)	Late convalescence phase (only AGP raised)
Ferritin ratios compared to no inflammation	1.30	1.90	1.36
Proposed correction factors for ferritin concentrations	0.77	0.53	0.75

Table 3. Effect of different phases of inflammation on ferritin concentration, and proposed factors to correct for the effect of inflammation on ferritin concentrations. Adapted from (Thurnham et al. 2010).

3. Interventions to reduce the prevalence of anemia

Unfortunately, efforts in the last decades to reduce the prevalence of anemia and iron deficiency have not been too successful. As anemia has a multi-factorial etiology, reasons for success or failure of interventions are also many. One striking feature of all public health interventions is the huge difference between the efficacy of studies done in a controlled research setting and the effectiveness of strategies implemented on a national scale. Unfortunately, anemia and iron deficiency interventions also demonstrate this difference compellingly. Whereas there are many studies published showing excellent efficacy of interventions to improve iron status in pregnant women or other risk groups, the few studies reporting effectiveness of large-scale iron interventions show little or no impact. Indeed, even the INACG (International Nutritional Anemia Consultative Group) was forced to conclude that although both daily and weekly iron supplementation regimens have been demonstrated to be efficacious in vulnerable population groups, existing data do not demonstrate that large-scale programs with iron supplementation are generally effective (INACG 2004).

3.1 Evidence-based intervention development and implementation: Moving policy forward

Globally, most efforts to reduce anemia have focused on pregnant women, with millions of iron and folic acid tablets being provided to pregnant women all over the world annually. There are several reasons for this specific attention during pregnancy. Looking more closely at the reasons shows how science, health care and policy interact together resulting in the development and implementation of interventions. First of all, iron requirements during pregnancy increase by more than two-fold, to >4 mg Fe/day (Steer 2000), an amount that is almost impossible to meet with a diet with low available iron (Yip 1996). Indeed, it is even difficult to meet this requirement with a Western-style diet (with meat) with high iron-availability. Thus interventions would be useful in this situation, and direct effects can be expected. Furthermore by targeting pregnant women, one hopes to break the negative inter-generational vicious circle of poor intra-uterine growth leading to low adult height predisposing to poor intra-uterine growth. . So interventions in this target group can also contribute more indirect, long-term effects. Thirdly, during pregnancy women are encouraged to access health services, offering opportunities for targeted interventions such as iron supplementation. Often, health care access for pregnant women is already part of national public health policy, with encouraging antenatal care programs and registration in place. Finally, most published studies have been done in pregnant women; hence most evidence on impact of interventions such as iron supplementation is available for pregnant women, driving policy towards strategies focusing on pregnant women. The available evidence informs and focuses policy interests, and as policy prefers predictable results this encourages policy development in this field. However, other closely linked groups also at risk for anemia such as young infants and children or women of reproductive age (WRA) are thereby often sidelined, as the available evidence for these groups is less complete and less clear, and effects less well documented. This results in less interest from policy, and less momentum to advocate and develop interventions for these groups. In this way, policy interests may drive science but science also steers policy interests. To remain updated on latest policy developments, specific sites such as eLENA from the WHO (www.who.int/elena/en) are available.

3.2 Interventions for pregnant women

A meta-analysis on the effects of iron and folic acid supplementation in pregnancy was recently done by Pena-Rosas and Viteri (Pena-Rosas and Viteri 2009). Their meta-analyses comprises 49 trials with >23,000 women. Data on anemia and IDA was available for 1108 women from 6 trials. In women taking iron supplements, 30.7% were still anemic at term, whereas only 4.9% had IDA. For women not receiving iron these figures were 54.8% and 15.5%. These findings clearly demonstrate the multi-factorial etiology of anemia. Iron deficiency and folic acid deficiency are only part of the problem. Hence, providing only iron and folic acid can only be expected to give a partial improvement in anemia prevalence, depending on the extent of the pre-existing deficiency of iron. Despite this remaining prevalence of anemia, the intervention significantly increased hemoglobin concentrations in the pregnant women, and thereby reduced the risk at term for anemia (RR 0.27 CI 0.17 – 0.42). Surprisingly, the authors found no significant effects on important health outcomes such as premature delivery, low birth weight (RR 0.79 CI 0.61 – 1.03), birth weight (+36.1 g CI -4.8 – 77.0), perinatal death or infant hemoglobin concentrations at 6 mo of age. It is important to consider these conclusions. Currently, blanket iron and folic acid supplementation programs for pregnant women are in place in many countries, with the expectation that it will substantially improve maternal and infant health (Bhutta et al. 2008). But apparently, the benefits of only iron and folate supplementation during pregnancy are less substantial and not as clear-cut as hoped for.

One explanation for the lack of improvement in maternal and infant health outcomes could be that the number of studies providing data on outcomes such as perinatal mortality was too low to draw consistent conclusions. Dibley and colleagues examined Indonesian demographic data with >40,000 pregnancies and showed that the iron and folic acid supplementation program protected against neonatal death in the first week after birth (RR: 0.53; 95% CI: 0.36–0.77) (Titaley et al. 2010b). And this beneficial effect also holds true in countries with endemic malaria, provided that it is combined with intermittent malaria treatment (Titaley et al. 2010a). Another explanation could be that other nutritional deficiencies, such as vitamin A deficiency or zinc deficiency, hampered a beneficial effect of the intervention. Perhaps, providing only iron (and folic acid) is not enough. Are multiple micronutrient supplements during pregnancy more effective? It is known that multiple micronutrient deficiencies often coexist (Dijkhuizen et al. 2001). Indeed, deficiency of multiple micronutrients in one individual is more common than single micronutrient deficiency (Thurlow et al. 2006). And given the multi-factorial etiology of anemia, a greater benefit might be expected from multiple micronutrient supplementation than from supplementation with iron and folic acid alone.

In the last decade, several large studies on the efficacy of multiple micronutrient supplementation during pregnancy on improving anemia and health outcomes have been conducted. However, results have been conflicting or confusing, partly because studies used different combinations of micronutrients, different amounts of micronutrients or different outcomes. An 2006 Cochrane review of 9 trials with >15,000 women showed that multiple micronutrient supplementation decreased the prevalence of low birth weight and maternal anemia (RR 0.61 CI 0.52 – 0.71) (Haider and Bhutta 2006). However, the effect of multiple micronutrient supplementation was not different from iron (+folic acid) supplementation alone and there was no effect on preterm births or peri-natal mortality. Hence, from this review, there appears to be no additional benefit of multiple micronutrient supplementation over only iron + folic acid during pregnancy. However, more recently, another meta-analysis using different criteria and inclusion of 2 recently published large trials, concluded that prenatal multi-micronutrient supplementation was associated with a significantly reduced risk of low birth weight and improved birth weight per se when compared with iron–folic acid supplementation (Shah and Ohlsson 2009). Some studies suggest that different combinations of micronutrients have different effects on the birth weight distribution curve, with iron and folic acid affecting the lower end of the distribution curve, meaning that there is only a specific effect on low-birth weight, without a change in overall birth weight. In contrast, supplementation with multiple micronutrients appears to shift the whole distribution curve to higher birth weights (Katz et al. 2006). Although this seems more beneficial, this could also have a downside. The shift towards higher birth weights after multiple micronutrient supplementation could possibly also increase the number of obstructed deliveries. Hence, the potential benefits on infant survival by reducing the number of low birth weight infants, might be nullified by increasing the number of large-for-gestational age infants (Katz et al. 2006). Also, there are indications that supplementation with micronutrients (especially zinc and vitamin A) during pregnancy might affect the immune system of the newborn, and that these effects might be long-lasting and may not be only beneficial (Raqib et al. 2007; Wieringa et al. 2010; Wieringa et al. 2008). It is unclear at present whether these concerns also hold true with a weekly multiple micronutrient supplement given during pregnancy, with supplements given before conception, or with food-based interventions such as fortification, but these strategies, by being more physiological, could well have less negative or nullifying effects and therefore be more effective overall. However, results of such interventions are scarce and not very clear yet at this moment.

Besides safety concerns, there are other aspects of supplementation programs which need to be taken into account. In a study in China, effects of micronutrient supplementation during pregnancy on outcomes such as birth weight were only significant when supplementation started *before 12 weeks* of gestation (Zeng et al. 2009). Neither iron + folic acid nor multiple micronutrient supplementation started after 12 weeks of gestational age had an effect on birth weight. Other studies confirm that hemoglobin concentrations early in pregnancy are related to low birth weight in a U-shaped curve. Women between 4 and 8 weeks of pregnancy with hemoglobin concentration between 90 and 99 g/L had a 3.27 (CI 1.09 – 9.77) higher risk for a low birth weight baby than the reference category (110 – 119 g/L), whereas risks for low birth weight and preterm birth also increased with hemoglobin concentrations >130 g/L (Zhou et al. 1998). However, it is unlikely that the conditions of the study (high compliance, very early start of supplementation) can be met by standard national programs, where women are more likely to report to the health system for the first time at around 16 weeks of pregnancy. Based on the above observations, it can be expected that the effects of supplementation programs for pregnant women, whether providing iron, iron + folic acid or multiple micronutrients, will be disappointingly small or absent.

3.3 Interventions for women of reproductive age

Surprisingly, only few studies have investigated the effects of pre-conception supplementation with iron or multiple micronutrients on maternal or neonatal health, even though improving micronutrient status before or early in pregnancy seems to be most effective, and nutritional status around conception is a very important determinant of pregnancy health and outcome. This is especially clear for folic acid, where pre-conceptual increases in status have a strong effect on the reduction of neural tube defects, with possibly >70% of neural tube defects prevented by adequate intakes of folic acid. For other micronutrients such as iron, the exact effect of pre-conception status on maternal and child health is less clear, mainly due a lack of studies in humans. To meet iron needs during gestation, women need an iron reserve of at least 300 - 500 mg prior to conception so as not to become iron deficient after the first trimester (Milman et al. 2005; Viteri and Berger 2005). Many women in developing countries will have much lower iron reserves than this and hence are at risk of becoming iron deficient during pregnancy. Indeed, even many women in affluent countries fail to enter pregnancy with adequate iron stores. Studies suggest that

56% of non-pregnant women in the USA had iron stores <300 mg (Viteri and Berger 2005) and <20% of Danish women were estimated to have adequate (>500 mg) iron stores before pregnancy (Milman et al. 2005). A multi-country trial in SE-Asia examined long-term effects of supplementing women of reproductive age with iron and folic acid by following the women through pregnancy and delivery (Cavalli-Sforza et al. 2005). In the non-pregnant women, iron status significantly improved over the intervention period. In Vietnam for example, anemia prevalence decreased from 45% at baseline to <20% after 9 months to 1 year. Moreover, longer pre-pregnancy supplementation was associated with less anemia and better iron status during the first and second trimester of pregnancy. Indeed, there was no IDA in the first and second trimester of pregnancy in women who started taking supplements >3 months before conception (Berger et al. 2005). Another important observation was that although anemia prevalence rose in the 3rd trimester of pregnancy, there was almost no severe anemia (Hb< 95 g/L). Severe anemia is directly associated with increased perinatal risk for mothers and newborns, whereas mild anemia is often physiological in the third trimester and is a sign of the hemodilution normally seen in pregnancy. Unfortunately, data on birth weight was available for only 200 infants, but there was a tendency towards higher birth weights per se (+81 g) in the weekly supplementation group (P=0.15) and towards lower prevalence of low birth weight (<2500 g; 3% and 9% respectively, P=0.08) (Berger et al. 2005). In Vietnam, weekly supplementation of iron and folic acid in combination with deworming has been continued as pilot to improve iron status of WRA and has been shown to be successful as such: provision of weekly iron and folic acid for free has resulted in significant reductions in anemia (from 38% to 19%) and ID (ferritin<15 µg/L) (23% to 9%) prevalence in Vietnamese WRA (Casey et al. 2009). Nowadays, the World Health Organization (WHO 2009) recommends weekly iron and folic acid in WRA as one of the strategies to reduce anemia during pregnancy.

Similar to pregnant women, deficiencies of more than one micronutrient are also likely in women of reproductive age. However, until now no studies have documented the long-term effects of providing women of reproductive age with multiple micronutrients.

3.4 Interventions for young children

Infants and young children are especially at risk of anemia and iron deficiency as growth increases nutrient requirements. Iron deficiency not only leads to anemia, but may, even before the onset of anemia, cause impairment of psycho-motor development which is in part irreversible (Beard 2001; Black 2003). In many developing countries, over 50% of infants are anemic by 1 year of age (Dijkhuizen et al. 2001). Although blanket iron supplementation for young children has being considered as an option to reduce anemia prevalence in childhood, studies comparing the effects of iron supplementation on infants in Sweden and Honduras suggested that iron supplementation in iron-replete infants may not be beneficial, and can cause growth faltering (Dewey et al. 2002). Furthermore iron supplementation in children living in malarious areas increased morbidity and mortality (Sazawal et al. 2006), iron supplementation may negatively influence zinc uptake and zinc status (Wieringa et al. 2007a), and iron supplementation in infancy may cause a redistribution of vitamin A (Wieringa et al. 2003) . Therefore, as public health interventions must operate from the 'Non Nocere' (Do No Harm) principle, these potential adverse effects make global blanket iron supplementation for under-five children unfeasible.

Four parallel studies on iron and zinc supplementation in infants were conducted in South-East Asia (Thailand, Vietnam and Indonesia) to investigate effects on micronutrient status and growth. These studies showed that although iron status and anemia prevalence were significantly improved, no overall effect on growth could be found (Dijkhuizen et al. 2008). Also, despite iron supplementation for 6 mo, at least 25% of the infants remained anemic in the iron-supplemented groups. The prevalence of iron deficiency anemia, however, was less than 2.5% after iron supplementation. Hence, the anemia remaining after supplementation may be due to unresolved deficiencies of other nutrients such as vitamin B_{12} or folic acid, to chronic inflammation, or to hereditary hemoglobinopathies. Estimates of for example α-thalassemia prevalence in the region ranges from 3 to 11% (Weatherall and Clegg 2001) and could explain at least part of the remaining anemia. However the data itself could also be interpreted differently perhaps. As discussed earlier, cut-off values for anemia in infancy are being reconsidered, and using other newly proposed (lower) cut-offs on these study results will give lower estimates of the prevalence of anemia. This is an important consideration whenever cut-off thresholds are used, the threshold that is used determines the prevalence found. Cut-off values for anemia that are currently used may not be appropriate for infants and may thus lead to an overestimation of anemia prevalence in this age group (Domellof et al. 2002a). Another interesting finding in the 4 studies in SE Asia, is that the effect of iron supplementation on hemoglobin concentrations was almost twice as large in boys than in girls (Wieringa et al. 2007b). Although hemoglobin concentrations differed between genders at recruitment, the differences were not as large as at the end of the study. Hence the largest part of the difference in hemoglobin concentrations between boy and girl infants developed during the second half of infancy. One possible explanation for these gender differences may be the higher growth rate of boy infants, leading to increased iron requirements. An important implication is that boy infants are more at risk for anemia and iron deficiency (Table 4), a finding that has been reported elsewhere also (Domellof et al. 2002b). We estimated that daily iron intake of boy infants should be almost 1 mg/d higher than that of girl infants to achieve similar iron body stores (Wieringa et al. 2007b). These considerations on age and gender related differences in iron status complicate the development of interventions, and together with the potential adverse effects of iron, make appropriate dosing and targeting important aspects to consider in intervention strategies for infants and under-five children. Also, approaches with lower, more physiological dosing such as weekly dosing and food based interventions such as fortification may have significant advantages here, as will be discussed below.

	Relative Risk for Boy infants
Anemia	1.6 (1.3 – 2.1)
Iron Deficiency Anemia	3.3 (2.1 – 5.0)

Table 4. Relative risk for boy infants to be anemic or have iron deficiency anemia at 11 months of age when not receiving iron supplements. Table adapted from (Wieringa et al. 2007b).

Besides supplementation, other strategies to improve anemia prevalence and micronutrient status of young children need to be considered. One noteworthy strategy is the provision of complementary foods fortified with micronutrients. In a series of studies in Vietnam, we showed that micronutrient-fortified complementary foods significantly improved iron status and reduced the prevalence of anemia (Phu et al. 2010). Importantly, the intervention showed that when infants received fortified complementary food from 5 months of age onwards, iron status remained at the same level, whereas iron status in the control group deteriorated over the 6 month intervention period. Other important strategies are delayed cord-clamping and the promotion of exclusive breastfeeding during the first 6 months of life (Dewey and Chaparro 2007). Indeed, iron stores can be increased by 33% by a 2-minute delay in clamping the umbilical cord (Dewey and Chaparro 2007)! De-worming is probably a less effective strategy in this age-group in Vietnam as the prevalence of parasitic infestation is still low, and only increases rapidly when the child starts to venture outside. However, large differences in the prevalence of parasitic infestation exist among cultures, so this intervention is also worth considering, and often added as an adjuvant measure in older children.

To conclude, although iron supplementation benefits hemoglobin concentrations and reduces the prevalence of anemia in infancy, potential adverse effects such as increased morbidity and mortality and growth-faltering in iron-replete infants make blanket supplementation unfeasible. Therefore, targeting is warranted, e.g. by screening infants prior to implementing iron supplementation. Appropriate and more physiological dosing is another important concern. Provision of high-quality complementary foods improves micronutrient status and reduces the prevalence of anemia, probably without the risk of detrimental effects on health or growth as seen with supplementation.

3.5 Interventions for school-aged children

School-age children are a neglected group with regard to interventions to reduce the prevalence of anemia or improve micronutrient status. One of the few interventions widely implemented is deworming. Helminthic infections have been shown to be major contributors to anemia and malnutrition in the developing world through effects on digestion and absorption, chronic inflammation and increased nutrient losses (Stoltzfus et al. 2000; Stoltzfus et al. 1997). However, many children only receive deworming every 6 months, a frequency which might not be enough to bring down parasite infestation if the infection rate is high. And only deworming might not be enough to restore depleted micronutrient stores (Hall 2007). Food provided at school that is fortified with multiple vitamins and minerals, in combination with regular deworming could be a more effective strategy to reduce anemia in school-aged children, and will supply the children with a whole range of nutrients necessary to grow and learn. The school food often also provides an additional motive for school attendance, which is an important concern in many countries. Indeed several studies have shown significant improvements in hemoglobin concentrations and micronutrient status from such combined programs (Faber et al. 2005; Nga et al. 2009; van Stuijvenberg et al. 1999). Besides improvements in micronutrient status, these studies also resulted in important improvements in cognitive function, thus showing also functional benefits of the intervention. Interestingly, in one study in Vietnam there was a high prevalence of anemia, but the prevalence of iron deficiency and iron deficiency anemia was low. Yet, biscuits fortified with multiple micronutrient decreased anemia prevalence by 40%, again highlighting the importance of other nutrients than only iron in the etiology of anemia (Nga et al. 2009). The same study reported an enhanced effect of deworming on Ascaris and Trichuris infection when combined with multi-micronutrient fortified biscuits, suggesting also improvements in immune function in school children who received fortified food (Nga et al. 2011). Given the low cost of food fortification (for example, fortifying a meal of rice per day for 1 school child would cost less than US$1/year), and the potential benefits, food fortification should be given high priority for this age group.

3.6 Interventions for adolescent girls

Finally, another often-forgotten age group is that of adolescent girls. Anemia prevalence is often high in adolescents girls due to blood loss through menstruation combined with an increase in growth rate. Reaching adolescent girls through existing health programs has been proven difficult, as often the most vulnerable groups are no longer attending school (Ahluwalia 2002), whereas anemia prevalence in these girls can be extremely high (Bulliyy et al. 2007). Otherwise, programs through schools have been shown to be effective in increasing hemglobin concentrations of adolescent girls (Tee et al. 1999), and as discussed above, multiple micronutrient supplementation is more beneficial than only iron and folic acid supplementation in reducing anemia prevalence as other nutritional causes of anemia are also addressed (Ahmed et al. 2010). The cultural context with regard to education, access to health care and other important aspects of the position of women play a disproportionally important role for this group, making the development and implementation of interventions especially challenging. However, as this group is poised to progress to WRA it is at the same time extremely urgent to reach this group.

There rests a special case for anemia in malaria endemic areas. This anemia is in part due to malaria infection, as there is an increased breakdown of erythrocytes. But as malaria itself is associated with poverty, nutritional deficiencies are also an important cause of anemia in these populations. However, interventions are not so easy, as the malaria infection is fuelled by iron and erythropiesis (Oppenheimer 2001). This makes for a dangerous combination, and indeed, many studies have found that iron supplementation increased morbibity and mortality in malaria endemic populations. The consensus for the moment is that iron supplementation interventions need to be combined with adequate bed-net usage and intermittent anti-malarial therapy (WHO/UNICEF 2007). Surprisingly, the increase in morbidity and mortality after iron supplementation in the study in Pemba was not only due to malaria but to a whole range of common childhood infections (Sazawal et al. 2006) suggesting a complex interplay between (sub-clinical) malaria infection, immune function and nutritional status. Again, food based interventions to improve iron status such as fortification and dietary diversification also seem to carry less risk to increase morbidity and mortality in malaria endemic areas, perhaps because the more physiological approach does not lead to an increase in the so-called non-transferrin bound iron (NTBI) (Troesch et al. 2011).

4. Conclusion

Anemia is major public health problem in many developing countries. Nutritional deficiencies of iron and also of other micronutrients underlie an important part of this, but are certainly not the sole contributor. Anemia is often regarded as nutritional anemia, however other causes of anemia include hemoglobinopathies (such as sickle cell trait and thalassemia), chronic infections (such as malaria and tuberculosis) and intestinal parasites. Anemia is also often equated to iron deficiency. However, WHO estimates that less than half of the anemia in the world is due to iron deficiency. Indeed, as shown by several studies from Vietnam, anemia prevalence remains high in vulnerable population groups whereas the prevalence of iron deficiency has decreased rapidly over the last decade. Other micronutrient deficiencies, such as vitamin B_{12}, folic acid or vitamin A deficiency, might underlie this paradox, although parasitic infestation certainly contributed to the anemia observed in this population. Many interventions with the potential to be effective in reducing anemia prevalence in vulnerable groups exist. Iron supplementation has been promoted for decades as a cost-effective strategy. However, care should be taken when implementing this intervention, as interactions with other micronutrients (zinc, copper, vitamin A) and infectious diseases (malaria) might lead to adverse effects, and correct timing of the intervention (early in pregnancy) appears to be of major importance for success. Interventions with multiple micronutrients have the benefit of addressing multiple causes of anemia, and have been shown to be successful in improving hemoglobin and micronutrient status of school children, with the additional benefit of improving cognition and immune function. Additional benefits of multiple micronutrient supplementation during pregnancy are unclear at the moment, with small gains in birth weight reported, but with no benefits for neonatal survival. New strategies such as weekly supplementation of women of reproductive age with multiple micronutrients need to be investigated urgently. For the long term, food fortification to improve overall micronutrient status of populations is the most cost-effective strategy, with adverse effects less likely to occur, and targeting or differential dosing often automatically incorporated in the choice of food vehicle. Effective interventions directed at all stages of the life cycle are urgently needed and both policy and science should work in concert. Not only to explore new approaches, but also to critically evaluate existing evidence and efforts, and gain understanding in the complex physiological, nutritional and social factors involved in anemia as a public health problem. This will allow the development of evidence-based effective strategies that are tailored to specific populations, vulnerable groups and cultural settings, providing improved and more accurate tools to reduce anemia.

5. References

Ahluwalia N. 2002. Intervention strategies for improving iron status of young children and adolescents in India. Nutr Rev 60:S115-117.

Ahmed F, Khan MR, Akhtaruzzaman M, Karim R, Williams G, Torlesse H, Darnton-Hill I, Dalmiya N, Banu CP, and Nahar B. 2010. Long-term intermittent multiple micronutrient supplementation enhances hemoglobin and micronutrient status more than iron + folic acid supplementation in Bangladeshi rural adolescent girls with nutritional anemia. J Nutr 140:1879-1886.

Ayoya MA, Spiekermann-Brouwer GM, Traore AK, Stoltzfus RJ, and Garza C. 2006. Determinants of anemia among pregnant women in Mali. Food Nutr Bull 27:3-11.

Baig-Ansari N, Badruddin SH, Karmaliani R, Harris H, Jehan I, Pasha O, Moss N, McClure EM, and Goldenberg RL. 2008. Anemia prevalence and risk factors in pregnant women in an urban area of Pakistan. Food Nutr Bull 29:132-139.

Bates CJ, Powers HJ, and Thurnham DI. 1989. Vitamins, iron, and physical work. Lancet 2:313-314.

Beard JL. 2001. Iron biology in immune function, muscle metabolism and neuronal functioning. J Nutr 131:568S-579S.

Berger J, Thanh HT, Cavalli-Sforza T, Smitasiri S, Khan NC, Milani S, Hoa PT, Quang ND, and Viteri F. 2005. Community mobilization and social marketing to promote weekly iron-folic acid supplementation in women of reproductive age in Vietnam: impact on anemia and iron status. Nutr Rev 63:S95-108.

Berry RJ, Bailey L, Mulinare J, and Bower C. 2010. Fortification of flour with folic acid. Food Nutr Bull 31:S22-35.

Bhutta ZA, Ahmed T, Black RE, Cousens S, Dewey K, Giugliani E, Haider BA, Kirkwood B, Morris SS, Sachdev HP and others. 2008. What works? Interventions for maternal and child undernutrition and survival. Lancet 371:417-440.

Black MM. 2003. Micronutrient deficiencies and cognitive functioning. J Nutr 133:3927S-3931S.

Bulliyy G, Mallick G, Sethy GS, and Kar SK. 2007. Hemoglobin status of non-school going adolescent girls in three districts of Orissa, India. Int J Adolesc Med Health 19:395-406.

Casey GJ, Phuc TQ, Macgregor L, Montresor A, Mihrshahi S, Thach TD, Tien NT, and Biggs BA. 2009. A free weekly iron-folic acid supplementation and regular deworming program is associated with improved hemoglobin and iron status indicators in Vietnamese women. BMC Publ Health 9:261.

Cavalli-Sforza T, Berger J, Smitasiri S, and Viteri F. 2005. Weekly iron-folic acid supplementation of women of reproductive age: impact overview, lessons learned, expansion plans, and contributions toward achievement of the millennium development goals. Nutr Rev 63:S152-158.

Cogswell ME, Looker AC, Pfeiffer CM, Cook JD, Lacher DA, Beard JL, Lynch SR, and Grummer-Strawn LM. 2009. Assessment of iron deficiency in US preschool children and nonpregnant females of childbearing age: National Health and Nutrition Examination Survey 2003-2006. Am J Clin Nutr 89:1334-1342.

Critchley J, and Bates I. 2005. Haemoglobin colour scale for anaemia diagnosis where there is no laboratory: a systematic review. Int J Epidemiol 34:1425-1434.

Dewey KG, and Chaparro CM. 2007. Iron status of breast-fed infants. Proc Nutr Soc 66:412-2

Dewey KG, Domellof M, Cohen RJ, Landa Rivera L, Hernell O, and Lonnerdal B. 2002. Iron supplementation affects growth and morbidity of breast-fed infants: results of a randomized trial in Sweden and Honduras. J Nutr 132:3249-3255.

Dijkhuizen MA, Wieringa FT, West CE, Muherdiyantiningsih, and Muhilal. 2001. Concurrent micronutrient deficiencies in lactating mothers and their infants in Indonesia. Am J Clin Nutr 73:786-791.

Dijkhuizen MA, Winichagoon P, Wieringa FT, Wasantwisut E, Utomo B, Ninh NX, Hidayat A, and Berger J. 2008. Zinc supplementation improved length growth only in anemic infants in a multi-country trial of iron and zinc supplementation in South-East Asia. J Nutr 138:1969-1975.

Domellof M, Dewey KG, Lonnerdal B, Cohen RJ, and Hernell O. 2002a. The diagnostic criteria for iron deficiency in infants should be reevaluated. J Nutr 132:3680-3686.

Domellof M, Lonnerdal B, Dewey KG, Cohen RJ, Rivera LL, and Hernell O. 2002b. Sex differences in iron status during infancy. Pediatrics 110:545-552.

Engmann C, Adanu R, Lu TS, Bose C, and Lozoff B. 2008. Anemia and iron deficiency in pregnant Ghanaian women from urban areas. Int J Gyn Obst 101:62-66.

Faber M, Kvalsvig JD, Lombard CJ, and Benade AJ. 2005. Effect of a fortified maize-meal porridge on anemia, micronutrient status, and motor development of infants. Am J Clin Nutr 82:1032-1039.

Grosse SD, Waitzman NJ, Romano PS, and Mulinare J. 2005. Reevaluating the benefits of folic acid fortification in the United States: economic analysis, regulation, and public health. Am J Public Health 95:1917-1922.

Haider BA, and Bhutta ZA. 2006. Multiple-micronutrient supplementation for women during pregnancy. Cochrane Database of Systematic Reviews(4):-.

Hall A. 2007. Micronutrient supplements for children after deworming. The Lancet infectious diseases 7:297-302.

Hercberg S, Preziosi P, and Galan P. 2001. Iron deficiency in Europe. Public Health Nutr 4:537-545.

INACG. 2004. Efficacy and effectiveness of interventions to control iron deficiency and iron deficiency anemia.

Kalaivani K. 2009. Prevalence & consequences of anaemia in pregnancy. Ind J Med Res 130:627-633.

Katz J, Christian P, Dominici F, and Zeger SL. 2006. Treatment effects of maternal micronutrient supplementation vary by percentiles of the birth weight distribution in rural Nepal. J Nutr 136:1389-1394.

Khambalia A, O'Connor DL, and Zlotkin S. 2009. Periconceptional iron and folate status is inadequate among married, nulliparous women in rural Bangladesh. J Nutr 139:1179-1184.

Koury MJ, and Ponka P. 2004. New insights into erythropoiesis: the roles of folate, vitamin B12, and iron. Annu Rev Nutr 24:105-131.

Lartey A. 2008. Maternal and child nutrition in Sub-Saharan Africa: challenges and interventions. Proc Nutr Soc 67:105-108.

Mejia LA, and Chew F. 1988. Hematological effect of supplementing anemic children with vitamin A alone and in combination with iron. Am J Clin Nutr 48:595-600.

Milman N, Bergholt T, Eriksen L, Byg KE, Graudal N, Pedersen P, and Hertz J. 2005. Iron prophylaxis during pregnancy -- how much iron is needed? A randomized dose-response study of 20-80 mg ferrous iron daily in pregnant women. Acta Obstet Gyn Scan 84:238-247.

Nga TT, Winichagoon P, Dijkhuizen MA, Khan NC, Wasantwisut E, Furr H, and Wieringa FT. 2009. Multi-micronutrient-fortified biscuits decreased prevalence of anemia and improved micronutrient status and effectiveness of deworming in rural Vietnamese school children. J Nutr 139:1013-1021.

Nga TT, Winichagoon P, Dijkhuizen MA, Khan NC, Wasantwisut E, and Wieringa FT. 2011. Decreased parasite load and improved cognitive outcomes caused by deworming and consumption of multi-micronutrient fortified biscuits in rural vietnamese schoolchildren. Am J Trop Med Hyg 85:333-340.

Oppenheimer SJ. 2001. Iron and its relation to immunity and infectious disease. J Nutr 131:616S-635S.

Pena-Rosas JP, and Viteri FE. 2009. Effects and safety of preventive oral iron or iron+folic acid supplementation for women during pregnancy. Cochrane Database Syst Rev(4):CD004736.

Phu PV, Hoan NV, Salvignol B, Treche S, Wieringa FT, Khan NC, Tuong PD, and Berger J. 2010. Complementary foods fortified with micronutrients prevent iron deficiency and anemia in Vietnamese infants. J Nutr 140:2241-2247.

Powers HJ. 2003. Riboflavin (vitamin B-2) and health. Am J Clin Nutr 77(6):1352-1360.

Raqib R, Hossain MB, Kelleher SL, Stephensen CB, and Lonnerdal B. 2007. Zinc supplementation of pregnant rats with adequate zinc nutriture suppresses immune functions in their offspring. J Nutr 137:1037-1042.

Roodenburg AJ, West CE, Hovenier R, and Beynen AC. 1996. Supplemental vitamin A enhances the recovery from iron deficiency in rats with chronic vitamin A deficiency. Brit J Nutr 75:623-636.

Sazawal S, Black RE, Ramsan M, Chwaya HM, Stoltzfus RJ, Dutta A, Dhingra U, Kabole I, Deb S, Othman MK and others. 2006. Effects of routine prophylactic supplementation with iron and folic acid on admission to hospital and mortality in preschool children in a high malaria transmission setting: community-based, randomised, placebo-controlled trial. Lancet 367:133-143.

Shah PS, and Ohlsson A. 2009. Effects of prenatal multimicronutrient supplementation on pregnancy outcomes: a meta-analysis. Can Med Assoc J 180:E99-108.

Sight_and_Life. 2007. Nutritional Anemia. In: Kraemer R, and Zimmermann M, editors. 1 ed. Basel: Sight and Life Press.

Steer PJ. 2000. Maternal hemoglobin concentration and birth weight. Am J Clin Nutr 71:1285S-1287S.

Stoltzfus RJ. 2008. Research needed to strengthen science and programs for the control of iron deficiency and its consequences in young children. J Nutr 138:2542-2546.

Stoltzfus RJ, Chwaya HM, Montresor A, Albonico M, Savioli L, and Tielsch JM. 2000. Malaria, hookworms and recent fever are related to anemia and iron status indicators in 0- to 5-y old Zanzibari children and these relationships change with age. J Nutr 130:1724-1733.

Stoltzfus RJ, Chwaya HM, Tielsch JM, Schulze KJ, Albonico M, and Savioli L. 1997. Epidemiology of iron deficiency anemia in Zanzibari schoolchildren: the importance of hookworms. Am J Clin Nutr 65:153-159.

Suharno D, West CE, Muhilal, Karyadi D, and Hautvast JG. 1993. Supplementation with vitamin A and iron for nutritional anaemia in pregnant women in West Java, Indonesia. Lancet 342:1325-1328.

Sukrat B, Suwathanapisate P, Siritawee S, Poungthong T, and Phupongpankul K. The prevalence of iron deficiency anemia in pregnant women in Nakhonsawan, Thailand. J Med Assoc Thai 93:765-770.

Tee ES, Kandiah M, Awin N, Chong SM, Satgunasingam N, Kamarudin L, Milani S, Dugdale AE, and Viteri FE. 1999. School-administered weekly iron-folate supplements improve hemoglobin and ferritin concentrations in Malaysian adolescent girls. Am J Clin Nutr 69:1249-1256.

Thurlow RA, Winichagoon P, Pongcharoen T, Gowachirapant S, Boonpraderm A, Manger MS, Bailey KB, Wasantwisut E, and Gibson RS. 2006. Risk of zinc, iodine and other micronutrient deficiencies among school children in North East Thailand. Eur J Clin Nutr 60:623-632.

Thurnham D, McCabe L, Wieringa F, Northrop-Clewes C, and McCabe G. 2010. Adjusting plasma ferritin concentrations to remove effects of sub-clinical inflammation in the assessment of iron deficiency: a meta-analysis. Am J Clin Nutr 92:546-55..

Thurnham DI, McCabe GP, Northrop-Clewes CA, and Nestel P. 2003. Effects of subclinical infection on plasma retinol concentrations and assessment of prevalence of vitamin A deficiency: meta-analysis. Lancet 362:2052-2058.

Titaley CR, Dibley MJ, Roberts CL, and Agho K. 2010a. Combined iron/folic acid supplements and malaria prophylaxis reduce neonatal mortality in 19 sub-Saharan African countries. Am J Clin Nutr 92:235-243.

Titaley CR, Dibley MJ, Roberts CL, Hall J, and Agho K. 2010b. Iron and folic acid supplements and reduced early neonatal deaths in Indonesia. Bull WIIO 88:500-8.

Trinh LT, and Dibley M. 2007. Anaemia in pregnant, postpartum and non pregnant women in Lak district, Daklak province of Vietnam. Asia Pacific J Clin Nutr 16:310-315.

Troesch B, Egli I, Zeder C, Hurrell RF, and Zimmermann MB. 2011. Fortification iron as ferrous sulfate plus ascorbic acid is more rapidly absorbed than as sodium iron EDTA but neither increases serum nontransferrin-bound iron in women. J Nutr 141:822-827.

Van Nhien N, Khan NC, Ninh NX, Van Huan P, Hop le T, Lam NT, Ota F, Yabutani T, Hoa VQ, Motonaka J and others. 2008. Micronutrient deficiencies and anemia among preschool children in rural Vietnam. Asia Pacific J Clin Nutr 17:48-55.

van Stuijvenberg ME, Kvalsvig JD, Faber M, Kruger M, Kenoyer DG, and Benade AJ. 1999. Effect of iron-, iodine-, and beta-carotene-fortified biscuits on the micronutrient status of primary school children: a randomized controlled trial. Am J Clin Nutr 69:497-503.

Vanderjagt DJ, Brock HS, Melah GS, El-Nafaty AU, Crossey MJ, and Glew RH. 2007. Nutritional factors associated with anaemia in pregnant women in northern Nigeria. J Health Pop Nutr 25:75-81.

Viteri FE, and Berger J. 2005. Importance of pre-pregnancy and pregnancy iron status: can long-term weekly preventive iron and folic acid supplementation achieve desirable and safe status? Nutr Rev 63:S65-76.

Weatherall DJ, and Clegg JB. 2001. Inherited haemoglobin disorders: an increasing global health problem. Bull WHO 79:704-712.

Weinberg ED. 1975. Nutritional immunity. Host's attempt to withold iron from microbial invaders. JAMA 231:39-41.

WHO. 2001. Iron Deficiency Anaemia Assessment, Prevention and Control. A guide for programme managers. Geneva: World Health Organization.

WHO. 2008. Worldwide prevalence of anaemia 1993–2005 : WHO global database on anaemia. Geneva: World Health Organization.

WHO. 2009. World Health Organization Position Statement. Weekly iron-folic acid supplementation (WIFS) in women of reproductive age: its role in promoting optimal maternal and child health. In: WHO, editor. Geneva: World Health Organization, 2009 (http://www.who.int/nutrition/publications/micronutrients/weekly_iron_folicacid.pdf (last accessed 20/09/2011).

WHO/UNICEF. 2007. Iron supplementation of young children in regions where malaria transmission is intense and infectious disease highly prevalent. p 1-2.

Wieringa FT, Berger J, Dijkhuizen MA, Hidayat A, Ninh NX, Utomo B, Wasantwisut E, and Winichagoon P. 2007a. Combined iron and zinc supplementation in infants improved iron and zinc status, but interactions reduced efficacy in a multicountry trial in southeast Asia. J Nutr 137:466-471.

Wieringa FT, Berger J, Dijkhuizen MA, Hidayat A, Ninh NX, Utomo B, Wasantwisut E, and Winichagoon P. 2007b. Sex differences in prevalence of anaemia and iron deficiency in infancy in a large multi-country trial in South-East Asia. Br J Nutr 98:1070-1076.

Wieringa FT, Dijkhuizen MA, Muhilal, and Van der Meer JW. 2010. Maternal micronutrient supplementation with zinc and beta-carotene affects morbidity and immune function of infants during the first 6 months of life. Eur J Clin Nutr 64:1072-1079.

Wieringa FT, Dijkhuizen MA, and van der Meer JW. 2008. Maternal micronutrient supplementation and child survival. Lancet 371:1751-1752.

Wieringa FT, Dijkhuizen MA, West CE, Northrop-Clewes CA, and Muhilal. 2002. Estimation of the effect of the acute phase response on indicators of micronutrient status in Indonesian infants. J Nutr 132:3061-3066.

Wieringa FT, Dijkhuizen MA, West CE, Thurnham DI, Muhilal, and Van der Meer JW. 2003. Redistribution of vitamin A after iron supplementation in Indonesian infants. Am J Clin Nutr 77:651-657.

Yip R. 1996. Iron supplementation during pregnancy: is it effective? Am J Clin Nutr 63:853-5.

Yip R. 2002. Iron supplementation: country level experiences and lessons learned. J Nutr 132:859S-861S.

Zeng L, Dibley M, Cheng Y, Chang S, and Yan H. 2009. What is the effect of starting micronutrient supplements early in pregnancy on birthweight, duration of gestation & perinatal mortality. Micronutrient Forum. Beijing.

Zhou LM, Yang WW, Hua JZ, Deng CQ, Tao X, and Stoltzfus RJ. 1998. Relation of hemoglobin measured at different times in pregnancy to preterm birth and low birth weight in Shanghai, China. Am J Epidem 148:998-1006.

Zimmermann MB, Biebinger R, Rohner F, Dib A, Zeder C, Hurrell RF, and Chaouki N. 2006. Vitamin A supplementation in children with poor vitamin A and iron status increases erythropoietin and hemoglobin concentrations without changing total body iron. Am J Clin Nutr 84:580-586.

11

Supplementation and Change of Nutritional Habits for the Prevention and Treatment of Iron Deficiency Anaemia in Gaza Children: A Case Study

Michele Magoni, Ghassam Zaqout, Omar Ahmmed Mady,
Reema Ibraheem Al Haj Abed and Davide Amurri
Terre des Hommes
Italy

1. Introduction

Iron deficiency anaemia (IDA) is one of the most severe and widespread nutritional disorders in the world. Children and pregnant women in resource-poor areas represent the most vulnerable groups. Iron deficiency impairs the cognitive development of children from infancy through to adolescence. It damages immune mechanisms and is associated with increased morbidity rates. Iron deficiency commonly develops after six months of age if complementary foods do not provide sufficient absorbable iron, even for exclusively breastfed infants (World Health Organization [WHO] et al, 2001). The WHO recommends universal iron supplementation when prevalence of anaemia is more than 40% (WHO, 2004).

In the Eastern Mediterranean regions there is an endemic high prevalence of iron-deficiency anaemia (Verster, 1996) due to low total iron intake, low bioavailability (in many diets over 80% of iron is of non-haem origin) and high intake of inhibitors of iron absorption (unleavened bread and tea are severe inhibitors of iron absorption and are consumed in large amounts everywhere). Anaemia and stunting prevalence in Gaza have always been found to be very high in recent years (Abdeen, 2002; Rahim et al 2009).

1.1 Emergency situation

In the Gaza Strip the basic living conditions of all the inhabitants have deteriorated constantly in recent years, particularly after the "Cast Lead" operation in January 2009: the blockade and the closure of terminals for the movement of goods and people created a very tense situation which severely affected the wellbeing of all the inhabitants: 98% of private businesses closed and the unemployment rate increased to 48.8%, while 80% of the population lives below the poverty line and 79% is aid-dependent. The rate of food insecure households in Gaza has also increased to 75%, up from 56% before the Cast Lead operation. Furthermore, the growing inability of the population to consume iron-rich animal proteins and fresh fruit and vegetables, which contain the vitamins required for iron absorption, is bound to have a critical impact on the already high prevalence of mild and moderate iron deficiency anaemia in the Gaza Strip, habitually already about 20% higher than in the West Bank (WHO, 2009; World Bank, 2009).

The National Nutrition Surveillance System Report (PNA, MOH, 2010) has confirmed a worsening level of anaemia and chronic malnutrition in the Gaza Strip, with an overall anaemia prevalence of 76.2% (45.5% in the West Bank) among children 9-12 months old and 58.6% (9.5% in the West Bank) among school children. Stunting prevalence in school children was 7.9% in the Gaza Strip and 4.4% in the West Bank. The national survey does not provide any data for children between the ages of 12 months and 5 years.

1.2 Present humanitarian intervention

Terre des Hommes Italy[1] (Tdh-It) and its Palestinian partner Palestinian Medical Relief Society[2] (PMRS) started operating with several humanitarian projects in Gaza in 2009, targeting pre-school children in a holistic way, where the prevention and treatment of anaemia have played a fundamental role. The projects were supported by the Italian Cooperation and other European donors.

It is worth pointing out that the Tdh-It and PMRS projects were designed and implemented as (and in the framework of) humanitarian interventions and not study; nevertheless, the projects have also been supported by a strong monitoring and evaluation system that has provided us with a massive and structured quantity of information allowing us to present the projects' impact and data as a case study, although the possibility of bias in the sample selections has to be borne in mind.

There is a strong need for a more evidence-based approach in humanitarian medical work and although a substantial body of knowledge has been accumulated regarding the effectiveness of interventions in acute emergencies, especially in refugee settings, the evidence base is much weaker for situations of protracted conflict with longer-term programmes in less controlled settings. (Banatvala and Zwi, 2000; Robertson et al, 2002; Roberts and Hofmann, 2004)

2. Method

2.1 Nutritional health projects

The interventions that Tdh-It and PMRS implemented included the following components:

-   screening for IDA and malnutrition in 22 kindergartens (South Gaza: Rafah and Khan Younis Governorates) and 4 paediatric clinics (North Gaza: Northern Governorate);
-   iron and vitamin supplementation based on therapeutic or preventive WHO protocols for all children contacted;
-   medical follow-up for anaemic and malnourished children;
-   provision of a home visit service for anaemic and malnourished children in order to:
    -   assess families' and children's nutritional habits (24-hour recall questionnaire)

---

[1] Terre des Hommes Italia (Tdh-It) was founded in 1989 in Milan (Italy) and is part of the Terre des Hommes International Federation. It is a non-profit non-governmental organisation (ONLUS) whose mission it is to carry out humanitarian relief and international development projects for the benefit of children, their families and communities.

[2] Palestinian Medical Relief Society (PMRS) is a grassroots, community- based Palestinian health organization founded in 1979. PMRS operates with 4 Primary Health Care Centres (PHCCs) in the Gaza Strip, providing preventive and curative services, and specialized health care for women and children.

Supplementation and Change of Nutritional Habits for the Prevention and Treatment of Iron
Deficiency Anaemia in Gaza Children: A Case Study

173

- provide family nutritional counselling
- support behavioural health change;
- health education sessions for mothers and fathers - held at the clinics, in kindergarten and during home visits.

Children who were still anaemic after intervention underwent further clinical investigation, treatment and longer follow-up.

The following table summarizes the activities and treatment protocols for the different projects.

Period	Area	Target	Intervention for anaemics	Treatment for anaemics*
September 2009 - June 2010	South Gaza (1)	Children in 12 kindergartens and their siblings	Screening and treatment, monthly follow-up with haemoglobin control after 4 months, health education, home visit for anaemic children	Iron polymaltose complex 5mg/kg and multivitamins daily for 4 months, followed by preventive iron (1mg/kg daily)
January 2010 - December 2010	North Gaza	Children from 3 local communities invited to local clinics	Screening, treatment, follow-up after 3 months with haemoglobin test, health education, home visit only for some anaemic children	Iron polymaltose complex 3-6mg/kg and multivitamins daily for at least 3 months, followed by multivitamin including iron (1mg/kg daily)
September 2010 - June 2011	South Gaza (2)	Children in 11 kindergartens and their siblings	Screening and treatment, monthly follow-up with haemoglobin control after 4 months, health education, home visit for anaemic children	Iron polymaltose complex 5mg/kg and multivitamins daily for 4 months, followed by preventive iron (1mg/kg daily)

*A paediatrician or medical doctor changed the dosage and length of treatment when required by the child's clinical condition.

Table 1. Summary of Tdh-It/ PMRS nutritional projects in Gaza.

2.2 Data collection

Data were collected using two questionnaires, which were also used during the monitoring process:

1. CHILD FILE (annex-1): basic information about family and screened children gathered in the kindergarten during screening and follow-up visits. 10,445 children were screened for anaemia (blood test), including the main anthropometric indicators (height, weight), between October 2009 and March 2011: 3,941 (37.7%) children were screened at 3 paediatric clinics in northern Gaza (Izbet Beit Hanoun, Umm El Nasser, Jabalia/Beit Lahia) while the other 6,504 were screened in the kindergartens (including siblings aged less than 6 years) in southern Gaza (eastern areas of Khan Younis and western areas of Rafah City).

FAMILY INFORMATION

1) Name of the family's head (four names) _____

    a. Name in Arabic _____

2) ID number of the family's head: _____ **Family code** _ _/_ _ _ _

3) Full Address: _____ 4) Telephone n. _____

5) Number of family's members: ___;   below 5 years: _ _;   5-18 years: _ _;

6) Mother's personal status: Living with husband   divorced   Widow
    Married but living alone   Married but living with her family   Dead mother

7) Mother's education: Illiterate   can read & write   elementary
    Preparatory   secondary   lower diploma   bachelor and more

8) Father's education: Illiterate   can read & write   elementary
    Preparatory   secondary   lower diploma   bachelor and more

9) Father Job:
(1) Worker   (2) Government/Municipality employee   (3) Self employee
(4) Business (employing others)   (5) Peasant   (6) Shepherd
(7) Driver   (8) Unemployed   (9) Other

10) Mother age _____ **11) n. of pregnancy** _____ **12) n. of deliveries** _____

13) Pregnant now   Yes   Not   **N° of death children**

		<1 year	1-5 years
N° of death children	M		
	F		

CHILD FILE

14) Date of visit _ _/_ _/_ _ _ _ Family code_ _/_ _ _ _ CODE of the Child _ _ _

15) Name of the Child .... 16) Date of birth _ _/_ _/_ _ _ _

17) ID number of the child: .... 18) attending KG   Yes   Not

19) Sex: M F   20) Weight (kg) _ _, _ _   21) Height (cm) _ _ _

22) Percentile weight for age _____   23) Hb level _ _, _

24) Referred for doctor visit Yes   Not   25) Referred to clinic Yes Not

Reason ....   Reason ....

25b) does the child suffer from a chronic disease? Thalassaemia   G6PD   Other ....

26) Already receiving fortified food?   Yes   Not comments................................

27) N° of iron bottles given: _ _ (ml/day_____)   28) N° of MULTIVITAMIN given: _ _

FOLLOW UP FILE

CODE of the Child   Date of follow up _ _/_ _/_ _ _ _   visit N° 1

Medication taken: regularly (>=5days/week)   irregularly (4-2days/week)   not taken (<=1)

Have drugs given been finished? YES NO why? _____
    Weight (kg) _ _, _ _   Height (cm) _ _ _ C° weight for age _____   Hb level _ _, _

N° of iron bottles given: _____   **N° of MULTIVITAMIN given:** _____

ANNEX 1. Extract from the CHILD FILE.

2.   HOME VISIT (annex-2): details of the families of anaemic children were collected twice
      during home visits (coinciding roughly with the start and end of treatment) and
      concerned mother's knowledge, nutritional habits of all the children, iron treatment
      compliance and adoption of healthy life styles.

In the project implemented in northern Gaza only some families received home visits and
there was also a problem with coding of the children, so the link between data collected
during screening and the home visit was not available; for this reason we analysed only data
from the kindergarten visits carried out in southern Gaza. A total of 1,733 families of
anaemic children screened in kindergartens were visited at home.

NUTRITIONAL QUESTIONNAIRE

Is the child presently breastfed?

Child 1	Child 2	Child 3	Child 4
Yes No	Yes No	Yes No	Yes No
if yes no. of times_____	if yes no. of times_____	if yes no. of times_____	if yes no. of times_____

How many meals the child has on average per day?   Child 1_____ Child 2_____

Child 3_____ Child 3_____

	Child 1	Child 2	Child 3	Child 4		Child 1	Child 2	Child 3	Child 4
Indicate number of "portion" of the following food (or number of items where indicated) that the CHILD has eaten in the last 24 h? (One portion is big as the person's fist)									
Vegetables					Cheese and dairy products				
Fruits					Bread				
Legumes					Rice				
Nuts and Seeds					Pasta				
Meat					Potatoes				
Chicken					Biscuits/cake				
Fish					Chocolate bars (n.)				
Eggs (n.)					Sweets and candies (n)				
Chips (n. of sachet)					Jam/ cream (n. of big spoon)				
Indicates how many cups/glasses the CHILD had of the following drinks in the last 24 h? (mark with X)									
Milk (with sugar)					Tea (outside meal)				
Milk (without sugar)					Tea (with main meal)				
Water					Fresh Juice				
Soft drink					Packed Juice				

How many times is the child eating junk food outside main meals? Child 1_____ Child 2_____

KNOWLEDGE OF THE MOTHER ASSESSMENT (don't prompt the mother before she has finished to answer the all questions)

– **Why anaemia is bad for the child?** Doesn't know____; mental retard ____; weakness____; infection vulnerability____; poor school performance____; other answers____; AHA......?????

– **What are the causes of anaemia is bad for the child?** Doesn't know____; tea___; Tea with meal____; lack of meat/chicken /fish ____, lack of rich iron vegetable (she can mention one) ____; some diseases ____; poverty____; other answers____;

– **What can be done to prevent or treat anaemia?** Doesn't know____; good diet___; iron supplementation ____. food fortification ____, wrong answer____;

– **What is the GOOD food for the child growth?** doesn't know____; Breast feeding___; Vegetables____; Legumes____; Fruits____; Meat____; Chicken ____; Fish____; Eggs____; Milk___; Cheese and milk products____; fresh juice ____; other answers____;

– **What are the food BAD for the child growth?** doesn't know____; Sugar____; Soft drinks___; Chips____; Salted biscuits___; Butter___; Biscuits___; Cakes ____; Chocolate bars ___; Sweets and candies ____; ice cream____; jam and cream ____; other answers____;

ANNEX 2. Extract from the HOME VIST FILE (nutritional questionnaire and mother's knowledge assessment).

Data were collected for 3,619 children (2,024 anaemics and 1,595 non-anaemic siblings) of these families concerning:
- drug adherence, tolerance, storage and administration
- mother's knowledge of anaemia and nutrition
- nutritional habit (24-hour recall nutritional questionnaire)

The second visit took place on average 111 days (SD=46) after the first visit.
The home visit data included children on iron preventive treatment, not only anaemics.

2.3 Haemoglobin assessment
Blood samples taken at kindergarten were analysed using the Haemocue rapid test.
Blood samples in clinics were tested using an aXE-2100D automated haematology analyser (Sysmex).

2.4 Definition of anaemia and malnutrition
Anaemia. Children with a haemoglobin level below 11g/dl were considered anaemic. Anaemia was defined as mild for a haemoglobin level of 10-11g/dl, moderate for 7-9.9 gm/dl and severe for less than 7gm/dl.
Malnutrition. The software used to calculate Z score was "WHO ANTHRO, Software for Calculating Anthropometry, Version 2.0" and "WHO ANTHROPLUS". Segments of the population below -2 Z score (2SD) were considered as suffering from wasting (acute malnutrition, weight/height), underweight (weight/age) and stunting (chronic malnutrition, height/age). Segments of the population above 2Z of body mass index for age were considered as overweight (WHO, 2009).

2.5 Statistical analyses

Statistical analyses were performed using STATA software (Stata Statistical Software release 9.2, 2007; Stata Corporation, College Station, Texas). Uni- and multivariate binary regression and chi square test were used where appropriate. All statistical tests were two sided, and P values of < 0.05 were considered significant.

2.6 Main objectives

As already mentioned, the intervention was not conceived or performed as a study, thus the monitoring and evaluation (M&E) system was a tool for correct activity management and for evaluating the impact of the project, but it did allowed us to gather useful information:

- for comparing the prevalence of anaemia and malnutrition before and after the project in the pre-school child population;
- for identifying risk factors for anaemia;
- for assessing compliance and tolerability of treatment and their association with lack of improvement;
- for assessing change in the families' knowledge of anaemia and nutrition (mothers);
- for assessing nutritional habits and evaluating changes promoted by intervention;
- for evaluating anaemia prevalence 1 year after intervention (long-lasting impact);
- for monitoring and evaluating anaemic children who did not improve during the first phase of the project, including identification of non-iron deficiency anaemia (e.g. thalassaemia).

2.7 Ethical approval

The Helsinki Committee of Palestinian Ministry of Health gave approval for publication of present paper.

3. RESULTS

3.1 Anaemia prevalence at screening

10,445 children were screened for anaemia between October 2009 and March 2011: 3,941 (37.7%) of them were screened at the PMRS paediatric clinics in northern Gaza, while the other 6,504 (including siblings) were screened at the 22 kindergartens in southern Gaza.

51.6% (5,391) of the screened children were male. The mean age of the screened children was 39.7 months (SD=18.0), with no difference between the sexes.

5.877 (56.3%) of the tested children were not anaemic and 4,568 (43.7%) were anaemic (HB level <11g/dl); 421 of the anaemics (4.1%) had a haemoglobin level below 9g/dl.

The prevalence of anaemia was similar in males (44.0%) and females (43.4%, p=0.5) and strongly and inversely associated with age, as shown in Figure 1 and Table 1: anaemia had a very high prevalence in children below 24 months, peaking at 6-11 months (76.2%) and 12-23 months (72.2%). The percentage was much lower in older children (17.0% for children > 5 years old).

When considering only the under-5 population, the prevalence of anaemia was 49% (4,271/8,709), but it should be noted that children below 12 months of age were under-represented and our sample did not adequately represent the under-5 population of Gaza.

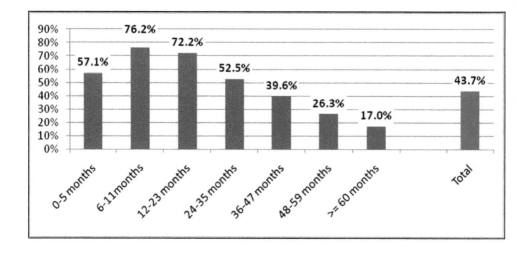

Fig. 1. Prevalence of anaemia by age group.

Age groups	N° of screened	N° of anaemics	% of anaemics	% of stunting	% of underweight	% of wasting	% of overweight
0-5 months	56	32	57.1%	0.0%	3.6%	8.9%	5.4%
6-11 months	513	391	76.2%	6.9%	2.7%	5.5%	5.7%
12-23 months	2,026	1,462	72.2%	10.7%	2.9%	2.9%	7.2%
24-35 months	1,973	1,036	52.5%	10.8%	2.2%	3.6%	8.2%
36-47 months	1,967	778	39.6%	9.6%	2.5%	3.2%	6.3%
48-59 months	2,174	572	26.3%	6.6%	2.6%	2.7%	5.3%
≥ 60 months	1,726	294	17.0%	6.2%	2.1%	1.8%	3.8%
Total	10,435	4,565	43.7%	8.7%	2.5%	3.1%	6.2%

Table 2. Prevalence of anaemia and malnutrition by age group.

As shown in Table 3, anaemia was also associated with:
- mother's poor education, regardless of child's age (p<0.0001)
- stunting in children over 24 months of age
- not having received fortified food (data collected for kindergarten children only).

		Children below 24 months (2,595)	Children over 24 months (7,850)
Mother's education	No education (278)	88%	54%
	Primary (1,380)	82%	49%
	High school (5,887)	71%	31%
	University (2,423)	69%	30%
Stunting	No (9,495)	73%	33%
	Yes (901)	73%	45%
Received fortified food (only children screened at kindergarten)	No (2,172)	73%	30%
	Yes (4,312)	60%	24%

Table 3. Anaemia prevalence by age group and other variables.

A multivariate logistic analysis showed that being anaemic was associated with:
- child's younger age (odds ratio=0.95 for every month of age, p<0.0001)
- mother's education (OR=0.73 for each level, p<0.0001)
- stunting (OR=1.36, p<0.0001)
- not having received fortified food (OR=1.35, p<0.0001).

No association was found between anaemia and: mother's age, number of pregnancies, father unemployment or sex of the child.

Prevalence of underweight and wasting (acute malnutrition) were low (around 2-3%), similar to the level registered in the normal healthy population according to WHO standards; prevalence of stunting was high (8.7%), and overweight was moderately higher (6.2%) than in the healthy population.

3.2 Anaemia improvement after intervention

4,077 of the anaemic children were monitored until a second haemoglobin test was performed, on average after 175 days (SD=43) of treatment. Table 4 below shows that:
- of 4,077 children anaemic at enrolment 2,690 (66.0%) were no longer anaemic and 1,387 (34.0%) were still anaemic after 4-6 months of treatment;
- severe and moderate anaemia was reduced from 9.4% to only 1.7%;
- of the 1,387 children still anaemic 360 (26.0%) had an improvement in haemoglobin $\geq$1g/dl, a clinically significant result, bringing to 74.8% the percentage of anaemic children with improved status;
- the mean haemoglobin level increased from 9.99 g/dl to 11.0 g/dl.

Type of anaemia	Admission		Last follow-up		p value
	n.	%	n.	%	
Severe and moderate anaemia <9g	383	9.4%	71	1.7%	
Mild anaemia	3,694	90.6%	1,316	32.3%	<0.0001
No anaemia	0		2,690	66.0%	
Mean haemoglobin level among 1,211	9.99 g/dl		11.09 g/dl		<0.0001

Table 4. Anaemia status before and after treatment.

Anaemic children at screening were classified as "improved" if they recovered from anaemia or if they had at least a >1g/dl increase in haemoglobin level. A strong link between improvement and child age was noticed: improvement was much lower for younger children (less than 60%) compared to older ones (around 80%), as shown in Figure 2.

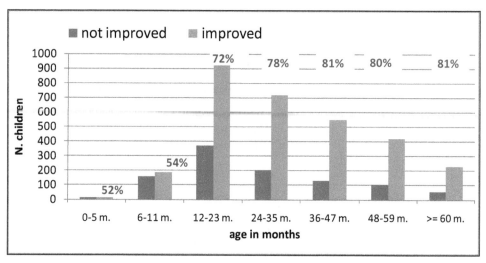

Fig. 2. Anaemia improvement after treatment by age group (number of children and % of improved).

Improvement was not associated with mother's education or other family variables collected.

In order to investigate the reasons for not improving we linked data collected via the CHILD FILE and HOME VISIT file to establish whether improvement was associated with:

- drug adherence
- drug tolerance
- mother's level of knowledge
- change in nutritional habits.

The above information was not available for all the children enrolled and is presented in detail in the following subsections (3.3 to 3.6).

3.3 Adherence to iron supplementation

In the first two phases of the project (South Gaza-1 and North Gaza) we were unable to associate improvement with good adherence to iron supplementation; this was due to the fact that almost all the mothers reported having given the iron as prescribed. A more careful investigation in a subsample of still anaemic children showed that in order to obtain more reliable answers:

- the questions on adherence had to be more precise and more specific
- the investigator was not to blame the mothers.

For this reason a more precise and more sensitive data collection method was introduced in SOUTH GAZA-2; therefore, with regard to drug adherence, we present data limited to this project. Information on drug adherence was collected for all the 2,804 children enrolled, during each distribution at the kindergarten and during the home visit. Specific questions were asked, such as whether the drugs had been taken regularly (≥ 5 days/week), irregularly (4-2 days/week) or not at all (≤ 1/week) during the previous week. Figure 3 below shows that:

- drugs were taken regularly by 57% of the children after one month, the percentage decreasing constantly to 45.7%;
- the percentage of children who took drugs irregularly rose with time from 21.7% to 32.8%;
- the percentage of children not taking drugs or not showing for follow-up increased with time.

The major reason mentioned for not taking drugs regularly were careless mother and/or child's refusal.

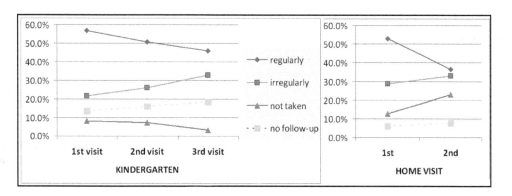

Fig. 3. Reported adherence among anaemic children.

To allow a better comparison we created a comprehensive index of drug adherence by combining all assessments performed, giving a score of 2 when the drugs were taken regularly, 1 when taken irregularly and 0 when not taken or the follow-up was missed. As shown in Table 5, there were 136 children who always took the drugs regularly, (score=10) and 31 who never took the medicine. We can further classify in 3 categories the level of adherence

Adherence category	Adherence score	No.	%	Cumulative %
POOR	0	31	3.6%	3.6%
	1	35	4.1%	7.7%
	2	49	5.7%	13.5%
	3	39	4.6%	18.1%
	4	72	8.4%	26.5%
FAIR	5	77	9.0%	35.5%
	6	99	11.6%	47.1%
	7	93	10.9%	58.0%
GOOD	8	116	13.6%	71.6%
	9	106	12.4%	84.1%
	10	136	15.9%	100.0%

Table 5. Adherence scores for anaemic children.

We found a significant association (p<0.0001) between improvement of anaemia and the treatment adherence score (as previously described). The percentage of improvement after adjustment for age was:
- *68.0% for children with good adherence (score 8-10)*
- *64.2% for children with fair adherence (score 5-7)*
- *60.5% for children with poor adherence (score <5)*

3.4 Drug tolerance, storage and administration
In the previous subsection we presented data on drug adherence recorded for anaemic children; the data here include non-anaemic children undergoing preventive treatment (prophylaxis).

There were very few reported complaints related to drug intake: around 2% in children with anaemia who received a higher dosage of iron and less than 1% for children on preventive treatment.

Vomiting and diarrhoea were the most common symptoms reported.

Drug storage was adequate in more than 90% of the cases during the first visit, the figure dropping slightly declined at the second visit. A similar pattern was noticed with regard to correct drug administration.

		1st visit	2nd visit
Drug-related complaints	anaemics	1.8% (38 cases)	1.8% (37 cases)
	non-anaemics	0.7% (11 cases)	0.4% (7 cases)
Adequate drug storage	anaemics	94.32%	93.08%
	non-anaemics	92.75%	89.33%
Correct drug administration	anaemics	89.65%	87.54%
	non-anaemics	86.26%	81.89%

Table 6. Drug tolerance, storage and administration among anaemic and non-anaemic children.

3.5 Mother's knowledge of anaemia and nutrition

A total of 1,724 mothers answered a questionnaire on anaemia and nutrition (annex-2) twice during the two home visits. The questions were open-ended and the social workers did not prompt any answers to them.

Considering the average number of good/correct answers given by mothers, it is clear for each section that there was a significant increase in knowledge (p-value paired t-test was always <0.0001).

The average number of good answers increased by 35%, from 7.7 to 10.4. The number of mothers improving their score was 1,205 (70%), while 247 showed the same and 272 a lower score.

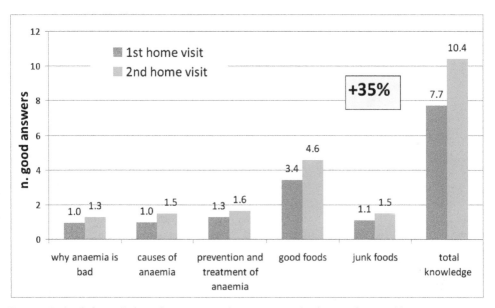

Fig. 4. Mother's knowledge of anaemia and nutrition at the first and second home visit.

When we considered as having a "good basic knowledge" women with a score of ≥ 10 with at least one good answer for every section, we found that the percentage of mothers with a good basic knowledge was only 20.2% at the first home visit, rising to 51.6% at the second home visit (p<0.0001).

The level of "good basic knowledge" was strongly related to mother's education at the first home visit, ranging from 10% in women with primary education to 28% for the highly educated (p>0.0001). At the second visit no difference in good basic nutritional knowledge was seen between mothers with different standards of education (apart from the 12 illiterate subjects).

This is particularly important since:

- less educated mothers displayed a proportionally higher increase in knowledge than highly educated ones;
- disparity was reduced at the end of the project;
- we proved that the nutritional messages given were well understood even by the less advantaged, who are more in need,

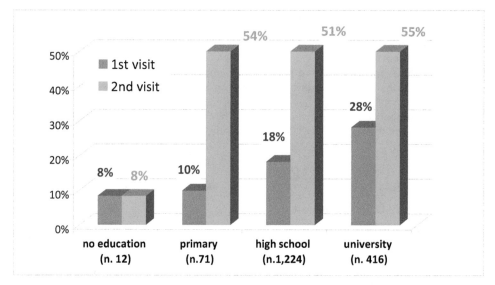

Fig. 5. Good-basic knowledge at the first and second home visit by mother's education level.

We found an association between improvement in anaemic status and mother's good basic knowledge at the second home visit: after adjustment for child's age, mothers with a good-basic knowledge were 24% more likely to have a child with improved status than mothers without a good basic knowledge (odds ratio=1.24, p=0.013).

Furthermore, in a sub-sample of children with available data, we found a significant association (p=0.016) between improvement of anaemia with mothers' and fathers' participation in awareness sessions at the kindergarten. The percentages of improvement stratified for participation were:

- 78.3% for the 69 children whose mother and father both participated in the awareness session
- 69.1% for the 162 children whose mother participated in the awareness session
- 62.3% for the 533 children whose parents did not participate in the awareness session.

3.6 Change in children's nutritional habits

In order to appreciate a possible impact in nutritional habit we compared the results of the 24-hour recall nutritional survey done during the first home visit with those of the same survey repeated 3-4 months later.

Since children below 2 years of age, who are at the weaning stage, can have a substantial change in their nutritional habit independently of the project, we analysed in a stratified way the results for children below 24 months of age (where considerable change is naturally expected) and those for older children (where changes can reflect project impact).

The specific messages of nutritional counselling were:

- stop tea consumption during meals;
- increase vegetable and fruit consumption;
- increase haem-rich animal food consumption (meat, fish, chicken);
- reduce junk food consumption.

3.6.1 Children over 24 months of age at screening

The overwhelming majority of children were having an average of 3 meals a day before and after the project.

When considering the average number of portions consumed the previous day, we noticed a 25% increase in the consumption of fruit and vegetables, +29% for staple food, +19% for animal products and +25% for haem-rich animal food.

Table 7a			Anaemic children ≥ 24 months			
			1st visit	2nd visit	change	p value paired t-test
Number of children			1,251			
Average no. of meals			2.93	2.96		
% of children having fewer than 3 meals			10.27%	6.59%	-36%	0.0001
Average number of portions* consumed the previous day		Vegetables, fruits and legumes	2.26	2.83	25%	<0.0001
		Staple food	2.11	2.73	29%	<0.0001
		Animal foods	2.42	2.88	19%	<0.0001
		Of which haem-rich food	0.56	0.71	25%	<0.0001
		Junk food	2.24	2.01	-10%	<0.0001
		Of which chips	0.82	0.57	-30%	<0.0001
		Of which candies	0.21	0.24	18%	0.03
		Of which soft drinks	0.11	0.08	-28%	0.026
Average number of times child eats junk food between meals			2.04	1.93	-6%	0.0001
Average cups/glasses consumed the previous day		Water	4.17	5.07	22%	<0.0001
		Tea No. of cups	1.18	0.76	-35%	<0.0001
		(Percentage drinking tea)	(67%)	(54%)	-19%	<0.0001
		Of which tea outside meals	0.90	0.61	-33%	<0.0001
		Of which tea with meals	0.28 (16.3%)	0.15 (10.6%)	-45% -35%	<0.0001 <0.0001
Table 7b			Non-anaemic children ≥24 months			
			1st visit	2nd visit	change	p value paired t-test
Number of children			1451			
Average no. of meals			2.95	2.99		
% of children having fewer than 3 meals			6.72%	4.56%	-32%	
Average number of portions* consumed in the previous day		Vegetables, fruit and legumes	2.26	2.77	23%	<0.0001
		Staple food	2.21	2.79	26%	<0.0001
		Animal foods	2.44	2.89	19%	<0.0001
		Of which haem-rich food	0.58	0.69	19%	<0.0001
		Junk food	2.26	2.12	-6%	0.003
		Of which chips	0.87	0.63	-27%	<0.0001
		Of which candies	0.21	0.29	37%	<0.0001
		Of which soft drinks	0.10	0.11	16%	0.13
Average number of times child eats junk food between meals			2.04	2.01	2%	-3%
Average cups/glasses consumed the previous day		Water	4.53	5.30	17%	<0.0001
		Tea No. of cups	1.18	0.78	-34%	<0.0001
		(Percentage drinking tea)	(65%)	(53%)	-18%	<0.0001
		Of which tea outside meals	0.92	0.64	-30%	<0.0001
		Of which tea with meals	0.26 (14.9%)	0.14 (10.2%)	-46% -32%	<0.0001 <0.0001

Table 7. Food consumption during previous 24 hours as recorded during first and second home visit for children over 24 months of age, anaemic (7a) and not anaemic (7b).

The increase in fruit and vegetable consumption may not be an effect of the project since we recorded at the same time an increase in staple food that the project did not promote.

Junk food consumption declined slightly, with chips and soft drinks up and candies down.

Tea consumption decreased by 35%, and tea with meals decreased even more (-45%). At the same time water consumption increased. Similar results were recorded in the non-anaemic population.

As shown in Table 8, the children of parents who participated in awareness sessions seem to have had a better improvement of nutritional habits, particularly in terms of reducing tea consumption during meals: -72% versus -32% when considering cups; -55% versus -10% when considering the percentage of children drinking tea.

			843 children with parents who did not attended awareness sessions			362 children with parents who attended awareness sessions		
			1st visit	2nd visit	Change	1st visit	2nd visit	Change
Average number of portions consumed the previous day		Vegetables, fruit and legumes	2.66	2.94	11%	2.77	3.48	26%
		Staple food	2.54	3.16	24%	2.49	3.34	34%
		Animal foods	2.60	2.76	6%	2.45	2.92	19%
		Of which haem-rich food	0.61	0.69	13%	0.48	0.64	33%
		Junk food	2.67	2.79	4%	2.29	2.26	-1%
Average number of times child eats junk food between meals			2.02	2.16	7%	1.94	1.86	-4%
Average cups/glasses consumed the previous day		Tea	1.37	0.87	-36%	1.43	0.89	-38%
		Of which tea with meals No. of cups	0.25 (13.3%)	0.17	-32%	0.25 (14.0%)	0.07	-72%
		(% drinking tea)		(12.0%)	-10%		(6.3%)	-55%

Table 8. Food consumption during previous 24 hours stratified for participation of parents in awareness sessions.

3.6.2 Children below 24 months of age at screening

The overwhelming majority of children were having an average of 3 meals a day and the percentage was stable. However, the percentage of children receiving fewer than 3 meals a day was reduced from 15.5% to 8.4.% (breast feeding was not considered).

As expected, the consumption of all types of food increased, with the exception of junk food, which remained stable. The consumption of soft drinks and candies, however, increased significantly.

Tea consumption was high, even among small children, half of whom had drunk it the previous day. There was an 18% decrease in quantity, and tea with meals decreased even more (-40%). At the same time water consumption increased.

Similar values were found in the non-anaemic population (144 children).

		Anaemic children <24 months			
		1st visit	2nd visit	change	P
N. of children		773			
Average no. of meals		2.90	2.96		
% of children having fewer than 3 meals		**15.5%**	**8.4%**	**-46%**	**<0.0001**
Average number of portions consumed the previous day	Vegetables, fruit and legumes	2.04	2.61	28%	0.0014
	Staple food	1.85	2.27	23%	<0.0001
	Animal foods	3.00	3.28	9%	0.0014
	Of which rich haem food	*0.53*	*0.64*	*21%*	*0.002*
	Junk food	1.92	1.86	-3%	0.4
	Of which chips	*0.62*	*0.50*	*-20%*	*<0.0001*
	Of which candies	*0.17*	*0.23*	*39%*	*0.001*
	Of which soft drinks	*0.06*	*0.09*	*49%*	*0.07*
Number of times child eats junk food between meals		1.91	1.88	-2%	0.4
Average cups/glasses consumed the previous day	Water	3.73	4.69	26%	<0.0001
	Tea no. of cups	0.82	0.67	-18%	0.0008
	(Percentage drinking tea)	(49%)	(47%)	-4%	0.3
	Of which tea between meals	*0.63*	*0.55*	*-12%*	*0.06*
		0.19	0.12	-40%	0.0007
	Of which tea with meals	*(12.2%)*	*(8.1%)*	*-34%*	*0.002*

Table 9. Food consumption during previous 24 hours as recorded during first and second
home visit for anaemic children below 24 months of age.

*WE COULD NOT FIND ANY ASSOCIATION BETWEEN IMPROVEMENT OF ANAEMIC
STATUS AND CHANGE IN NUTRITIONAL HABIT*

3.7 Anaemia prevalence after 1 year of intervention: a random sample of Phase 1 KGs children

One of the biggest challenges of any medical intervention is to maintain the benefit obtained
in the short term also in the long term. This is particularly important for nutritional
supplementation intervention, such as treatment for iron deficiency anaemia: it is
reasonable to have an improvement after iron supplementation, but what happens then? It
is true that even a temporary improvement in anaemia at a crucial age with regard to
growth can have long-lasting benefits, but our task was to assess the level of anaemia 1 year
after the end of the intervention.

3.7.1 Methods

We randomly selected 178 children who were anaemic when enrolled in October 2009
during the SOUTH GAZA-1 project and had improved by the end of the project (May
2010),   and we re-tested them in May 2011, one year after the end of the project. To
evaluate improvement we compared anaemia prevalence and haemoglobin level at the
three different time points using the pair t-test (comparison of each subject with
himself/herself).

3.7.2 Results

It can be seen from Table 10 below and Figure 6 that:

- at the end of phase 1 only 8 children were still anaemic (all of them had an improvement in Hb level ≥1g/dl; none had moderate or severe anaemia);
- 1 year later the vast majority of children (88.2%) were still not anaemic and only 21 had regressed to mild anaemia;
- the level of anaemia increased significantly after 1 year (from 5.5% to 11.8%; p=0.011) but was still much lower than found at baseline;
- none of the 21 anaemic cases in May 2011 had moderate or severe anaemia and only 2 had an Hb level below 10g/dl, meaning that even the children who were still anaemic were at the limit of normality. The average haemoglobin level among the children was lower than in May 2010, yet much higher than the level recorded at the beginning of the SOUTH GAZA 1 project.

Type of anaemia	October 2009		May 2010		May 2011		P value
	No.	%	No.	%	No.	%	
Severe and moderate anaemia <9g	18	10.1%	0	0%			<0.0001
Mild anaemia	160	89.9%	8	5.5%	21	11.8%	
No anaemia	0		170	95.5%%	157	88.2%	
Mean Hb level among 178 children	9.94 g/dl		11.98 g/dl		11.85 g/dl		<0.0001
Mean Hb level among 21 children still anaemic in May 2011	9.89 g/dl		11.71 g/dl		10.42 g/dl		<0.0001

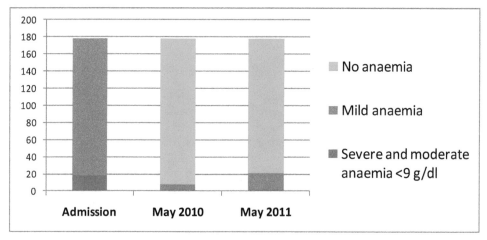

Table 10. and Fig. 6. Anaemia prevalence at three different time points.

Conclusions drawn:

- anaemia improvement achieved during the SOUTH GAZA 1 project persisted after 1 year;
- the overwhelming majority of children were still not anaemic after 1 year;

- there was still a fraction of children who regressed to anaemia after stopping supplementation, but their Hb levels were much higher than before project implementation.

3.8 Follow-up of still anaemic children

Children who were still anaemic after intervention underwent a more thorough clinical investigation, treatment and a longer follow-up.

Only 50 were diagnosed as having thalassaemia: the 0.48% of the 10.445 children screened and the 1.01% of the children found to be anaemic.

Out of the 296 children found to be still anaemic during follow-up screening at the end of the SOUTH GAZA-1 project, 159 (from 140 families) were still attending kindergarten in October 2010 and were enrolled in Phase 2 activities; the others had left, mainly to go to school. One hundred and twenty-nine of them were tested again; the other 33 refused to enter the new program.

After intensive counselling, the majority of children with no improvement in anaemic status were found to:

- have had poor drug adherence and/or
- have high tea consumption during meals and/or
- drink large amounts of tea.

Extra counselling was given to the mothers of these children.

The results for the 129 children re-tested in October 2010 showed a substantial change from their previous status (Table 11):

- 50.4% of children were no longer anaemic;
- the number of children with severe/moderate anaemia dropped from 17 to 3;
- 19 children were still anaemic, but improved their Hb value by at least 1g/dl;
- only 45 children did not improve.

Type of anaemia	June 2010		October 2010		p value
	No.	%	No.	%	
Severe and moderate anaemia <9gr	17	13.2%	3	2.3%	
Mild anaemia	111	86.2%	61	47.3%	<0.0001
No anaemia	1	0.8%	65	50.4%%	
Mean Hb level among 129 children	9.62 g/dl		10.91 g/dl		<0.0001

Table 11. Haemoglobin level and anaemic status of children not improving in the first phase.

4. Discussion

4.1 Anaemia prevalence

Our sample cannot be considered as fully representative of the under-5 population of the Gaza Strip because they were not randomly selected, and because children below 12 months of age were under-represented. We found an anaemia prevalence at screening of 43.7%, which was strongly associated with children's younger age (from 76.2% at 6-11 months to 17.0% for children over 5 years of age).

The prevalence we found is very similar to that reported by the local Ministry of Health (PNA MOH, 2011) for children below 12 months (prevalence 76.2% among children aged 9-12 months) but much lower for the oldest age group (prevalence 58.6% among school children in 2009). The lower prevalence noticed in our children over 5 years of age could be explained by the fact that there have been several instances in the last 2 years of iron-fortified-food distribution in kindergartens, and we found that children receiving fortified food had a significantly lower level of anaemia. However the fortified food distribution, which was not implemented within a public health scheme, does not seem to be able to tackle completely the problem and several kids were found anaemic despite it.

In addition to child's age and utilisation of fortified food, we found a significant association of anaemia with mother's poor education (an indication that low-social-status subjects are more vulnerable) and with stunting (not surprising since anaemia and stunting both reflect poor quality nutrition).

It is worth noting that children aged between 12 and 48 months, particularly those below 24 months, have very high prevalence of anaemia but are particularly difficult to reach because they do not attend the health clinic regularly (the vaccination program ends in the first year) or go to kindergarten: specific actions to target them should be implemented because anaemia can have very negative consequences for them (Walter, 2003).

Universal growth monitoring at least once a year for all under-5s, including haemoglobin level testing, could be one of the measures to take in the Palestinian context, where medical facilities and health workers are readily available and could easily provide this service. This would also provide the opportunity to monitor and contrast stunting, an age-old chronic problem, at an early stage, and also obesity, the new rampant one.

4.2 Anaemia improvement

Overall performance for anaemia was very good. Nearly 70% of the children treated were cured within 4-6 months. A review of the literature shows that this rate is in line, if not better, with what has been achieved in specific studies elsewhere (Rosadoet al, 2010) or in the region where children received iron daily or weekly (Faqih et al, 2006; Tavil et al, 2003), but these were clinical trials with a small number of participants and effectiveness in the field is always more complicated.

One good result seen is an impact of the supportive counselling, including home visits: this is backed up by the fact that mothers who gained a better knowledge had an additional 24% chance of having a child who recovered from anaemia. The effect of well-motivated parents - something rarely studied in trials, where almost all participants are well motivated - is confirmed by the better results achieved when parents participated in awareness sessions.

Of course we have to be careful in considering this difference as a result of the awareness sessions, since it is likely that we had a strong selection bias: parents most interested in "nutritional" topics even before the project probably attended more awareness sessions, and they were also more attentive in monitoring their children's adherence and nutritional habits.

The lower rate of improvement in children below 24 months of age confirms the high vulnerability of this age group.

The use of more palatable iron with fewer side effects, such as that used in our projects (Toblli et al, 2007), can explain the relatively good adherence and impact: and the link between adherence and improvement was clearly proven during our interventions.

Supplementation and Change of Nutritional Habits for the Prevention and Treatment of Iron
Deficiency Anaemia in Gaza Children: A Case Study

191

As found in another study (Zlotkin et al, 2003), further supplementation is not needed to maintain non-anaemic status in most children previously treated for anaemia: almost all the children who recovered from anaemia were not anaemic 1 year later.

4.3 Nutritional habits: knowledge and practice
Knowledge of anaemia and nutrition was quite low, particularly for less educated mothers, but health education achieved a substantial increase in the level of knowledge, particularly in the less educated.

The 24-hour nutritional questionnaire was designed as a tool for diagnosis and family counselling, not for gathering information, but it provided some interesting data on food consumption:

- high prevalence of junk food in the under-5s, as also noticed for school children (PNA MOH, 2011);
- low consumption of fruit and vegetables;
- high consumption of tea, half of the children below 24 months of age having drunk some during the previous day.

During the second home visit we found a consistent decrease in tea consumption in all age categories, particularly during meals, but we were unable to establish a real reduction in junk food consumption and there was only a minimal increase in the intake of fruit and vegetables.

It is important to point out that food consumption was reported by the mothers, so the reported "good change" should be treated with caution because this could in part be the result of the mother's desire to give the (counselling) interviewer a good impression.

Our data confirm that increased knowledge did not immediately result in improved feeding habits, a constraint found in many interventions that try to address chronic nutritional problems such as obesity in children (Branca et al, 2007).

Little change in nutritional habits and the weakness of having only two monitoring measures of habits could explain why we were unable to establish a significant association between change in nutritional habit and anaemia improvement.

5. Acknowledgment

The article preparation was not funded by the donors in any way, and all its contents are published under the responsibility of Terre des Hommes Italia and the Palestinian Medical Relief.
Thanks go to the staff of PMRS, Tdh-It and kindergarten who implemented the projects

6. References

Abdeen, Z., Greenough, G., Shahin, M., Tayback M; 2002. Nutritional Assessment of the West Bank and Gaza Strip. Accessed on the internet on the 07/07/2007 at: http://www.usaid.gov/wbg/reports/Nutritional_Assessment.pdf

Azeredo CM, Cotta RM, Sant'Ana LF, Franceschini Sdo C, Ribeiro Rde C, Lamounier JA, Pedron FA. Greater effectiveness of daily iron supplementation scheme in infants. Rev Saude Publica. 2010 Apr;44(2):230-9.

Faqih AM, Kakish SB, Izzat M. Effectiveness of intermittent iron treatment of two- to six-year-old Jordanian children with iron-deficiency anemia. Food Nutr Bull. 2006 Sep;27(3):220-7.

Palestinian National Authority, 2011. National Nutrition Surveillance System. 2010 Report. Ministry of Health, Nutrition Department

Rahim HF, Wick L, Halileh S, Hassan-Bitar S, Chekir H, Watt G, Khawaja M. Maternal and child health in the occupied Palestinian territory. Lancet. 2009 Mar 14;373(9667):967-77. Epub 2009 Mar 4. Erratum in: Lancet. 2009 Jun 27;373(9682):2200.

Roberts, L. and Hofmann, C.A.; 2004. Assessing the impact of humanitarian assistance in the health sector. Emerg Themes Epidemiol. 1:3. Available from: http://www.ete-online.com/content/1/1/3

Robertson, D.W., Bedell, R., Lavery, J.V., Upshur. R.; 2002. What kind of evidence do we need to justify humanitarian medical aid? Lancet. 360, 330-333

Rosado JL, González KE, Caamaño Mdel C, García OP, Preciado R, Odio M. Efficacy of different strategies to treat anemia in children: a randomized clinical trial. Nutr J. 2010 Sep 23;9:40.

Rychetnik, L., Frommer, M., Hawe, P., Shiell, A.; 2002. Criteria for evaluating evidence on public health interventions. J Epidemiol Community Health. 56,119-127.

Tavil B, Sipahi T, Gökçe H, Akar N. Effect of twice weekly versus daily iron treatment in Turkish children with iron deficiency anemia. Pediatr Hematol Oncol. 2003 Jun;20(4):319-26.

Toblli JE, Brignoli R. Iron(III)-hydroxide polymaltose complex in iron deficiency anemia / review and meta-analysis. Arzneimittelforschung. 2007;57(6A):431-8. Review

Verster, A.; 1996. Guidelines for the control of iron deficiency in countries of the Eastern Mediterranean, Middle East and North Africa. World Health Organization, Regional Office for the Eastern Mediterranean. WHO-EM/NUT/177, E/G/11.96/1000.

Walter T. Effect of iron-deficiency anemia on cognitive skills and neuromaturation in infancy and childhood. Food Nutr Bull. 2003 Dec;24(4 Suppl):S104-10. Review.

WHO and UNICEF; 2004. Focusing on anaemia. Towards an integrated approach for effective anaemia control. Accessed on the internet on the 05/10/2011 at: http://www.who.int/medical_devices/publications/en/WHO_UNICEF-anaemiastatement.pdf

Francesco Branca, Haik Nikogosian and Tim Lobstein, 2007. The challenge of obesity in the WHO European Region and the strategies for response. WHO Regional Office for Europe, Copenhagen, Denmark

WHO, 2009. Multicentre Growth Reference Study Group. WHO Child Growth Standards: Growth velocity based on weight, length and head circumference: Methods and development. Geneva: World Health Organization, 2009.

WHO, UNICEF, United Nations University; 2001. Iron deficiency anaemia: assessment, prevention, and control. Geneva, World Health Organization. WHO/NHD/01.3.

WHO; 2009. Health conditions in the occupied Palestinian territory, including east Jerusalem, and in the occupied Syrian Golan. Provisional agenda item 14 A62/24: Provisional agenda item 13 A59/INF.DOC./21 May 2009. Accessed on the internet on the 05/08/2011 at: h http://apps.who.int/gb/ebwha/pdf_files/A62/A62_R2-en.pdf

12

Acceptance and Effect of Ferrous Fumarate Containing Micronutrient Sprinkles on Anemia, Iron Deficiency and Anthropometrics in Honduran Children

Teresa M. Kemmer[1], Preston S. Omer[2],
Vinod K. Gidvani-Diaz[3] and Miguel Coello[4]
[1]*Health and Nutritional Sciences, SDSU Extension
and Agricultural Experiment Station
South Dakota State University, Brookings,*
[2]*U.S. Army, U.S. Army Medical
Command, Fort Riley,*
[3]*U.S. Air Force San Antonio Uniformed
Services Health Education Consortium,
Pediatric Residency San Antonio,*
[4]*U.S. Medical Element, Joint Task
Force-Bravo, Soto Cano Air Base*
[1,2,3]*USA*
[4]*Honduras*

1. Introduction

Anemia is reflective of global inequalities between developing and developed countries and is an endemic problem (Balarajan et al., 2011). Global Iron deficiency anemia (IDA) is one of the top ten risk factors contributing to the global burden of disease and economic costs are estimated at 4.05% of gross domestic product per capita from loss in productivity and $14.46 (U.S.) per capital in lost cognitive function (World Bank, 2004). One-quarter of the world's population is affected by anemia (McLean et al., 2009). Using data from the World Health Organization (WHO) Vitamin and Mineral Nutrition Information System for 1993-2005 (WHO, 2008), McLean et al. estimated an anemia prevalence of 47.4% (293 million) in preschool-aged children (2009). Iron deficiency (ID) is attributed annually to 20,854 global deaths in children under 5 years of age (Black et al., 2008), anemia affects 1.62 billion people (24.8% of the population) and anemia prevalence is highest in preschool-age children (47.4%) (WHO, 2008). The WHO categorizes the prevalence of anemia as a public health problem as follows: <5% – no problem, 5–19% – mild public health problem, 20–39% – moderate public health problem, and >40% – severe public health (Badham, 2007). According to the 2011 World Bank World Development Indicators, in children less five years of age, the prevalence of anemia is greatest in South Asia at 71% and is estimated at

66% in low income areas of the world (World Bank, 2011). The average prevalence of anemia in Europe and Central Asia is 30%, Latin America and the Caribbean is 38%, and Middle East and North Africa is 48% (World Bank, 2011).

Iron deficiency anemia contributes to poor growth and cognitive impairment which in turn has a negative effect on learning potential and productivity (Lozoff et al., 2006; Grantham-McGregor & Ani, 2001). At school entry, children that had chronic, severe ID during infancy are at a behavioral disadvantage as compared to their peers (Corapci et al., 2006). Hemoglobin has been shown to be associated with a decrease in verbal short-term memory and the severity of anemia has an impact on neurocognitive deficits, indicating reduced oxygen delivery to the brain as an etiological mechanism (Hijmans et al., 2011). Iron deficiency anemia in infancy results in children and young adults with poorer inhibitory control and executive functioning as well as other negative effects on neurotransmitters, myelination, dendritogenesis, neurometabolism in hippocampus and striatum, gene and protein profiles, and there associated behaviors (Lozoff, 2011). The long term affects of iron deficiency during infancy on poorer cognitive, motor, affective, and sensory system functioning highlight the requirement to focus on early intervention strategies that minimize the long-term effects (Lozoff, 2011). In a review by Madan, et al. (2011) ID resulted in negative developmental and neurophysiologic deficits and lower scholastic achievement. Results from an inner-city study revealed poorer object permanence and short-term memory problems in infants with IDA at 9 months and concluded that these cognitive effects were partially due to IDA related deficits in socioemotional function (Carter et al., 2010). Analysis of multiple trials found 1.73 lower IQ points per 1 g/dL decrease in hemoglobin (Stoltzfus et al., 2004). The predicted rate of mental retardation in a population with hemoglobin distribution shifted 1 g/dL downward due to iron deficiency is estimated at 2.94% (Stoltzfus et al., 2004).

Indirectly, ID negatively impacts the earning potential and entire economy of third world countries throughout the world. It was estimated that 0.2% of deaths and 0.5% of disability-adjusted life-years (DALYs) in children under 5 years of age are attributed to ID (Black et al., 2008). Iron deficiency results in 0.5% of maternal and child deaths in the world and 1.3% of DALYs and are higher in low income countries at 0.8% and 1.6% respectively. Estimated attributable DALYs to maternal and child iron deficiency are 19.7 million (WHO, 2009).

Approximately a quarter of children under five years of age in the developing world are undernourished based on the Millennium Development Goals (MGD) Report (United Nations, 2011), and progress in reducing the proportion of people suffering from hunger is insufficient to reach the target goal by 2015. If this MDG is to be achieved, nutrition must be given higher priority and should include simple, cost-effective measures delivered particularly from conception to two years after birth such as improved maternal nutrition and care, breastfeeding within one hour of birth, exclusive breastfeeding for the first 6 months of life, and timely, adequate, safe, and appropriate complementary feeding and micronutrient intake between 6 and 24 months of age (United Nations, 2011).

According to the Oxford Poverty and Human Development Initiative for Honduras (2010), 18% of the population are poor according to the $1.25 a day poverty line and 51% are poor according to the national poverty line. Inequities in under-5 mortality rate exist within Honduras where the mortality rate spans from 20 deaths per 1000 live births in the wealthiest to 50 per 1000 in the poorest (WHO, 2011). Anemia is very prevalent in

Acceptance and Effect of Ferrous Fumarate Containing Micronutrient Sprinkles on Anemia,
Iron Deficiency and Anthropometrics in Honduran Children

195

Honduras. A study by Nestel et al. (1999) showed that the prevalence of anemia in Honduran children ages 12 to 71 months was approximately 30%. Albalak and colleagues reported anemia prevalence in Honduran children at 40% in ages 12 to 36 months and 18% in children 36 to 60 months (Albalak et al., 2000). As a developing country, Honduras suffers from the negative impact anemia has on health, growth, and cognitive development, which indirectly decreases the productivity of the country. The estimate of economic loss from IDA as a percent of gross domestic product in Honduras is 2% (Horton & Ross, 2003). Programs within Honduras have tried to decrease the prevalence of anemia through different methods that include fortification of staples as well as supplementation (Dewey et al., 1998, 2004; Darnton-Hill et al., 1999; Darnton-Hill, 1998; Venkatesh Mannar, 2006). In addition, studies by Dewey et al. support the Honduran Ministry of Health's efforts to improve the iron status of breast-fed infants (Dewey et al., 1998, 2004).

The prevalence of ID can be reduced by increasing the consumption of iron-containing foods in the diet, supplementation with iron, or fortification of foods with iron (Finch & Cook, 1984; Provan, 1999; Trowbridge, 2002). The International Nutritional Anemia Consultative Group (INACG), WHO, and United Nations International Children's Emergency Fund (UNICEF) recommend introducing iron supplementation to healthy term infants with normal birth weight at 6 to 12 mo of age if the prevalence of anemia is less than 40% in the population, and supplementing the infants onward until 24 mo of age if the prevalence of anemia is 40% or higher in the population (Zlotkin & Tondeur, 2007). Ferrous sulfate is mainly used to supplement food stuffs (Dary, 2007). An alternative supplement method is adding iron into the diet with "Micronutrient Sprinkles" which were developed at the Hospital for Sick Children (Schauer & Zlotkin, 2003). Sprinkles refer to a blend of micronutrients in powder form that are added to foods to target susceptible populations at higher risk of anemia and micronutrient deficiencies (Sprinkles Global Health Initiative, 2008). Sprinkles may contain any combination of micronutrients and are packaged in a small sachet, the contents of which can be added to any semi-solid food. Sprinkles can be designed and produced based on the population needs and allow susceptible populations to fortify home cooked foods.

The objectives of this randomized case-control study in non-anemic rural Honduran children ages 6 to 60 months were to determine if micronutrient sprinkles 1) are an effective method of preventing anemia and reducing ID, 2) result in improved growth parameters, and 3) are acceptable to the population.

2. Methods

This randomized case-control nutritional assessment study in rural Honduras was conducted in collaboration with the Honduran Ministry of Health (MoH); medical liaison officers at Joint Task Force Bravo, Medical Element, Soto Cano, Honduras; the San Antonio Military Pediatric Center; and South Dakota State University in 2006-2007. Immunization records obtained from the local health centers of children within the age range of 6 to 60 months were used for randomization of the household. Immunization records were used for the randomization since 98% of 1-year-old children in Honduras are immunized against Hepatitus B; measles; diphtheria, pertussis and tetanus (DPT); and tuberculosis (TB) and 94% of newborns are protected against tetanus (UNICEF, 2010). A minimum of 10% of the children within each health center were randomly selected for participation. Each child's household was visited with the assistance of local volunteers from the MoH clinics and community. Data collection included anthropometrics, survey data, blood collection, and altitude. Written consent was obtained from one of the primary care providers prior to participation. Completion of the survey required approximately 15 to 20 minutes and was administrated by a fluent Spanish speaker. The household was excluded if consent was not obtained or the household did not have children within the specified age range. No eligible family refused study participation. Officials of the Honduran Ministry of Health approved and supported this project and the protocol was approved through Wilford Hall Medical Center, San Antonio, TX; and the Office of Research/Human Subjects Committee, South Dakota State University, Brookings, SD. Research was conducted in compliance with the Declaration of Helsinki guidelines.

2.1 Anthropometric measurements

Weight and height/length were recorded during home visits using standardized equipment and procedures (WHO, 2006). Child weight was measured without clothing to the nearest 10th of a kilogram of body weight using a Seca® scale (Seca, Vogel & Halke, Germany). A child who was unable to stand on the scale was held and weight was obtained using the tare weight function. Child length was measured without shoes to the nearest 0.1 cm if the child was younger than 2 years using the infant/child Shorrboard® (Shorr Productions, Olney, MD). Height was obtained for children $\geq$ 2 years of age. World Health Organization Anthro program (WHO, 2005) was used to calculate anthropometrics. The cut-off values used to identify children as stunted was length/height-for-age < -2 z-scores (HAZ), underweight was weight-for-age < -2 z-scores (WAZ), and wasted was weight-for- length/height < -2 z-scores (WHZ) using the WHO standards (WHO, 2006). Following anthropometric data analysis, there were no outliers based on the following definitions: height-for-age < -6.0 and > +6.0, weight-for-age < -6.0 and > +5.0, and weight for height < -5.0 and > +5.0 (WHO, 2006).

2.2 Blood analysis

On-the-spot hemoglobin (Hb) was used to determine study eligibility. Hemoglobin was measured using the HemoCue Hemoglobin Photometer (HemoCue US, Mission Viejo, CA) and was adjusted for altitude (Ruiz-Arguelles, 2006). Altitude adjusted age-specific cutoff Hb values of <11.0 g/dL were used to determine anemia (WHO, 2001). The households of non-anemic children were randomly assigned to the sprinkles or non-sprinkles arm. All non-anemic children of the household in the target range were enrolled. All eligible children in one household were randomized to the same arm of the study. Anemic children were not enrolled in the study, were treated with ferrous sulfate, and their names were provided to the local MoH clinic personnel for follow-up.

Finger prick blood samples were obtained from the children. A global positioning system (GPS) was used at the household to determine altitude.

Analysis of transferrin receptor (TfR) to determine iron status was obtained using dried blood spot (DBS) samples on filter paper. The use of DBS is a convenient way of collecting samples in the field compared to venous blood sampling that would require a phlebotomist, centrifugation of samples, and immediate cold storage (Flowers & Cook, 1999). Care was taken not to touch the pre-printed circles on the filter paper before, during, and after blood collection and to avoid having one blood spot flow into another spot. Following blood spot collection, filter papers were exposed to air for a short period of time to allow drying, were placed in an airtight/watertight container with a desiccant, were stored away from light and

Acceptance and Effect of Ferrous Fumarate Containing Micronutrient Sprinkles on Anemia,
Iron Deficiency and Anthropometrics in Honduran Children

197

heat, and were dried overnight in the drying box. Following the drying process, the filter papers were stored in a zip-closure plastic freezer bag with desiccant and were kept at refrigerator or freezer temperature until analysis. The analysis of TfR from DBS was completed by The Craft Technologies, Inc., Wilson, NC, using the quantitative sandwich enzyme linked immunoassay (ELISA) (Erhardt et al., 2004). Iron deficiency was defined based on the manufacture's TfR assay reference. Iron deficiency anemia was defined as anemia in combination with ID.

Participants were enrolled during three separate trips to Honduras over the span of 12 months. A four month supply of sprinkles packets and pictorial and verbal instructions for use were provided for each child assigned to the sprinkles arm. The micronutrient sprinkle formula for this study contained iron (12.5 mg), zinc (5 mg), folic acid (150 µg), vitamin A (1600 I.U.), vitamin C (50 mg), and vitamin D (300 I.U.) and cost $0.025 (U.S.) per packet. Parents were asked to save the empty sachets and to return the empty and unused sachets during the four month follow-up visit as a measure of usage compliance. Measurements of Hb and TfR as well as anthropometric measurements were obtained at the initial visit and at the four and eight month intervals. Enrollees were provided Albendazol for helminthes infestation at each visit. Children found to be anemic at 4 months were started on supplemental iron therapy and were not included in the 8 month follow-up. A survey was administered at the four month follow-up visit to assess compliance, acceptability, side effects, and any logistical problems.

Statistical analysis was performed using SPSS computer software. Differences between the groups were assessed by independent samples t-test. Paired t-test was used to analyze change within groups. Chi-square test was used to compare the proportion of change in prevalence. The acceptable level of statistical significance was $P < 0.05$.

3. Results

In the households visited, there were 220 children. Of these, 21 were diagnosed with anemia and were ineligible for the study. Those found to be anemic were treated and referred directly to the MoH clinic. The remaining 199 children were enrolled in the study and randomized into the sprinkles (n=114) and non-sprinkles (n=85) groups.

3.1 Baseline characteristics

The mean age was 34.66 months (± 15.31 SD), mean Hb was 12.47 g/dL (± 0.81 SD), mean TfR was 7.02 mg/L (± 2.52), mean altitude was 5,023.98 ft (± 558.57 SD) and 55% were male. The groups did not differ significantly at base-line in age, gender, Hb, TfR, weight or height; however, average altitude was significantly different (P < 0.001). Children within the sprinkles group were at a higher mean altitude (5134 ft vs 4876 ft). Within this study population, Hb and TfR were not significantly correlated with altitude. Of the 199 children enrolled in the study, four children (2%) did not return for the four month follow-up visit, an additional 3 children did not provide a blood sample to evaluate Hb. At the 4 month follow-up visit 20.3% of participants were anemic, treated with iron, referred to the MoH clinic and were removed from the study. At the 8 month follow-up, an additional 15.2% were anemic.

3.2 Primary outcome measures

There was no significant difference seen in mean Hb between the sprinkles and non-sprinkles groups between visits (Table 1). At the 4 and 8 month visits, 4.4% and 2.4%

respectively had IDA. The prevalence of anemia and IDA by visit for the sprinkles and non-sprinkles groups is presented in Table 2. There was no significant difference between groups for ID or IDA at 4 or 8 months.

At baseline, 23.8% of the sprinkles group and 22.8% of the non-sprinkles group were iron deficient (ID). Within children that were ID at baseline, 58.3% of the sprinkles group and 55.6% of the non-sprinkles group were no longer ID at 4 months and 60.9% of the sprinkles group and 77.8% of the non-sprinkles group were no longer ID at 8 months. There was no significant difference in TfR change from baseline to 4 or 8 months between groups (Table 1). At 8 months, 24.5% of the sprinkles group and 20.0% of the non-sprinkles group were ID. Paired T-test results for change in Hb from baseline to 4 months was 0.20 (p=0.13) for the sprinkles group and 0.31 (p<0.05) for the non-sprinkles group respectively. From baseline to 4 months there were significant paired T-test differences in TfR of -1.37 within the sprinkles group (p< 0.001) and -.076 within the non-sprinkles group (p< 0.05).

	Sprinkles (SD)	Non-Sprinkles (SD)	P-value*
Initial Hb (gm/dL)	12.45 (0.80)	12.55 (0.83)	
4 months	12.13 (1.19)	12.22 (1.26)	0.63
8 months	12.46 (1.35)	12.47 (1.17)	0.73
Overall change			0.56
Initial TfR	7.02 (2.07)	7.02 (2.39)	
4 months	8.39 (2.93)	7.78 (2.29)	0.98
8 months	7.19 (1.64)	7.02 (1.81)	0.12
Overall change			0.52

* Significance determined at P <0.05.

Table 1. Change in Mean Hemoglobin (Hb) and Serum Transferrin Receptor (TfR) between Visits for Sprinkles vs Non-Sprinkles.

	Anemia (%)*	IDA (%)*
Initial	n=199	n=182
Sprinkles	0	0
Non-Sprinkles	0	0
4 Months	n=192	n=180
Sprinkles	16.5	4.0
Non-Sprinkles	25.3	5.0
8 Months	n=132	n=123
Sprinkles	17.5	4.1
Non-Sprinkles	11.5	0

* No significant differences was seen in prevalence between Sprinkles and non-Sprinkles groups. Significance determined at P<0.05.
Note: No anemic children were enrolled in the study. If children were anemic at 4 months, they were treated and removed from the study.

Table 2. Prevalence of Anemia and Iron Deficiency Anemia (IDA) by visit for Sprinkles vs. non-Sprinkles groups.

3.3 Anthropometric measurements

There was no significant difference between baseline and 4 and 8 months in the sprinkles group compared to the non-sprinkles group when comparing change in mean height, weight, weight-for-age Z-score, height-for-age Z-score, or weight-for-height Z-score (Tables 3 & 4). There was also no significant change between groups in the prevalence of stunting, underweight or wasting (Table 5).

	Sprinkles	Non-Sprinkles	P-value*
Initial weight (kg)	11.74	12.25	
4 months	12.54	12.89	0.63
8 months	13.01	13.59	0.27
Overall change			0.25
Initial height (cm)	84.45	85.94	
4 months	87.05	88.65	0.62
8 months	89.82	91.07	0.35
Overall change			0.35

*Significance determined at P <0.05.

Table 3. Change in Mean Weight and Height between Visits for Sprinkles vs Non-Sprinkles.

	Sprinkles	Non-Sprinkles	P-value*
Initial weight-for-age Z-score	-0.99	-0.91	
4 months	-0.98	-1.0	0.89
8 months	-1.09	-0.98	0.73
Overall change			0.68
Initial height-for-age Z-score	-2.04	-1.99	
4 months	-2.09	-2.05	0.75
8 months	-2.07	-2.09	0.94
Overall change			0.96
Initial weight-for-height Z-score	0.20	0.31	
4 months	0.29	0.25	0.84
8 months	0.17	0.34	0.66
Overall change			0.48

*Significance in mean change between time intervals for Sprinkles vs non-Sprinkles. Significance determined at P<0.05.

Table 4. Change in Mean Weight-for-Age Z-score, Height-for-Age Z-score, and Weight-for-Height Z-score by Visit.

	Stunting (%)*	Underweight (%)*	Wasting (%)*
Initial (n=195)			
Sprinkles	48.6	16.2	0.9
Non-Sprinkles	54.8	14.3	0
All	51.3	15.4	0.5
4 Months (n=187)			
Sprinkles	51.9	13.5	0
Non-Sprinkles	54.2	10.8	0
8 Months (n=168)			
Sprinkles	46.3	14.7	0
Non-Sprinkles	58.9	9.6	1.4

* No significant difference was seen in prevalence between Sprinkles and non-Sprinkles groups. Significance determined at P<0.05.

Table 5. Prevalence of Stunting, Underweight and Wasting by Visit for Sprinkles vs. Non-Sprinkles groups
Stunting = height-for-age Z-score <-2; Underweight = weight-for-age <-2 Z-scores; wasting = weight-for-age <-2 Z-scores.

3.4 Sprinkles use and acceptability

Based on parental responses and counting of the returned empty sprinkles packets, children who received sprinkles used an average 108 of 120 (90%) packets. The number of packets consumed ranged from 24 to 120. Of children who received sprinkles, 55% used all 120 packets, and 86% used more than 100 packets. The majority of families, 92%, used seven packets per week with a range from 3 to 7 packets per week. Parents reported that only 3 children (2.75%) disliked food with sprinkles added, 1 child had diarrhea, and one had difficulty in administering sprinkles. Rice, beans and soup were the foods most commonly mixed with the sprinkles. Sprinkles in food were not noticed by 54.1% of the children, 32.1% liked the food better with the sprinkles and 13.8% did not like the food with sprinkles. They were found easy to use in food preparation by 98.2% of the families and one parent reported that it was difficult to use daily and another reported that it took added time. All of the participants reported that they would continue to use the sprinkles if they were delivered free through the MoH clinic.

4. Discussion

4.1 Anemia and iron status

Only three other studies were located that reported information on sprinkles trials in subjects that were not anemic at the beginning of the study (Lundeen et al., 2010; Giovannini et al., 2006; Zlotkin et al., 2003a). Daily use of sprinkles for 2 months in anemic (72%) and non-anemic children ages 6 to 36 months revealed that within the non-anemic children receiving sprinkles 28% became anemic compared to 50% in the non-sprinkles group (Lundeen et al., 2010).

A 12 month double-blind, placebo-controlled trial in children aged 6 months by Giovannini et al. (2006) included both anemic and non-anemic children within the analysis (mean

Acceptance and Effect of Ferrous Fumarate Containing Micronutrient Sprinkles on Anemia,
Iron Deficiency and Anthropometrics in Honduran Children

201

baseline Hb $\geq$ 10.1 g/dL) and did not report results for non-anemic children only. Prevalence of anemia was significantly reduced in infants receiving either of the sprinkles supplements (Giovannini et al., 2006). A 6 month study performed by Zlotkin et al. looked at the effectiveness of microencapsulated iron (II) fumarate sprinkles with and without vitamin A, iron (II) sulfate drops or placebo sprinkles in preventing the recurrence of anemia in non-anemic (Hb $\geq$ 10.0 g/dL) children between the ages of 8-20 months (2003a). From baseline to the end of the supplementation period, there were no significant changes seen in the mean Hb or ferritin within the four groups and the children that became anemic were equally distributed among groups (Zlotkin et al., 2003a). Within the study, 82.4% of the children from all four groups remained in their non-anemic status, while 77.1% of children maintained their non-anemic status during the post-supplementation period (Zlotkin et al., 2003a). Zlotkin et al. (2003a) concluded that their findings do not support the continued use of long-term prophylactic iron supplementation to maintain iron status in children treated previously for IDA. Within the current study, there were also no significant changes in Hb or iron status between the sprinkles or non-sprinkles groups. Though the change in Hb over the study and the anemia prevalence was not significantly different between groups, a decrease in Hb is a late finding in IDA (Provan, 1999). An additional study being conducted by Bilenko et al. (2010) is similar to the current study in that the objective is to evaluate the efficacy of sprinkles in primary prevention of iron and other micronutrient deficiencies; however, results of the study are pending.

Studies performed in several countries have shown that sprinkles are effective in treating IDA, and that sprinkles are more effective and more easily administered than iron drops due to less side effects (Hirve et al., 2007; Schauer & Zlotkin, 2003; Zlotkin et al., 2004). Efficacy has been shown with sprinkles including formulations containing relatively low amounts of iron, and better results were achieved with daily dosing versus weekly dosing (Christofides et al., 2006; Giovannini et al., 2006; Menon et al., 2007; Shareiff et al., 2006). An analysis of studies that used dispersion of micronutrients in sachets completed by Horton et al. (2010) resulted in an increase in Hb concentration of 0.057 g/dL and IDA was reduced as compared to controls. When allowing flexible administration of micronutrient sprinkles compared to daily administration Hb was significantly higher in the group allowed flexible administration and resulted in an anemia prevalence decrease by 65% vs. 51% (Ip et al., 2009).

In comparison with other studies (Adu-Afarwuah et al., 2008; Giovannini et al., 2006; Zlotkin et al., 2003a), this study attempted to determine the utility of sprinkles to prevent anemia in non-anemic children. The prevention of anemia within children can lower the risk of developing cognitive and physical impairments (Grantham-McGregor & Ani, 2001). Giovannini et al. compared the efficacy of iron plus folic acid and zinc, iron plus folic acid alone, or a placebo and within the two sprinkle supplement groups there was no significant change in the rate of ID; however, the occurrence of ID increased in the placebo group (Giovannini et al., 2006).

A study completed by Adu-Afarwuah et al. compared the effectiveness of sprinkles, crushable Nutritabs, fat-based Nutributter, or a placebo on Ghanaina infants from 6 to 12 months of age (2008). This study showed that the risk of ID or anemia was significantly lower in the three intervention groups compared to the control group (Adu-Afarwuah et al., 2008). A meta-analysis evaluating the effect of multiple micronutrients in micronutrient deficient children, resulted in small but significant improvements in Hb (effect size=0.39) (Allen et al., 2009). In a randomized comparison of the effects of sprinkles, foodlets and iron drops, iron status improved in all treatment groups though there was no difference in change in anemia prevalence; however, drops resulted in significantly greater changes in Hb and serum ferritin (Samadpour et al., 2011).

Other studies determined the effectiveness chewable tablets in the prevention of iron deficiency (Smuts et al., 2005; Lopez de Romaña et al., 2005). Children from South Africa, Peru, Vietnam, and Indonesia were randomly assigned to one of four intervention groups: a daily placebo, a weekly multiple micronutrient supplement, a daily multiple micronutrient supplement, or a daily iron supplement and results showed that the overall prevalence of anemia decreased over the course of the study in all four intervention groups (Smuts et al., 2005). Iron deficiency increased in the placebo and weekly micronutrient supplement groups while decreasing in the daily iron and daily micronutrient supplement groups (Smuts et al., 2005). Lopez de Romaña et al. determined the efficacy of different micronutrient supplements in preventing growth failure, anemia, and other micronutrient deficiencies in Peruvian infants (2005). Infants between the ages of 6 to 12 months were randomly assigned to receive a placebo, a weekly dose of multiple micronutrients, a daily dose of multiple micronutrients, or a daily dose of iron (Lopez de Romaña et al., 2005). The prevalence of anemia decreased in all intervention groups; however, the decrease was not significant in the placebo group and anemia was best controlled by daily micronutrient supplements containing iron (Lopez de Romaña et al., 2005).

Additional studies have included treatment for anemic children (Rosado et al., 2010; Christofides et al., 2006; Menon et al., 2007; Zlotkin et al., 2004; Zlotkin et al., 2001). The use of sprinkles in the treatment of anemia has been shown to be successful within children and infants (De-Regil et al., 2011; Zlotkin et al., 2001; Zlotkin et al., 2003b). In a compilation of six studies, home fortification with sprinkles resulted in anemia reduction by 31% (RR 0.69) and in four studies, iron deficiency was reduced by 51% (RR 0.49) (De-Regil et al., 2011). In an efficacy study of different strategies to treat anemia in children, all treatments significantly increased Hb and total iron concentration; however, ferritin did not change significantly (Rosado et al., 2010). A study by Zlotkin et al. looked at the treatment of anemic children ages between 6 months to 18 months in Ghana and demonstrated that over 50% of children treated with sprinkles were successfully cured (Zlotkin et al., 2001). Menon et al. showed a drop in anemia prevalence from 52.3% to 28.3% in children receiving sprinkles with the fortified wheat-soy blend (WSB) compared to the WSB only, which showed an increase in anemia prevalence from 37% to 45% (2007). Christofides et al. found that various doses of sprinkles and iron drops garnered significant changes in Hb concentration and the prevalence of IDA decreased significantly over the course of the study (2006).

4.2 Anthropometric measurements

Higher rates of stunting are seen in Honduras than in its neighboring countries and income peers (World Bank, 2010). Within Honduran children under five years of age, 29% suffer from stunting, 11% from underweight and 1% from wasting (UNICEF, 2010). Growth parameters measured in Honduran children ages 12 to 71 months during the 1996 National Micronutrient Survey revealed that 38% were stunted, 24% were underweight, and 1% were wasted (Nestel et al., 1999). The prevalence of stunting, underweight and wasting within rural Honduran children ages 6 to 60 months was 57%, 33%, and 3.5% respectively (Tolson et al., 2010). Analysis of the 2006 Honduran Demographic and Health Survey data revealed that children that were wanted and had adequate parental care resulted in significant effects on children's height-for-age growth status (Sparks, 2011).

In a pooled analysis of 55 studies completed by Horton et al. (2010) they noted no benefit of iron supplementation on growth. Multi-micronutrient fortified energy-dense, fat-based Nutributter resulted in significantly greater WAZ and HAZ, than the use of micronutrient home fortification in either sprinkles or crushed tablets (Adu-Afarwuah et al., 2007). Even though sprinkles was successful in treating anemia in infants and young children, it did not promote catch-up growth in a stunted and wasted population in Ghana (Zlotkin et al., 2003a). Prevention of growth faltering was not noted in a double-blind, masked, controlled trial in infants provided iron or multiple micronutrients as compared to placebo (Lopez de Romana et al., 2005). When pooling data from four countries, a daily micronutrient supplement proved the most effective in promoting significant weight gain; however, there was no difference in height gain (Smuts et al., 2005). A compilation of eight trials (3748 participants) on the use of micronutrient powders in home fortification of foods showed no effect on growth (De-Regil et al., 2011). A four month evaluation of iron supplements in varying forms provided to anemic children also resulted in no difference in growth parameters (Rosado et al, 2010). In a meta-analysis evaluating the effect of multiple micronutrients on child growth, the intervention resulted in small but significant improvements in height/length (effect size=0.13) and weight (effect size= 0.14) (Allen et al., 2009). In a 4 month trial comparing efficacy of sprinkles, foodlets and drops, there was no significant difference in anthropometric measurements, or change in prevalence of underweight, stunting and wasting between treatment groups (Samadpour et al, 2011).

4.3 Sprinkles use and acceptability

The overall use of sprinkles within this study was well accepted with 55% of participants using all of the packets provided for the 4 month intervention. Lundeen et al. (2010) found that on average 45 of 60 sprinkles packets were consumed with 38.8% of participants consuming all 60 packets and 83.1% of children eating the entire portion of food mixed with the sprinkles. In a study conducted by Loechl et al. (2009), 63% of mothers reported using the sprinkles every day based on survey results and 86% based on exit interview results.

Other studies have compared alternative treatments of anemia to sprinkles (Christofides et al., 2006). One study showed that 92.9% of children had a strong dislike for the iron drops while only 6.5% objected to the consumption of sprinkles (Zlotkin et al., 2003a). Hirve et al. (2007) found that the side effects such as diarrhea, vomiting, staining of teeth, and stool discoloration were all significantly higher in the iron drops group than compared to sprinkles. In a study conducted by Adu-Afarwuah et al. (2008), 96.9% of mothers thought it was easy to give the sprinkles supplement, 89.6% said that the child accepted the food well, 95.9% did not have any major problems feeding the sprinkles to the child and 100% had a good impression of the sprinkles supplement. Allowing flexible administration vs. daily administration of micronutrient sprinkles improved adherence and was more acceptable (Ip et al., 2009). In an evaluation of iron drops vs. sprinkles, both groups had generally pour adherence and overall, there was no significant difference between groups (Geltman et al., 2009). Eighty percent of respondents in the sprinkles group vs. 69% in the drops group would use them again; however, the difference was not significant. There was a significant difference between the sprinkles vs. the drops group of respondents being concerned about using a new products and about the product's safety (Geltman et al., 2009).

4.4 Use of anti-parasitic medication

At each home visited anti-parasitic medication for children > 2 years of age was provided per MoH protocol. Because helminth infection is common in Honduras (Smith et al., 2001) and is a significant contributing factor to anemia (Bethony et al., 2006; Brooker et al., 2006), this intervention itself likely impacted the prevalence and severity of anemia in both groups (Stoltzfus et al., 1998) thus confounding results focused on the effect of sprinkles. It is important to note that at end of the study, the percentage of children with anemia in each group was less than the general prevalence of anemia among Honduran children.

Study strengths included the large number of participants in this randomized design used to determine efficacy of sprinkle supplements for the prevention of anemia in children ages 6 to 60 months. The large number of participants helps to prove the reliability of the effectiveness of the sprinkles compared to no treatment (Brooker et al., 2006). Altitude was collected at the household for accurate determination of the participants altitude adjusted Hb. Household data collection was convenient for participants. As a measure of compliance, participants were required to turn in empty and leftover sprinkle packets at the 4 month follow-up visit. The field friendly DBS method allowed measurement of iron status and eliminated the requirements for venipucture, a highly trained phlebotomist, centrifugation, and immediate ultra cold storage. Limitations of the study include the DBS were obtained in a field environment and they were not available for all participants due to parental refusal or inadequate blood sample size for analysis. Regarding sprinkle acceptability, parent reports were relied upon and may not be entirely accurate. The areas where the study was conducted were assigned by the Honduran MoH and included rural homes with low socioeconomic status. While this may be a representative sample for much of the population in Honduras, our results may not be applicable to children in different settings.

5. Strategies to address anemia and iron deficiency

If the MDG of reducing the proportion of people suffering from hunger is to be achieved by 2015, nutrition must be given higher priority and should include simple, cost-effective measures delivered particularly from conception to two years after birth (United Nations, 2011). These measures should incorporate improved maternal nutrition and care, breastfeeding within one hour of birth, exclusive breastfeeding for the first 6 months of life, and timely, adequate, safe, and appropriate complementary feeding and micronutrient intake between 6 and 24 months of age (United Nations, 2011).

A lifecycle approach to the problem is required to control iron deficiency and should include effective public health programs that consider the whole reproductive cycle and create a combination of strategies that are complementary and comprehensive across vulnerable periods (Stoltzfus, 2011). Anemia prevention and control strategies include: 1) increased food diversity with increased iron bioavailability and improved dietary quality and quantity; 2) biofortification, fortification of staples with iron, open market fortification of processed food, targeted fortification; 3) iron and folic acid supplementation to high-risk groups; 4) disease control; and 5) improved knowledge and education on anemia prevention and control for policy makers and the general public (Balarajan et al., 2011).

When implementing large-scale programs it is essential to assess the coverage, compliance and effectiveness and the programs should promote a food-based approach, including fortification of staple foods and condiments for the general population as well as home fortificants for specific target groups, since they are more sustainable, less perceived as treatment of a condition and are applicable for use in malaria-endemic areas (Badham et al., 2007). Prevention of ID requires policy and program guidance and working closely with decision makers about the what, when and how to implement and manage the program (Lutter, 2008). The widespread endemic of iron deficiency can be approached through a number of options which include dietary measures, fortification, supplementation, and treatment of infections/infestations and it is essential to consider that an effective resolution may vary by population subgroups, region and country (Milman, 2011). Using existing maternal and child health and nutrition programs to distribute micronutrient sprinkles and educate parents on their use is feasible and acceptable (Loechl et al., 2009).

Several recommendations from the World Bank Scaling up Nutrition paper (Horton et al., 2010) that can be implemented in partnership with the health sector in support of reducing the prevalence of anemia and iron deficiency include: 1) the use of multiple micronutrient powders and deworming drugs in children under the age of five years of age; 2) complimentary and therapeutic feeding interventions that provide micronutrient fortified and/or enhanced complementary foods for the prevention and treatment of moderate malnutrition among children 6-23 months of age; 3) promotion of breastfeeding, appropriate complementary feeding practices, and proper hygiene; and 4) iron fortification of staple foods for the general population.

Public health interventions addressing iron deficiency are one of the most cost effective with a cost-benefits ratio for iron programs estimated at 200:1 (Badham et al., 2007). On a worldwide scale, it would take an additional $10.3 billion (U.S.) in public resource support to begin successfully alleviating undernutrition on a worldwide scale benefiting over 360 million (Horton et al., 2010). On a nationwide basis in Honduras, it is estimated that it would take $6 million (U.S.) per year to scale up core micronutrient nutrition interventions and the costs are as low as $0.05-8.46 per person annually with a return on investment as high as 6-30 times the cost (World Bank, 2010; Horton et al., 2010). To alleviate much of iron deficiency's burden, iron fortification of staple foods would cost $0.20 (U.S.) per person per year, deworming cost would be $0.25 (U.S.) per child 24–59 month per round per year, and iron-folic acid supplements for pregnant women would cost approximately $2.00 (U.S.) per pregnancy (Horton et al., 2010). For sprinkles supplementation targeted to children 6–12 mo, it is estimated that cost per DALY saved could be as low as $12 with a benefit: cost ratio of 37:1 (Horton, et al., 2006). When determining the cost effectiveness of home-fortification programs in a low income country with a high infant mortality rate and high prevalence of anemia, it is estimated that cost per DALY saved is $12.2 and the present value of the gain in earnings is $37 for each dollar spent on the micronutrient sprinkles program (Sharieff et al., 2006).

Iron fortification continues to be evaluated in a variety of food stuffs for efficacy and acceptance (Karn et al., 2011; Angeles-Agdeppa et al., 2011; Varma et al., 2007; Andersson et al., 2008; Adu-Afarwuah et al., 2008; Wegmuller et al., 2006; Hurrell et al., 2010; Faber et al., 2005; Torrejon et al., 2004); however, it is essential that the fortification efforts are supported politically, adequately marketed, cost effective and have long-term commercial commitment (Angeles-Agdeppa et al., 2011). Iron supplementation and fortification are effective in controlling iron deficiency in populations and bioavailability of the iron is an important factor, iron status should be used and monitored to assess fortification requirements and efficacy (Zimmermann & Hurrell, 2007).

When implementing anemia prevention strategies the focus should be on preschoolers and adolescent women and on integrated public health programs (Boy et al., 2009). Lutter (2008) recommends iron prevention programs targeted during pregnancy, at birth, the immediate postnatal period and during the first 24 months of life and to not underestimate the challenges of delivery through the public health systems. Recommended practices for children ages 6-24 months include iron rich complementary foods, micronutrient supplements (medicinal iron supplements, micronutrient sachets, fortified complementary foods, lipid-based spreads) and deworming (Lutter, 2008).

National decision makers in each country are responsible to select the type and quantity of micronutrients added to foodstuffs and their decision should be based on their country's situation. The WHO recommends designing flour fortification programs based on four average wheat flour consumption ranges, the type of iron fortification compound (NaFeEDTA, ferrous sulfate, ferrous fumarate, or electrolytic iron) and flour extraction rate (low or high) (Hurrell et al., 2010). Wheat flour fortification programs were evaluated in 78 countries and only nine of the national programs could potentially result in a significant positive impact on iron status and that updated legislation is required to maximize the potential of meeting iron needs through fortification of wheat flour (Hurrell et al., 2010).

Genetic engineering of grains to increase iron content and bioavailability and selective plant breeding are also avenues being explored to combat iron deficiency (Zimmermann & Hurrell, 2007; Lucca et al., 2001 & 2006). Biofortified crops complement fortification and supplementation programs and are an option that provides a rural-based intervention that reaches more remote populations and then transfers into urban populations as production surpluses are marketed (Bouis et al., 2011). New iron fortification technologies that eliminate detrimental effects on taste, appearance, and product stability and that do not interfere with iron bioavailability show promising results (Mehansho, 2006).

Sustainable strategies for the prevention and control of iron deficiency require food based and non food based approaches incorporating agriculture, health, commerce, industry, education, communication and local nongovernmental organizations (Lokeshwar et al., 2011). Barriers to effective implementation of anemia prevention and control strategies include insufficient political priority, lack of resource commitment, lack of institutional and operational capacity, restricted financial access, poor awareness of the magnitude of disease burden, and lack of knowledge and education (Balarajan et al., 2011).

Strategic research is required to address the effective prevention and control of iron deficiency and its consequences in young children living in low-income countries and should address: 1) scaling up known effective interventions, 2) evaluating cost-effective alternatives that are likely to work, 3) efficacy research to discover promising practices that lack proven interventions, and 4) determining physiological processes and mechanisms underlying the risks and benefits of supplemental iron for children exposed to infectious diseases (Stoltzfus, 2008).

6. Conclusions

Within this study of non-anemic rural Honduran children ages 6 to 60 months, there were no statistically significant differences between the sprinkles and non-sprinkles groups when comparing change in mean Hb, TfR, and anthropometric measurements or prevalence in anemia, iron deficiency, stunting, underweight and wasting. However, at the end of the study, prevalence of anemia in each study group was less than the general prevalence of anemia for Honduran children. Sprinkle compliance was good; they were well tolerated by children and were accepted among the participating families. Additional research is

Acceptance and Effect of Ferrous Fumarate Containing Micronutrient Sprinkles on Anemia,
Iron Deficiency and Anthropometrics in Honduran Children

207

required to determine efficacy of sprinkles for anemia prevention in larger populations and over longer periods of time.

7. Acknowledgements

Funding was provided by Wilford Hall Medical Center, San Antonio, TX; South Dakota State University Agricultural Experiment Station, Brookings, SD; and the Center for Disaster and Humanitarian Assistance Medicine, Uniformed Services University of the Health Sciences, Bethesda, MD. Micronutrient sprinkles were provided by Heinz Company, Canada.

8. References

Adu-Afarwuah S, Lartey A, Brown, KH, Zlotkin S, Briend A, Dewey K. (2008). Home fortification of complementary foods with micronutrient supplements is well accepted and has positive effects on infant iron status in Ghana, *Am J Clin Nutr*, 87:929-38

Adu-Afarwuah S, Lartey A, Brown, KH, Zlotkin S, Briend A, Dewey K. (2007). Randomized comparison of 3 types of micronutrient supplements for home fortification of complementary foods in Ghana: Effects on growth and motor development, *Am J Clini Nutr*, 87:929-38

Albalak R, Ramakrishnan U, Stein AD, Van der Haar F, Haber MJ, Schroeder D, Martorell R. (2000). Co-Occurrence of Nutrition Problems in Honduran Children, *J Nutr*, 130:2271-2273

Allen LH, Peerson JM, Olney DK. (2009). Provision of multiple rather than two or fewer micronutrients more effectively improves growth and other outcomes in micronutrient-deficient children and adults, *J Nutr*, 139(5):1022-30

Andersson M, Thankachan P, Muthayya S, Goud RB, Kurpad AV, Hurrell RH, Zimmermann MB. (2008). Dual fortification of salt with iodine and iron: a randomized, double-blind, controlled trial of micronized ferric pyrophosphate and encapsulated ferrous fumarate in southern India, *Am J Clin Nutr*, 88(5):1378-1387

Angeles-Agdeppa I, Saises M, Capanzana M, Juneja LR, Sakaguchi N. (2011). Pilot-scale commercialization of iron-fortified rice: effects on anemia status, *Food Nutr Bull*, 32(1):3-12

Badham J, Zimmermann MB, Kraemer K (ed). (2007). *The Guidebook Nutritional Anemia.* Sight and Life Press, Basel, Switzerland. (51 pages)

Balarajan Y, Ramakrishnan U, Ozaltin E, Shankar AH, Subramanian S. (2011). Anaemia in low-income and middle-income countries, *Lancet.* 2011 Aug 1, [Epub ahead of print]

Bethony J, Brooker S, Albonico M, Geiger SM, Loukas A, Diemert D, Hotez PJ. (2006). Soil-transmitted helminth infections: ascariasis, trichuriasis, and hookworm, *Lancet*, 367:1521-32

Bilenko N, Belmaker I, Vardi H, Fraser D. (2010). Efficacy of multiple micronutrient supplementations on child health: study design and baseline characteristics, *Isr Med Assoc J*, 12(6):342-7

Black RE, Allen LH, Bhutta ZA, Caulfield LE, de Onis M, Ezzati M, Mathers C, Rivera J. (2008) Maternal and child undernutrition: global and regional exposures and health consequences, *Lancet*, 371:243-60

Bouis HE, Hotz C, McClafferty B, Meenakshi JV, Pfeiffer WH. (2011). Biofortification: a new tool to reduce micronutrient malnutrition, *Food Nutr Bull*, 32(1 Suppl):S31-40

Boy E, Mannar V, Pandav C, de Benoist B, Viteri F, Fontaine O, Hotz C. (2009). Achievements, challenges, and promising new approaches in vitamin and mineral deficiency control, *Nutr Rev*, 67:S24-30

Brooker S, Clements ACA, Hotez PJ, Hay SI, Tatem AJ, Bundy DAP, Snow RW. (Nov 2006). The co-distribution of Plasmodium falciparum and hookworm among African schoolchildren, *Malaria Journal*, 5(99), Accessed July 7, 2009, Available at http:www.malaria journal.com/ content/5/1/99

Carter RC, Jacobson JL, Burden MJ, Armony-Sivan R, Dodge NC, Angelilli ML, Lozoff B, Jacobson SW. (2010). Iron deficiency anemia and cognitive function in infancy, *Pediatrics*, 126(2):e427-34. Epub 2010 Jul 26

Christofides A, Asante KP, Schauer C, Sharieff W, Owusu-Agyei S, Zlotkin S. (2006). Multi-micronutrient sprinkles including a low dose of iron provided as microencapsulated ferrous fumarate improves haematologic indices in anaemic children: a randomized clinical trial, *Matern Child Nutr*, 2(3):169-80

Corapci F, Radan A, Lozoff B. (2006). Iron deficiency in infancy and mother-child intereaction at 5 years, *J Dev Behav Pediatr*, 27(5):371-378

Darnton-Hill I, Mora JO, Weinstein H, Wilbur S, Ritu Nalubola P. (1999). Iron and folate fortification in the Americas to prevent and control micronutrient malnutrition: An analysis, *Nutrition Reviews*, 57(1): 25-31

Darnton-Hill I. (1998). Overview: Rationale and elements of a successful food-fortification programme, *Food Nutr Bull*, 19(2):92-100

Dary O. (2007). The importance and limitations of food fortification for the management of nutritional anemia. In: Badham J, Zimmermann MB, Kraemer K (eds). *The Guidebook Nutritional Anemia*. Sight and Life Press, (pages 42-43)

De-Regil LM, Suchdev PS, Vist GE, Walleser S, Peña-Rosas JP. (2011). Home fortification of foods with multiple micronutrient powders for health and nutrition in children under two years of age, *Cochrane Database Syst Rev*, Sep 7;9:CD008959 (83 pages)

Dewey KG, Cohen RJ, Rivera LL, Brown KH. (1998). Effects of age of introduction of complementary foods on iron status of breast-fed infants in Honduras, *Am J Clin Nutr*, 67: 878-84

Dewey KG, Cohen RJ, Brown KH. (2004). Exclusive breast-feeding for 6 months, with iron supplementation, maintains adequate micronutrient status among term, low-birthweight, breast-fed infants in Honduras, *J Nutr*, 134:1091-98

Erhardt, JG, Estes, JE, Pfeifer, CM, Biesalski, HK, Craft, NE. (2004). Combined measurement of ferritin, soluble transferrin receptor, retinol binding protein, and C-reactive protein by an inexpensive, sensitive, and simple sandwich enzyme-linked immunosorbent assay technique, *J Nutr*, 134: 3127-32

Faber M, Kvalsvig JD, Lombard CJ, AJ Spinnler Benadé. (2005). Effect of a fortified maize-meal porridge on anemia, micronutrient status, and motor development of infants, *Am J Clin Nutr*, 82(5):1032-1039

Finch CA, Cook JD. (1984). Iron Deficiency, *Am J Clini Nutr*, 39:471-77

Flowers CH, Cook JD. (1999). Dried plasma spot measurements of ferritin and transferrin receptor for assessing iron status, *Clini Chem*, 45(10):1826-32

Acceptance and Effect of Ferrous Fumarate Containing Micronutrient Sprinkles on Anemia,
Iron Deficiency and Anthropometrics in Honduran Children
209

Geltman PL, Hironaka LK, Mehta SD, Padilla P, Rodrigues P, Meyers AF, Bauchner H. (2009). Iron supplementation of low-income infants: a randomized clinical trial of adherence with ferrous fumarate sprinkles versus ferrous sulfate drops, *J Pediatr*, 154(5):738-43

Giovannini M, Sala D, Usuelli M, Livio L, Francescato G, Braga M, Radaelli G, Riva E. (2006). Double-blind, placebo-controlled trial comparing effects of supplementation with two different combinations of micronutrients delivered as sprinkles on growth, anemia, and iron deficiency in cambodian infants, *J Pediatr Gastroenterol Nutr*, 42(3):306-12

Grantham-McGregor S, Ani C. (Feb 2001). A review of studies on the effect of iron deficiency on cognitive development in children, *J Nutr*, 131(2S-2):649S-666S; discussion 666S-668S

Hijmans CT, Grootenhuis MA, Oosterlaan J, Heijboer H, Peters M, Fijnvandraat K. (2011). Neurocognitive deficits in children with sickle cell disease are associated with the severity of anemia, *Pediatr Blood Cancer*, 57(2):297-302

Hirve S, Bhave S, Bavdekar A, Naik S, Pandit A, Schauer C, Christofides A, Hyder Z, Zlotkin S. (2007). Low dose 'Sprinkles'-- an innovative approach to treat iron deficiency anemia in infants and young children, *Indian Pediatr*, 44(2):91-100

Horton S, Shekar M, McDonald C, Mahal A, Brooks JK. (2010). *Scaling Up Nutrition: What Will it Cost?* World Bank (136 pages)

Horton S. (2006). The economics of food fortification, *J Nutr*, 136:1068–1071

Horton S, Ross J. (2003). The economics of iron deficiency, *Food Policy*, 28:51-75

Hurrell R, Ranum P, De Pee S, Biebinger R, Hulthen L, Johnson Q, Lynch S. (2010). Revised recommendations for iron fortification of wheat flour and an evaluation of the expected impact of current national wheat flour fortification programs, *Food Nutr Bull*, 31(1) S7-S21

Ip H, Hyder SM, Haseen F, Rahman M, Zlotkin SH. (2009). Improved adherence and anaemia cure rates with flexible administration of micronutrient sprinkles: a new public health approach to anaemia control, *Eur J Clin Nutr*, 63(2):165-72

Karn SK, Chavasit V, Kongkachuichai R, Tangsuphoom N. (2011). Shelf stability, sensory qualities, and bioavailability of iron-fortified Nepalese curry powder, *Food Nutr Bull*, 32(1):13-22

Loechl CU, Menon P, Arimond M, Ruel MT, Pelto G, Habicht JP, Michaud L. (2009). Using programme theory to assess the feasibility of delivering micronutrient Sprinkles through a food-assisted maternal and child health and nutrition programme in rural Haiti, *Maternal Child Nutr*, 5:33-48

Lokeshwar MR, Mehta M, Mehta N, Shelke P, Babar N. (2011). Prevention of iron deficiency anemia (IDA): How far have we reached? *Indian J Pediatr*, 78(5):593-602

López de Romaña G, Cusirramos S, López de Romaña D, Gross R. (2005). Efficacy of multiple micronutrient supplementation for improving anemia, micronutrient status, growth, and morbidity of Peruvian infants, *J Nutr*, 135(3):646S-652S

Lozoff B. (2011). Early iron deficiency has brain and behavior effects consistent with dopaminergic dysfunction, *J Nutr*, 141: 740S–746S

Lozoff B, Beard J, Connor J, Barbara F, Georgieff M, Schallert T. (2006). Long-lasting neural and behavioral effects of iron deficiency in infancy, *Nutr Rev*, 64(5 Pt 2):S34-43; discussion S72-91

Lucca P, Hurrell R, Potrykus I. (2001). Genetic engineering approaches to improve the bioavailability and the level of iron in rice grains, *Theor Appl Genet*, 102:392–397

Lucca P, Poletti S, Sautter C. (2006). Genetic engineering approaches to enrich rice with iron and vitamin A. *Physiologia Plantarum*, 126: 291-303

Lundeen E, Schueth T, Toktobaev N, Zlotkin S, Ziauddin Hyder SM, Houser R. (2010). Daily use of Sprinkles micronutrient powder for 2 months reduces anemia among children 6 to 36 months of age in the Kyrgyz Republic: a cluster-randomized trial, *Food Nutr Bull*, 31:446-460

Lutter CK. (2008). Iron deficiency in young children in low-income countries and new approaches for its prevention, *J Nutr*, 138:2523-2528

Madan N, Rusia U, Sikka M, Sharma S, Shankar N. (2011). Developmental and neurophysiologic deficits in iron deficiency in children, *Indian J Pediatr*, 78(1):58-64

McLean E, Cogswell M, Egli I, Wojdyla D, de Benoist B. (2009). Worldwide prevalence of anaemia, WHO vitamin and mineral nutrition information system, 1993–2005, *Public Health Nutr*, 12: 444–54

Mehansho H. (2006). Iron fortification technology development: New approaches, J Nutr, 136:1059-1063

Menon P, Ruel MT, Loechl CU, Arimond M, Habicht JP, Pelto G, Michaud L. (2007). Micronutrient sprinkles reduce anemia among 9- to 24-mo-old children when delivered through an integrated health and nutrition program in rural Haiti, *J Nutr*, 137(4):1023-30

Milman N. (2011). Anemia- still a major health problem in many parts of the world! *Ann Hematol*, 90:369-377

Nestel P, Melara A, Rosado J, Mora JO. (1999). Vitamin A deficiency and anemia among children 12-71 months old in Honduras, *Pan Am J Public Health*, 6(1): 34-43

Oxford Department of International Development. (2010). Oxford Poverty and Human Development Initiative (OPHI). Country Briefing: Honduras

Provan D. (1999). Mechanisms and management of iron deficiency anemia, *Br J Haem*, 105:19-26

Rosado JL, González KE, Caamaño Mdel C, García OP, Preciado R, Odio M. (2010). Efficacy of different strategies to treat anemia in children: a randomized clinical trial, *Nutr J*, 9:40

Ruiz-Arguelles G (2006). Altitude above sea level as a variable for definition of anemia. *Blood*, 108, 2131-2132

Samadpour K, Long KZ, Hayatbakhsh R, Marks GC. (2011). Randomised comparison of the effects of Sprinkles and Foodlets with the currently recommended supplement (Drops) on micronutrient status and growth in Iranian children, *Eur J Clin Nutr*, doi: 10.1038/ejcn.2011.124. [Epub ahead of print]

Schauer C, Zlotkin SH. (2003). "Home-fortification" with micronutrient sprinkles – A new approach for the prevention and treatment of nutritional anemias, *J Paediatr Child Health*, 8:87–90

Sharieff W, Yin SA, Wu M, Yang Q, Schauer C, Tomlinson G, Zlotkin S. (2006). Short-term daily or weekly administration of micronutrient sprinkles has high compliance and does not cause iron overload in Chinese schoolchildren: a cluster-randomized trial, *Public Health Nutr*, 9(3):336-44

Sharieff W, Horton SE, Zlotkin S. (2006). Economic gains of a home fortification program: evaluation of "Sprinkles" from the provider's perspective, *Canadian J Pub Health*, 97:20-23

Smith HM, DeKaminsky RG, Niwas S, Soto RJ, Jolly PE. (Apr 2001). Prevalence and intensity of infections of Ascaris lumbricoides and Trichuris trichiura and associated socio-demographic variables in four rural Honduran communities, Mem Inst Oswaldo Cruz, Rio de Janeiro, 96(3):303-14

Smuts CM, Lombard CJ, Spinnler Benade AJ, Dhansay MA, Berger J, Hop LT, Lopez de Romaña G, Untoro J, Karyadi E, Erhardt J, Gross R. (2005). Efficacy of a foodlet-based multiple micronutrient supplement for preventing growth faltering, anemia, and micronutrient deficiency of infants: the four country IRIS trial pooled data analysis, *J Nutr*, 135:631S-638S

Sparks CS. (2011). Parental investment and socioeconomic status influences on children's height in Honduras: an analysis of national data, *Am J Hum Biol*, 23:80-88

Sprinkles Global Health Initiative. (2008). Micronutrient sprinkles for use in infants and young children: guidelines on recommendations for use and program monitoring and evaluation. Accessed Sept 20, 2011, Available from: http://sghi.org/resource_centre/GuidelinesGen2008.pdf

Stoltzfus RJ, Albonico M, Chwaya HM, Tielsch JM, Schulze KJ, Savioli L. (1998). Effects of the Zanzibar school-based deworming on iron status of children, *Am J Clin Nutr*, 68:179-86

Stoltzfus RJ, Mullany L, Black RE. (2004). Iron deficiency anaemia. In: Ezzati M, Lopez AD, Rodgers A, Murray CLJ, eds. Comparative quantification of health risks: global and regional burden of disease attributable to selected major risk factors. Geneva: World Health Organization, 163–209

Stoltzfus RJ. (2008). Research needed to strengthen science and programs for the control of iron deficiency and its consequences in young children, *J Nutr*, 138:2542-2546

Stoltzfus RJ. (2011). Iron interventions for women and children in low-income countries, *J Nutr*, 141:756S-762S

Tolson DJ, Kemmer TM , Lynch J, Lougee D, Aviles R, Amador WE, Duron CA, Guifarro Fino RO. (2010). Identifying children at risk for nutritional crisis in rural Honduras, *J Hunger Env Nutr*, 5:1, 13-22

Torrejon CS, Duran-Castillo C, Hertrampf E, Ruz M. (2004). Zinc and iron nutrition in Chilean children fed fortified milk provided by the Complementary National Food Program, *Nutrition*, 20:177-80

Trowbridge, F. (2002). Prevention and control of iron deficiency: priorities and action steps, *J Nutr*, 132:880S-882S

United Nations. (2011). *Millennium Development Goals Report*. New York (72 pages). Accessed Sept 10, 2011, Available from: http://www.un.org/millenniumgoals/pdf/(2011_E)%20MDG%20Report%202011_Book%20LR.pdf

UNICEF. (2010). *UNICEF Honduras Statistics*. Accessed Sept 10, 2011, Available from: <http://www.unicef.org/infobycountry/honduras_statistics.html>

Varma JL, Das S, Sankar R, Venkatesh Mannar MG, Levinson FJ, Hamer DH. (2007). Community-level micronutrient fortification of a food supplement in India: a controlled trial in preschool children aged 36-66 mo, *Am J Clin Nutr*, 85:1127-1133

Venkatesh Mannar MG. (2006). Successful food-based programmes, supplementation and fortification, *J Ped Gastro and Nutr*, 43:S47–S53

Wegmüller R, Camara F, Zimmermann MB, Adou P, Hurrell RF. (2006). Salt dual-fortified with iodine and micronized ground ferric pyrophosphate affects iron status but not hemoglobin in children in Côte d'Ivoire, *J Nutr*. 136:1814-1820

World Bank. (2011). *2011 World Development Indicators*, Accessed Sept 1, 2011, Available from: <http://data.worldbank.org/data-catalog/world-development-indicators>

World Bank. (2010). *Nutrition at a Glance: Honduras*. Accessed September 20, 2011, Available from:
<http://siteresources.worldbank.org/NUTRITION/Resources/281846-1271963823772/Honduras.pdf>

World Bank. (2004). *Public Health at a Glance: Anemia-World Bank Group*. Accessed September 17, 2011, Available from:
<http://siteresources.worldbank.org/INTPHAAG/Resources/anemiaAAG.pdf>

World Health Organization. (2001). *Iron deficiency anaemia: assessment, prevention and control. A guide for programme managers*. (114 pages)

World Health Organization. (2005). WHO Anthro, Accessed June 20, 2011, Available from: http://www.who.int/childgrowth/software/en/

World Health Organization Multicentre Growth Reference Study Group. (2006). WHO Child Growth Standards: Length/height-for-age, weight-for-age, weight-for-length, weight-for-height and body mass index-for-age: Methods and development. Geneva: World Health Organization (312 pages)

World Health Organization. (2008). *Worldwide Prevalence of Anemia 1993-2005: WHO Global Data Base on Anemia*

World Heath Organization. (2009). *Global Health Risks; Mortality and burden of disease attributable to selected major risks*. (62 pages)

World Heath Organization. (2009). *Recommendations on Wheat and Maize Flour Fortification Meeting Report: Interim Consensus Statement* (3 pages)

World Heath Organization. (2011). *Honduras: health profile*. Accessed September 9, 2011, Available from http://www.who.int/gho/countries/hnd.pdf

Zimmermann MB, Hurrell RF. (2007). Nutritional iron deficiency, *Lancet*, 370:511-520

Zlotkin S, Arthur P, Antwi K, Yeung G. (2001). Treatment of anemia with microencapsulated ferrous fumerate plus ascorbic acid supplied as sprinkles to complementary (weaning) foods, *Am J Clin Nutr*, 74:791-5

Zlotkin S, Antwi KY, Schauer C, Yeung G. (2003a). Use of microencapsulated iron (II) fumarate sprinkles to prevent recurrence of anaemia in infants and young children at high risk, *Bull WHO*, 81:108-15

Zlotkin S, Arthur P, Schauer C, Antwi KY, Yeung G, Piekarz A. (2003b). Home-fortification with iron and zinc sprinkles or iron sprinkles alone successfully treats anemia in infants and young children, *J Nutr*, 133:1075-80

Zlotkin SH, Christofides AL, Hyder SM, Schauer CS, Tondeur MC, Sharieff W. (2004). Controlling iron deficiency anemia through the use of home-fortified complementary foods, *Indian J Pediatr*, 71(11):1015-9

Zlotkin S, Tondeur M. (2007). The importance and limitations of food fortification for the management of nutritional anemia: in Badham J, Zimmermann MB, Kraemer K, (eds). *The Guidebook Nutritional Anemia*. Sight and Life Press, 2007 (pages 36-37)

13

Risk Factors for Anemia in Preschool Children in Sub-Saharan Africa

Dia Sanou[1,*] and Ismael Ngnie-Teta[2]
*[1]Interdisciplinary School of Health Sciences,
Faculty of Health Sciences, University of Ottawa
[2]UNICEF – Haiti and Adjunct Professor,
Program of Nutrition, University of Ottawa
Canada*

1. Introduction

Iron is a mineral that is found in nature and foods. It is involved in many physiological functions in the body, and poor iron intake can lead to iron deficiency and later to anemia. Iron deficiency anemia (IDA) is the most prevalent nutritional disorder in the world despite iron being the fourth most common element on earth. Anemia is amongst the most important contributing factors to the global burden of disease. According to a recent WHO report on the global prevalence of anemia, one in four people is affected by anemia worldwide (McLean et al., 2009; WHO, 2008), with pregnant women and preschool-age children at the greatest risk. Two thirds of preschool-age children are affected in developing regions of Africa and South East-Asia, and about 40% of the world's anaemic preschool-age children reside in South-East Asia (McLean et al., 2009; WHO, 2008). Of the 293.1 million children who suffer from anemia worldwide, 83 million (28%) are in sub-Saharan Africa, representing 67% of the total population of children of this age group in the continent.

Adverse health consequences of anemia in preschool children include altered cognitive function, impaired motor development and growth, poor school performance, poor immune function and susceptibility to infections, decreased in responsiveness and activity, increased in body tension and fatigue. Even before clinical symptoms are visible, iron deficiency that leads to anemia is detrimental to children and may condemn one third of the world population to live permanently below their full mental and physical potential. Indeed, the impact of iron deficiency anemia on psychomotor development and cognitive function in children under the age of two years may be irreversible despite adequate therapy (Lozoff et al., 2000). Horton & Ross (2003) estimated the median productivity lost due to iron deficiency anemia alone to be about US$2.32 per capita or 4.05% of gross domestic product (GDP). The authors estimated an additional US$14.46 per capita lost in cognitive function, for a total annual loss (cognitive & productive) of about $50 billion in GDP worldwide from iron deficiency anemia. Due to its detrimental effects among children, effective interventions

---

*Corresponding Author

to improve iron status and reduce the burden of anemia will likely promote health and development.

Anemia is preventable, yet it remains the most widespread nutritional deficiency in the world. Countries, which realized significant progresses in the control of the problem have identified contextual risk factors and implement context relevant programs. In sub-Saharan African, conditions which increase the risk for anemia in children are complex and multidimensional. A first step for evidence-based interventions and policies towards the control and elimination of iron deficiency anemia is a better understanding of these risk factors. The current chapter discusses the determinants of iron deficiency anemia in sub-Saharan Africa children.

2. Definition and conceptual framework

In the literature, the terms anemia, iron deficiency, and iron-deficiency anemia are often used interchangeably, but are not equivalent. Anemia is defined as a significant reduction in hemoglobin concentration, hematocrit, or the number of circulating red blood cells at a level below that is considered normal for age, sex, physiological state, and altitude, without considering the cause of the deficiency (Nestel et al., 2002). Iron deficiency anemia is a condition in which there is anemia due to lack of available iron to support normal red cell production. It is the third and last stage of iron deficiency which starts with depletion of iron stores as reflected by a reduced serum ferritin concentration. The second stage is iron deficient erythropoiesis, characterized by decreased serum iron, transferrin saturation and serum ferritin concentration but with a normal hemoglobin concentration. Because anemia can arise from nutritional factors and from non-nutritional ones, several terms are used to classify anemia, including nutritional anemia, anemia of infection, anemia of chronic diseases, pernicious anemia. For the purpose of this chapter, we focus on the first three that are the most common in developing countries, have modifiable risk factors and can be prevented through appropriate behavioral tailored intervention.

Several factors contribute concurrently in childhood anemia, but their relationships to the onset of anemia are not identical. Therefore, from an epidemiological perspective, it is important to distinguish between the different factors. A causal factor is linked to the onset of a disease or the condition and precedes the disease. A risk factor is an element linked to a person (biologic or hereditary), a behaviour, lifestyle or environment that increases the likelihood of developing the condition and has been found correlated with the condition in epidemiological studies (Last, 2004). When an intervention targeting a factor can reduce the likelihood of the condition developing, the factor is considered a modifiable risk factor. A factor susceptible to increase the onset of a pathological condition is a determining factor or determinant. For example the major causal factors of iron deficiency that lead to anemia are low dietary iron intake, inadequate iron absorption, chronic blood loss, and increased iron demand. However, there are several other factors (non causal relationship) that contribute to anemia including among others sociocultural factors, poverty, maternal factors, chronic conditions secondary to AIDS, tuberculosis and genetic factors such as sickle cell and thalassemia. There are several levels of stratification of anemia risk factors for children including structural and environmental level factors, community level factors, household level factors and individual health and nutrition related factors. Figure 1 summarizes the multi-level risk factors of anemia in children in developing countries. There is an anthropological perspective that can be seen as a transverse risk factor.

3. Anthropological perspective

Anthropologists believed that agrarian revolution that resulted in changes in dietary behaviours and outbreak of infectious diseases about 10,000 years ago has played an important role in the emergence and spread of iron deficiency and anemia (Denic & Agarwal, 2008; Wander et al., 2009). According to this theory, meat was the main source of energy prior to agrarian revolution. When humans turned from hunting to agriculture, the diet became deficient in bioavailable iron, thus increased the prevalence of iron deficiency and its subsequent anemia. Cultivating plant-based foods has increased calorie intakes, but reduced meat consumption. As a result, iron intake became insufficient to meet individual daily requirements. According to Mann (2007), daily total iron intake decreased from 87 mg in the Palaeolithic age to 15 mg in the twentieth century. In addition, increased consumption of plant-based foods has reduced the intake of absorbable iron because the amount of non-heme iron and inhibitors of iron absorption has increased in the diet, while the amount of heme iron has decreased.

With sedentarization and animal husbandry, carriers of infectious diseases were able to be transmitted from animals to humans leading to emerging or re-emerging human infectious diseases. Thereafter, poor environmental and hygienic conditions, crowding and lifestyle changes have resulted in proliferation and spread of these carriers (Denic & Agarwal, 2007). Several studies suggested that mild to moderate iron deficiency may protect against acute infection (Oppenheimer, 2001; Prentice, 2008; Sazawal et al., 2006). Thus some authors put forward the hypothesis of a potential metabolic adaptation during which the human body self-regulates its iron to a deficiency status, the « iron-deficient phenotype », to prevent the severity of infections when re-infection is a continuous process (Denic & Agarwal, 2007). According to these authors, the important advancement in developed countries to control anemia are more likely due to the successful eradication of infections rather than the quality of diet. In malaria endemic areas such as Africa, the iron deficiency phenotype survived better over time (Denic & Agarwal, 2007; Wander et al., 2009). Therefore, iron substitution therapy in some population groups such as iron supplementation in children with no functional iron deficiency may cause more harm than good (Sazawal et al., 2006; WHO/UNICEF, 2006).

4. Dietary factors

The dietary risk factors for childhood anemia in developing countries include single or combined deficiency of micronutrients such as iron, folic acid, vitamin B6, vitamin B12, vitamin A and copper. Association has been found between anemia and deficiency of vitamin A, riboflavin, protein and other nutrients (Gamble et al., 2004, Semba & Bloem 2002; Thorandenya et al. 2006; Rock et al., 1988). Although nutritional factors are thought to be the most important contributing factors to childhood anemia, their exact contribution to the risk of anemia is not well established and may vary with the level of infection and the diet quality. Magalhaes & Clements (2011) estimated that about 37% of Anemia cases in preschool children in three West African countries namely; Burkina Faso, Ghana and Mali could be averted by treating nutrition related factors alone.

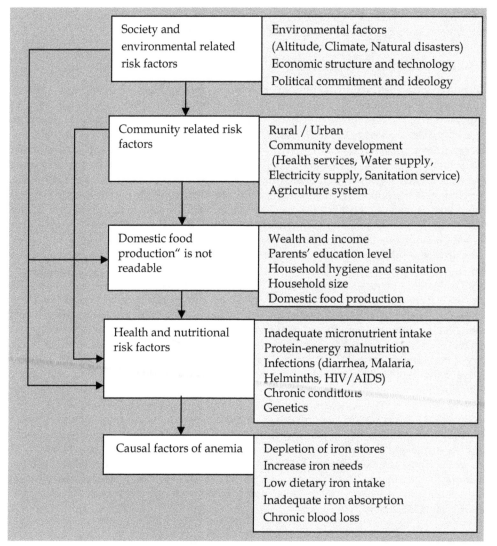

Fig. 1. Simplified conceptual framework for determinants of anemia among children (adapted from Ngnie-Teta et al, 2007).

4.1 Iron deficiency

The leading cause of anemia worldwide is iron deficiency due to inadequate intake or malabsorption of dietary iron. The adequacy of dietary iron depends on the intake and the bioavailability, which in turn are contingent to the nature of the food and the composition of the overall diet. In many developing countries, the amount of iron in the diet is usually enough to cover body needs, however because it is mainly provided by plant based food in the form of non-heme iron, its bioavailability is very low (Adish et al., 1998; Sanou et al., 2011; Zimmermann et al., 2005)

Iron is present in food in two forms: heme iron and non-heme iron. Heme is a component of hemoglobin and myoglobin and heme iron is mainly provided by animal tissues such as meat, poultry, fish and shellfish. Heme iron represents about 40% of animal tissue iron and is easily absorbed. However, it contributes to less than 15% of the total dietary iron, and may represent less than 1% in some countries where consumption of animal foods is very low (Monsen et al., 1978). Most of the dietary iron is provided in the form of non-heme iron that is comprised of non-heme iron component of animal tissues, iron from eggs, milk and plant-based foods. The absorption rate of non-heme iron is very low and depends on iron status and combined effects of enhancers and inhibitors of iron absorption (Monsen et al., 1978). Enhancers of iron absorption include animal tissues (meat, poultry, and fish) and vitamin C and organic acids (Diaz et al. 2003; Reddy et al. 2000). Dietary factors that can reduce the absorption of iron (inhibitors) are phytates and some groups of polyphenols such as tannins (Reddy et al., 2000; Sandberg et al., 1999), high intake of calcium and zinc (Lind et al., 2003; Lynch, 2000), and cow's milk (Kibangou et al. 2005). Studies conducted in different regions of the world with high prevalence of anemia showed strong correlation between iron stores and absorbable iron intakes while there is no evidence of association between total iron intake, iron deficiency and anemia (Zimmermann et al., 2005; Talata et al. 1998; Adish et al., 1998).

4.2 Other micronutrient deficiencies associated with anemia
Other micronutrients are directly or indirectly involved in red blood cell metabolism. Vitamin B_6 (pyridoxal phosphate) for example is required for activation of Δ-aminolevulinic acid synthase that is necessary for heme synthesis. Vitamine B_9 (folate) and B_{12} (cobalamine) deficiencies result in immature erythrocyte leading to macrocytic anemia (Gropper et al., 2005). Poor vitamin A status has been associated with Anemia (Gamble et al., 2004; Semba & Bloem 2002) and vitamin A supplementation has been shown to reduce the prevalence of Anemia (Semba et al., 2001). Copper is an enzymatic cofactor of ceruloplasmin (ferroxydase) that is involved in iron mobilisation during the hemoglobin synthesis. Therefore, a deficiency of copper may contribute to iron deficiency anemia (Gropper et al., 2005). It has been suggested that because of some similarities metabolic pathways of iron and zinc, high level zinc intake in the form of supplement may reduce the effectiveness of iron supplementation programmes aimed at reducing the burden anemia (Lind et al., 2003).

4.3 Severe acute malnutrition
Acute malnutrition resulting from inadequate dietary intake of nutrients and/or from acute infection and disease may also lead to mild to moderate anemia. Several hypotheses have been put forward to explain the relationship between anemia and protein-energy malnutrition; 1) adaptation to lower tissue-metabolic requirements for oxygen transport, 2) the reduction of protein required for hematopoiesis and 3) the reduction of survival time of red blood cells and the maturation of the erythroblasts (MacDougall et al., 1982). Some authors however consider that the anemia of PEM is the outcome of a complex haematological process in which iron and other micronutrient deficiencies interplay (Awasthi et al., 2003).

5. Infections

Infections are the second most important cause of anemia after iron deficiency and contribute in some settings to up to 50% of the cases (Asobayire et al., 2001; Stoltzfus et al., 2000). Children are particularly affected by infection-related anemia because of their lower immune response and their frequent exposure to poor sanitation and environmental conditions which favour the transmission and spread of parasites. Infections including malaria, hookworms, schistosomia, etc. are highly prevalent in developing countries and may negatively affect the nutritional status and growth of children. Studies conducted in many regions of Africa found positive associations between the presence and density of infection and chronic undernutrition, anemia and poor cognition (Brooker et al., 1999; Calis et al., 2008a; Friedman et al., 2005; Osazuwa et al. 2011; Sanou et al. 2008; Tolentino & Friedman, 2007). Regardless, the parasites or bacteria causing the anemia are different, all cases of anemia due to infection share some common pathways; 1) resulting iron deficiency through reduction of iron intake due to poor appetite and blood loss; 2) hemolysis i.e increased red blood cell destruction; 3) decreased red cells production and; 4) resulting inflammation. These mechanisms will be discussed later together with some pathways that are specific to each infection.

5.1 Malaria
The highest prevalence of childhood Anemia worldwide is found in malaria endemic regions. The WHO recent estimation of the global prevalence of anemia 1993-2005 suggested that between 31% and 90% of children in malaria-endemic areas of Africa suffer from anemia (WHO, 2008). Anemia is a common manifestation of the malaria infection and severe anemia can contribute to malaria mortality through hypoxia and cardiac failure (Memendez et al., 2000). Various *Plasmodium* species cause malaria, yet *P. falciparum* is the most critical for anemia in children. Contrary to iron deficiency anemia that develops slowly, *P. falciparum* causes severe and profound anemia within 48 hours of the onset of the fever. Other Plasmodium that can contribute to malaria include *P. vivax and P malariae*.

Table 1 shows the pathophysiology of malaria induced anemia. Philips and Pasvol (1992) summarized the pathophysiology of malarial anemia as follows, "anemia occurs when red cells are destroyed more rapidly than they can be replaced, or when red cell production falls below the minimal level required to maintain the steady state". Potential causes of increased red blood cell destruction include alteration of the red cell membrane rigidity and deformability, "loss of infected cells by rupture or phagocytosis, removal of uninfected cells due to antibody sensitization or other physico-chemical changes, and increased reticuloendothelial activity, particularly in organs such as the spleen" (Nuchsongsin et al., 2007; Park et al., 2008; Phillips & Pasvol, 1992). Factors leading to decreased red cell production include bone marrow hyploplasia and dyserythropoiesis. The severity of the malaria induced anemia is correlated with the density of the parasitaemia.

Although there is a consensus that clinical malaria causes severe anemia, there is limited evidence on the effect of asymptomatic malaria on severe anemia. While some authors reported that asymptomatic malaria does not significantly impact Haemoglobin level (Nkuo et al. 2002), some studies have demonstrated that asymptomatic malaria can cause homeostatic imbalance and lower Haemoglobin level in children (Kurtzhals et al. 1999); thus contributing to mild to moderate anemia (Price et al. 2001; Sowunmi et al., 2010; Umar et al. 2007). Imbalances of cytokines such as TNF-α, IL-6, IL-10 and IFN-γ resulting from malaria related-inflammation can induce changes in iron absorption and distribution, thus contributing to iron deficiency and subsequent iron deficiency anemia (Cercamondi et al., 2010; Shaw & Friedman, 2011). Bed net use is well documented as effective anemia prevention strategy (Korenromp et al., 2004, TerKuile, 2001). An exhaustive review of impact of malaria control on risk of anemia among children (Korenromp et al., 2004), estimates the protective effect of bed net on severe anemia to be 60%.

Mechanism	Comments
Increased erythrocyte destruction	
Non-immune mediated haemolysis	Rupture of parasitized red blood cells (PRBC) following invasion of RBC by malaria parasites
	Phagocytosis of parasitized (PRBC) and unparasitized red blood cells (NPRBC) due to proliferation and hyperactivity of macrophages in the reticuloendothelial system; thus shortening their life span
	Premature removal of NPRBC from the circulation due to reduce deformability and membrane binding of parasite components
	Increased clearance of parasitaemia due to splenic hypertrophy and hypersplenism (increased activity of the spleen that filters malaria infected RBC from the circulation)
Auto-immune haemolysis	Increased premature removal and clearance of unparasitized RBC due to immunoglobulin and complement activation leading to an extravascular haemolysis
	Hapten induced intravascular haemolysis due to the use of quinine that acts as a hapten combining with RBC protein to become antigenic
Decreased erythrocyte production	
Morphological abnormalities of the bone marrow	Aberrations of erythroblast morphology, macrophage hyperplasia, erythroid hypolasia and failure of reticulocyte release following a repeated attacks of malaria
Dyserythropoiesis	Morphological abnormalities of the eryhtroid series including multinuclearity of the normoblasts, intercytoplasmic bridging, karyorrhexis, incomplete and unequal mitotic nuclear divisions in some individuals with malaria
suppression of erythropoietin (EPO) synthesis	Suppression of EPO synthesis by inflammatory mediators such as TNF in some adults with malaria
Imbalances of cytokines (Inflammation induced anemia)	Bone marrow depression, dyserythropoeisis and erythrophagocytosis following low interleukine (IL-10 and IL-12) or excess of T helper cell type 1 (th1), cytokines THF-a et TNF-x, and nitric acid (NO)
Inflammation induced erythroid hypoplasia	Suppression of normal response to erythropoietin due to an autologous serum factor that may suppress the growth of early precursors of RBC including the burst-forming unit-erythron (BFU-E) and the colony-forming unit erythron (CFU-E).
Concomitant infections	Increased susceptibility to secondary infections due to reduced immune systems following malaria infection
Anti-malarial drugs	
Antifolate antimalarial	Megaloblastic anemia due to overdosing of pyremethamine and/or trimethoprim
	Quinine induced intravascular auto-immune haemolysis

Table 1. Pathophysiology mechanisms of malaria-related anemia (Memendez et al., 2000; Phillips & Pasvol, 1992).

Price et al. (2001) reported that treatment failure in uncomplicated malaria can lead to anemia. It has also been suggested that child undernutrition, particularly stunting modify the associations between malaria and anemia (Verhoef et al. 2002). Verhoef et al (2002) reported that stunting impairs host immunity, increases inflammation, and increases iron demand in developing erythroblasts, thus increasing the malaria-associated anemia.

5.2 Hookworms

Helminths are a group of intestinal nematodes that are recognized as a major public health problem in many developing countries. The effects on anemia are well documented for four species, namely trichomonas (*Trichuris trichiura),* ankylostoma (*Necator americanus, Ancylostoma duodenale*), hookworm (*Hymelolepis nana*) and ascaris (*Ascaris lumbricoides*). It is believed that the burden of hookworm is the most important particularly on severe anemia and is mostly due to extracorporeal blood loss in the stools resulting from a parasite release of a coagulase in the blood. *A. duodenale* was found more harmful than *N. americanum* and Skeletee (2003) for example estimated that it can cause approximately 0.25 mL blood loss per parasite per day during pregnancy.

According to a study done in Kenyan preschool children, hookworm contributed to 4% of anemia cases in children and heavy infection with hookworm increases the risk of anemia by 5 (Brooker et al., 1999). However, the authors did not find any association between hookworm and hemoglobin concentration likely due to the relatively low prevalence of the infection. Indeed, the burden of hookworm is directly related to the intensity of infection, the infecting species and the individual's nutritional status.

Calis et al. (2008a) also reported that the likelihood of developing severe anemia was increased by 4.8 in hookworm infected Malawian preschool children. In West Africa, a risk mapping approach using geostatistical models estimated that 4.2% of anemia cases in preschool children could be averted by treating hookworm (Magalhaes & Clements, 2011). *Trichomonas trichiura*, the causal agent of Trichuris Dysentery Syndrome has been associated with growth failure and Anemia. The anaemic effect of *T. trichiura* is thought to be linked to the blood consumption by the worm, inflammation induced anemia and reduced dietary iron intake due to decreased appetite (Shaw & Friedman, 2011).

Intervention studies have shown positive associations between mass deworming and decreased prevalence of anemia, physical performance, cognitive scores, growth and general morbidity among children from developing countries. Further, there is evidence that effectiveness of iron interventions such as supplementation and dietary approaches may be reduced when activities aiming at controlling infections are not part of the strategies (Davidson *et al.,* 2005). Therefore, it is recommended to include deworming in interventions targeting iron status at the community level.

5.3 Human schistosomiasis

Three major species of schistosomiasis have been identified as the most prevalent worldwide and cause human disease. These species that are endemic in some rural areas of Africa include *Schistosoma haematobium S. mansoni and S. japonica* (Friedman et al., 2005; Dianou *et al.,* 2004). Although most attention has been on schoolchildren, some studies have examined the relationship between schistosomiasis and anemia in preschool children (Brooker et al., 1999; Magalhaes & Clements, 2011; Talata et al., 1998). Friedman et al. (2005) described four mechanisms underlying the relationship between schistosome infections and anemia: 1) iron deficiency due to extracorporeal blood loss of iron; 2) splenic sequestration iii) auto-immune hemolysis and; 4) anemia of inflammation. It is also important to mention that infection may reduce appetite and disturb the intakes, absorption and metabolism of dietary iron.

5.4 HIV/AIDS

Anemia is a common hematological manifestation in Human immunodeficiency (HIV-infection), and has been identified as a marker for disease progression and survival (Calis et al., 2008b). A review of the global literature on HIV-related anemia in children by Calis et al. (2008b) revealed that mild to moderate anemia was more prevalent and hematocrit levels lower in HIV-infected children as compared to uninfected children. The authors also found that Anemia prevalence was higher in children with more advanced disease. However, blood loss and hemolysis are not common in HIV-infection. The suspected pathogenetic mechanisms for HIV-related anemia likely include decreased production of erythrocytes and subsequent inflammation. Further, based on findings from Uganda (Totin et al., 2002) and South Africa (Eley et al., 2002) that have suggested that iron deficiency anemia is equally affecting both HIV-infected and uninfected children, Shaw & Friedman (2011) concluded that HIV-related anemia is an Anemia of inflammation.

5.5 Bacteremia

The most common anemia inducing bacteria reported in the literature *is Helicobacter pylori* (Digirolamo *et al.* 2007; Dubois & Kearney 2005). *H. pylori* is thought to cause anemia through three mechanisms: 1) reduced iron absorption due to hypochlorhydria resulting from impaired secretion of gastric acid; 2) inflammation and; 3) competing iron demands of the bacteria and the host (Shaw & Friedman, 2011). Nontyphoid *Salmonella* has been also independently associated with anemia in children (Calis et al. 2008a; Dubois et al., 2005).

Although not investigated, it is possible that other species that can cause bloody dysentery such as *Shigella* and *Enteroinvasive E. coli* contribute to anemia. Comorbid conditions such as fever and respiratory infection often resulting from bacterial infection have been correlated with anemia (Stoltzfus *et al.,* 2000; Howard *et al.,* 2007). Diarrheal illness is associated with loss of iron and decreased absorption of nutrients needed to maintain normal Hb status. It is also likely that as demonstrated for other nutrient deficiencies, diarrhea shares many common causes with anemia (Tomkins, 1986).

Further due to the high susceptibility of HIV-infected children to opportunistic infection, bacteria may also act as synergetic factors in HIV-related anemia. A number of studies have reported biological synergisms between pathogens for disease progression (Ezeamama et al., 2008; Robertson et al., 1992). Ezeamama et al. (2008) investigated the effect of codistribution of schistosomiasis, hookworm and trichuris infection on paediatric anemia and found that hookworm and *S. japonicum* infections were independent risk factors for anemia and that co-infections of hookworm and either *S. japonicum* or *T. trichiura* were associated with higher levels of anemia than would be expected if the effects of these species had only independent effects on anemia. More recently, Magalhaes & Clements (2011) found that hookworm/S. haematobium coinfection significantly increased the likelihood of pediatric anemia as compared to individual infestation with one of these pathogens.

6. Inflammation and chronic diseases

Anemia of inflammation also termed the anemia of chronic disease (ACD) is the second most prevalent type of anemia after anemia of iron deficiency. It is observed in patients with chronic infectious disease (tuberculosis, meningitis, pulmonary infection to name a few), non-infectious chronic conditions (rheumatoid arthritis, Crohn disease, burn patients, etc.) or chronic neoplasic conditions (leukemia, carcinoma, Hodgkin disease, etc.) (Weiss & Goodnough, 2005). The pathophysiological mechanisms are not well understood, but it is believed that they are similar to the indirect pathways by which infection causes anemia. Anemia of chronic inflammatory diseases is immune driven and includes several pathways regulated by different immune and inflammatory mediators (Weiss & Goodnough, 2005):

- decreased red blood cell half-life because of dyserythropoiesis, red blood cell damage and increased erythrophagocytosis (TNF-α);
- inadequate erythropoietin responses for the degree of anemia in most, but not all (e.g. systemic-onset of juvenile chronic arthritis) (IL-1 and TNF-α);
- impaired responsiveness of erythroid cells to erythropoietin (IFN-γ, IL-1, and TNF-α);
- inhibited proliferation and differentiation of erythroid cells (IFN-γ, IL-1, TNF-α, and α-1-antitrypsin); and
- pathological iron homeostasis caused by increased DMT-1 (IFN-γ) and TfR (IL-10) expression in macrophages, reduced ferroportin 1 expression (IFN-γ and IL-6-induced high hepcidin levels) in enterocytes (inhibition of iron absorption) and macrophages (inhibition of iron recirculation), and increased ferritin synthesis (TNF-α, IL-1, IL-6, IL-10) (increased iron storage).

In a review published in New England Journal of Medicine, Weiss & Goodnough (2005) carefully discussed these mechanisms and summarized them in a single figure (Figure 2).

Recent studies have identified hepcidin as the main iron regulatory hormone in human (Andrews & Schmidt, 2007, Ganz, 2003). Hepcidin is an antimicrobial hormone that is synthesized in response to liver iron levels, inflammation, hypoxia and anemia. The persistence of inflammation results in excess hepcidin which in the circulation binds ferroportin on enterocytes and macrophages. The excess of hepcidin lowers iron absorption and prevents iron recycling, which results in hypoferremia and iron-restricted erythropoiesis, despite normal iron stores (functional ID), and anemia of chronic disease. In acute inflammation-related anemia (e.g. trauma or surgery), inflammatory responses are mediated by cytokine production mainly IL-6 and IL-8 (Weiss & Goodnough, 2005). Indeed, during inflammation, cytokines such as interleukin IL-6 stimulates the human hepcidin gene (HAMP) which in turns induces hepcidin secretion in the hepatocytes (Nicolas et al., 2002; Nemeth et al., 2004). In contrast, decreased hepcidin expression due to iron deficiency, anemia and hypoxia may lead to hereditary haemochromatosis (HH type I, mutations of the HFE gene) and type II (mutations of the hemojuvelin and hepcidin genes). In persisting iron deficiency due to decreased iron absorption and/or chronic blood loss, anemia of chronic disease evolves to anemia of chronic disease with a true iron deficiency (ACD + ID).

It is also important to keep in mind that the links between anemia and infection are bilateral and may be mutually beneficial. Indeed iron deficiency may protect against adverse effects of infections on iron status (Denic & Agarwal 2007; Sazawal et al., 2006; Oppenheimer, 2001; Weinberg 1984).

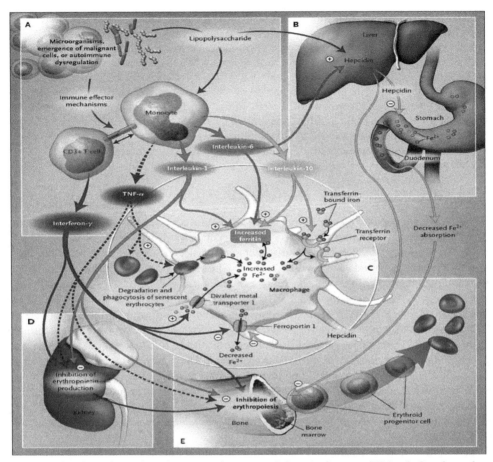

Fig. 2. Pathophysiological mechanisms of anemia of chronic diseases (Weiss & Goudnough, 2005) - reproduced with the permission from the authors and the New England Journal of Medicine -
In Panel A, the invasion of microorganisms, the emergence of malignant cells, or autoimmune dysregulation leads to activation of T cells (CD3+) and monocytes. These cells induce immune effector mechanisms, thereby producing cytokines such as interferon-γ (from T cells) and tumor necrosis factor α (TNF-α), interleukin-1, interleukin-6, and interleukin-10 (from monocytes or macrophages). In Panel B, interleukin-6 and lipopolysaccharide stimulate the hepatic expression of the acute-phase protein hepcidin, which inhibits duodenal absorption of iron. In Panel C, interferon-γ, lipopolysaccharide, or both increase the expression of divalent metal transporter 1 on macrophages and stimulate the uptake of ferrous iron ($Fe2+$). The antiinflammatory cytokine interleukin-10 up-regulates transferrin receptor expression and increases transferrin-receptor–mediated uptake of transferrin-bound iron into monocytes. In addition, activated macrophages phagocytose and degrade senescent erythrocytes for the recycling of iron, a process that is further induced by TNF-α through damaging of erythrocyte membranes and stimulation of phagocytosis. Interferon-γ and lipopolysaccharide down-regulate the expression of the macrophage iron

transporter ferroportin 1, thus inhibiting iron export from macrophages, a process that is also affected by hepcidin. At the same time, TNF-α, interleukin-1, interleukin-6, and interleukin-10 induce ferritin expression and stimulate the storage and retention of iron within macrophages. In summary, these mechanisms lead to a decreased iron concentration in the circulation and thus to a limited availability of iron for erythroid cells. In Panel D, TNF-α and interferon-γ inhibit the production of erythropoietin in the kidney. In Panel E, TNF-α, interferon-γ, and interleukin-1 directly inhibit the differentiation and proliferation of erythroid progenitor cells. In addition, the limited availability of iron and the decreased biologic activity of erythropoietin lead to inhibition of erythropoiesis and the development of anemia. Plus signs represent stimulation, and minus signs inhibition (Weiss & Goudnough, 2005).

7. Genetic polymorphisms

Some hemoglobinopathies such as sickle-cell disease, thalassaemias, glucose-6-phosphate deshydrogenase are common in many developing countries (Deyde et al., 2002; Simpore *et al.*, 2003; Thurlow *et al.*, 2005). These disorders are particularly found in malaria endemic areas and have been associated with Anemia. Glucose-6-phosphate deshydrogenase for example is correlated with chronic haemolytic Anemia (Lang *et al.*, 2002; van Bruggen *et al.*, 2002).

Sickle cell Anemia is highly prevalent in West Africa, with a frequency of the trait of 15% to 30% (WHO, 2006). Many studies suggested that these red cell polymorphisms are a human body adaptation against adverse effects of malaria. Sickle cell for example results from genetic mutation of allele A in allele S or C of the β chain to provide resistance against *Plasmodium* effect (Modiano *et al.* 2008; Kihet *et al.* 2004). In Gambia and Burkina Faso, it has been reported that sickle-cell trait is associated with protection against malaria, malaria Anemia and even cerebral Anemia (Hill, 1991; Modiano et al., 2008). In central Burkina Faso, the prevalence is expected to increase if the malaria prevalence does not decrease (Modiano et al., 2008).

Data from the National Health and Nutrition Examination Survey» (NHANES I, II et III) of the USA consistently show hemoglobin levels of Black Americans are usually lower than for their white and hispanic counterparts at all ages, regardless of the iron, health et socioeconomic status (Johnson-Spear & Yip, 1995). This finding has resulted in an adjustment of Haemoglobin cut-off for population origin 1 g/L below the normal cut-off for other population groups (Nestel et al., 2002). Although the causes of this difference is not well established, it is hypothesized that high prevalence of hemoglobinopathies such as thalassaemias and chronic inflammations as well as other genetic disorders may be important contributing factors (Beutler & West, 2005).

8. Socio-economic risk factors

The socioeconomic status, commonly measured by household income and/or household assets is a key determinant of anemia. There is strong evidence that that children living in low income household are at greater risk of anemia compared to those with higher income. Limited access to food and poor sanitation are often correlated to low income and to some extent, explain the higher risk of anemia among these children (Osorio et al., 2004). Moreover, the diet of children living in poor families is usually monotonous, even when there is enough food to eat. A study by Ag Bendech et al. (1996) in Burkina Faso showed that even though almost all the family enrolled were having three meals per day, only children from the wealthiest families were taken two or three different meals while their peers from middle income and poor households had the same meals for breakfast, lunch and dinner. The authors also reported that animal source foods which are rich in bioavailable iron were limited, contributing to only 9% of the total protein intake in poor households, 19% in middle income households and up to 41% in wealthiest households (Ag Bendech et al., 1996).

Parent's level of education constitutes another well documented determinant of anemia in children. Educated parents are more likely to have well paid job and also more likely to adopt healthier dietary behavior. In Brazil, Osorio's et al. (2004) found that mean hemoglobin level of children whose mothers attended secondary schools (9 years of schooling) was 11.5 g/dl, 11.2 for mothers with 5-8 years in school and 10.8 g/dl for mothers with less than 4 years of schooling. De Pee et al. (2002) report similar results among Palestinian children with risk of anemia twice higher for children from non-educated mothers. Even in developed countries, low level of education is associated with higher risk of anemia (Sargent et al., 1996; Soh et al., 2004).

Community level factors play an important role in the risk of anemia. Several studies have shown that living in rural areas increases the risk of child malnutrition (Kuate-Defo, 2001 ; Sommerfelt, 1991) and anemia (Bentley 2003; Osorio et al. 2001; Osorio et al., 2004; Ngnie-Teta et al., 2007). Altitude also affects the risk of anemia. Indeed, the amount of oxygen decrease with altitude, hence reducing the saturation ability of hemoglobin to capture oxygen (Cohen & Haas, 1999). This should be counterbalanced by an increased number of red blood cells. Therefore hemoglobin cut-offs have been adjusted for different age groups according to the altitude (Nestel *et al.*, 2002).

Due to increasing use of multilevel, modelling neighbourhood contribution to the risk of disease could now be quantified. A recent study in West Africa reported significant contribution of community factors of 14% to 19% to the prevalence of moderate-to-severe anemia (Ngnie-Teta et al., 2007; 2008). This reflects the variability in the risk of anemia attributable to the differences between communities, regardless of individual and households characteristics.

9. Conclusion

Anemia can result from deficiency of one or several micronutrients but also unfavourable environmental conditions and social determinants of health. Although quantitative and qualitative iron deficiency is thought to be the leading cause, infection such as malaria, schistosomiasis, hookworms, HIV and bacteria can contribute to up to 50% of the cases of anemia in developing regions where these conditions are common. Due to the multi-factorial conditions, the complexity of the risk factors of anemia, and potential interactions among them, a single strategy to control anemia in developing countries may have little success. Country level strategies to tackle anemia should include an emergency nutrition programme that will target severe anemia particularly in children under the age of two and children who live in rural areas, but also a broader nutrition and health programme that may to prevent and treat moderate to mild Anemia. Whatever strategy is used, nutrition education to increase animal sources in the diet where possible in order to enhance bioavailability of iron and to improve sanitation and basic hygiene are highly recommended as complementary measures.

10. Acknowledgement

We are grateful to Dr Weiss Gunter from the Medical University of Innsbruck, Austria and the Publishing Division of the Massachusetts Medical Society, publisher of the New England Journal of Medicine for granting us the permission to use their illustration. Our colleagues and friends who help with the editing of the earlier version of the manuscript namely Dr Nonsikelelo Mathe from the University of Alberta, Canada, Dr Reginald Annan from the International Malnutrition Task Force, University of Southampton, UK and Mrs Sabra Saleh from the Micronutrient Initiative, Dakar Senegal are kindly thanked.

11. References

Adish AA, Esrey ES, Gyorkos TW, Johns T, 1998. Risk factors for iron deficiency anemia in preschool children in northern Ethiopia. *Public Health Nutr* 2(3) : 243–252.

Ag Bendech M, Chauliac M and D Malvy Variability of home dietary habits of families living in Bamako (Mali) according to their socioeconomic status. Sante. 1996;6(5):285-297.

Andrews NC, Schmidt PJ, 2007. Iron Homeostasis. *Ann Rev Physiol* 69 : 69–85.

Awasthi S, Das R, Verma T, 2003. Anemia and undernutrition among preschool children in Uttar Pradesh, India. *Indian Pediatr* 40 : 985–990.

Asobayire FS, Adou P, Davidson L, Cook JD, Hurrell RF, 2001. Prevalence of iron deficiency with and without concurrent anemia in population groups with high prevalence of malaria and infections: a study in Côte d'Ivoire. *Am J Clin Nutr* 74 : 776-782.

Beutler E, West C, 2006. Hematologic differences between African-Americans and whites: the roles of Iron deficiency and α-thalassemia on hemoglobin levels and mean corpuscular volume. *Blood* 106(2) : 740–745.

Brooker S, Peshu N, Warn PA, Mosobo M, Guyatt H, Marsh K, Snow RW, 1999. Epidemiology of hookworm infection and its contribution to anemia among pre-school children on the Kenyan coast. *Trans Royal Soc Trop Med Hyg* 93: 240–246.

Calis JCJ, Phiri KS, Faragher EB, Brabin BJ, Bates I, Cuevas LE, et al., 2008a. Severe anemia in Malawian children. *N Engl J Med* 358(9) : 888-899.

Calis JCJ, Boele van Hensbroek MB, de Haan RJ, Moons P, Brabin BJ, Bates I, 2008b. Risk factors and correlates for anemia in HIV treatment-naïve infected patients: a cross-sectional analytical study. *AIDS*. 22(10):1099-112.

Cercamondi CI, Egli IM, Ahouandjinou E, Dossa R, Zeder C, Salami L, Tialsma H, et al. 2010. Afebrile Plasmodium falciparum parasitemia decreases absorption of fortification iron but does not affect systemic iron utilization: a double stable-isotope study in young Beninese women. *Am J Clin Nutr* 2010;92:1385–92.

Chandra J, Jain V, Narayan S, Sharma S, Singh V, Kapoor AK, Batra S, 2002. Folate and cobalamin deficiency in megaloblastic anemia in children. *Indian Pediatr* 39(5):453-7.

Cohen JH, Haas JD, 1999. Hemoglobin correction factors for estimating the prevalence of iron deficiency anemia in pregnant women residing at high altitudes in Bolivia. *Pan Am J Public Health* 6(6) : 392-399.

Davidson L, Nestel P et le comité de pilotage de l'INACG, 2005. *Efficacité et efficience des interventions dans la lutte contre la carence en fer et l'anémie ferriprive.* Washington 6 p.

De Pee S., Bloem M.W., Sari M., Kiess L., Yip R. The high prevalence of low hemoglobin concentration among indonesia infants aged 3-5 months is related to maternal anemia. J. Nutr 2002; 132:2215-21

Denic S, Agarwal MM, 2007. Nutritional iron deficiency: an evolutionary perspective. *Nutrition* 23(7-8) : 603-14.

Deyde V, Lo B, Khalifa I, Ball A, Fattoum S, 2002. Epidemiological profile of hemoglobinopathies in the Mauritanian population. *Ann Hemat* 81 (6): 320-321.

Dianou D, Poda JN, Savadogo LG, Sorgho H, Wango SP, Sondo B,2004. Parasitoses intestinales dans la zone du complexe hydroagricole du Sourou au Burkina Faso. *Vertigo* 5(2) : 1-8.

Diaz M, Rosado JL, Allen LH, Abrams S, García OP, 2003. The efficacy of a local ascorbic acid–rich food in improving iron absorption from Mexican diets: a field study using stable isotopes. *Am J Clin Nutr* 78 : 436–440.

Digirolamo AM, Perry GS, Gold BD, Parkinson A, Provost E, Parvanta I et al., 2007. Helicobacter pylori, anemia, and iron deficiency: relationships explored among Alaska native children. *Pediatr Infect Dis J* 26(10) : 927-934.

Dubois S, Kearney JD, 2005. Iron-deficiency anemia and Helicobacter pylori infection: A review of the evidence. *Am J Gastroent* 100(2) : 453–459.

Eley BS, Sive AA, Shuttleworth M, Hussey GD, 2002. A prospective, cross-sectional study of anemia and peripheral iron status in antiretroviral näive, HIV-1 infected children in Cape Town, South Africa. *BMC Infect Dis* 2(3) Epub 2002

Ezeamama AE, McGarvey ST, Acosta LP, Zierler S, Manalo DL, et al. (2008) The synergistic effect of concomitant schistosomiasis, hookworm, and trichuris infections on children's anemia burden. PLoS Negl Trop Dis 2: e245. doi

Friedman JF, Kanzaria HK, McGarvey ST, 2005. Human schistosomiasis and anemia: the relationship and potential mechanisms *Trends in Parasitology* 21(8):386-92.

Gamble MV, Palafox NA, Dancheck B, Ricks MO, Briand K, Semba RD, 2004. Relationship of vitamin A deficiency, iron deficiency, and inflammation to anemia among preschool children in the Republic of the Marshall Islands. *Eur J Clin Nutr* 58(10) :1396-401.

Ganz T, 2003. Hepcidin, a key regulator of iron metabolism and mediator of anemia of inflammation. *Blood* 102 : 783-788.

Gibson RS, Ashwell M, 2003. The association between red and processed meat consumption and iron intakes and status among British adults. *Public Health Nutr* 6(4) : 341-350.

Gleason GR. Iron deficiency anemia finally reaches the global stage of public health. Nutr Clin Care. 2002 (5):217-9

Gropper SS, Smith JL, Groff JL, 2005. *Advanced nutrition and human metabolism*. 14th ed. Thomson Wadsworth. Belmont CA.

Hill AV, Allsopp CE, Kwiatkowski D, Anstey NM, Twumasi P, Rowe PA, Bennett S, Brewster D, McMichael AJ, Greenwood BM, 1991. Common west African HLA antigens are associated with protection from severe malaria. *Nature* 352(6336):595.

Horton S, Ross J, 2003. The economics of iron deficiency, *Food Policy* 28:51-75.

Howard CT, de Pee S, Sari M, Bloem MW, Semba RD, 2007. Association of diarrhea with anemia among children under age five living in rural areas of Indonesia. *J Trop Pediatr* 53(4) : 238-244.

Jain SK, Williams DM, 1988. Copper deficiency anemia: altered red blood cell lipids and viscosity in rats. Am J Clin Nutr 48(3):637-40.

Johnson-Spear MA, Yip R, 1995. Hemoglobin difference between black and white women with comparable iron status: justification for race-specific anemia criteria. Am J Clin Nutr 60 : 117-121.

Kibangou IB, Bouhallab SH, Gwenaele BF, Allouche S, Blais A, Guerin P, Arhan P, Bougle DL, 2005. Milk proteins and iron absorption: contrasting effects of different caseino-phosphopeptides. Pediatric Res 58(4) : 731-734.

Korenromp EL, Armstrong-Schellenberg JR, Williams BG, Nahlen BL, Snow RW, 2004. Impact of malaria control on childhood anemia in Africa -- a quantitative review. Trop Med Int Health 9:1050-65.

Kuate-Defo B, 2001. Modelling hierarchically clustered longitudinal survival processes with applications to childhood mortality and maternal health. Canadian Studies Population 28 (2)

Kurtzhals JA, Addae M, Akanmori BD, Dunyo S, Koram KA, Appawu MA, Nkrumah FK, Hviid L, 1999. Anemia caused by asymptomatic Plasmodium falciparum infection in semi-immune African schoolchildren. Trans R Soc Trop Med Hyg 1999;93:623-627..

Lang K, Roll B, Myssina S, Schittenhelm M, Scheel-Walter HG, Kanz L, et al., 2002. Enhanced erythrocyte apoptosis in sickle cell anemia, thalassemia and glucose-6-phosphate dehydrogenase deficiency. Cell Phys Bioch 12 : 365-372.

Lind T, Lonnerdal B, Stenlund H, Ismail D, Seswandhana R, Ekstrom EC, Persson LA, 2003. A community-based randomized controlled trial of iron and zinc supplementation in Indonesian infants: interactions between iron and zinc. Am J Clin Nutr 77(4) : 883-890.

Lozoff B, Jimenez E, Hagen J, Mollen E, Wolf AW, 2000. Poorer behavioral and developmental outcome more than 10 years after treatment for iron deficiency in infancy. Pediatrics 105 : 1-11.

Lynch SR, 2000. The effect of calcium on iron absorption. Nutr Res Rev 13 : 141-158.

MacDougall LG, Moodley Gopal, Eyberg C, Quirk M, 1982. Mechanisms of anemia in protein-energy malnutrition in Johannesburg. Am J Clin Nutr 35 : 229-235.

Magalhães RJS, Clements ACA, 2011. Mapping the risk of anemia in preschool-age children: the contribution of malnutrition, malaria, and helminth infections in West Africa. PLoS Medicine, 8(6): e1000438 doi:10.1371/journal.pmed.1000438

Mann N, 2007. Meat in the human diet: an anthropological perspective. Nutr Diet 64 (Suppl. 4) : S102–S107.

Menendez C, Fleming AF, Alonso PL, 2000. Malaria-related anemia. Parasitol Today 16(11):469-76.

Mikki N, Abdul-Rahim HF, Stigum H, Holmboe-Ottesen G, 2011. Anemia prevalence and associated sociodemographic and dietary factors among Palestinian adolescents in the West Bank. East Medit Health J. 17 (3): 208-217.

McLean E, Coqswell M, Egli I, Wojdyla D, de Benoist B, 2009. Worldwide prevalence of anemia, WHO vitamin and mineral nutrition information system, 1993-2005. Public Health Nutr. 12(4):444-54.

Modiano D, Bancone G, Ciminelli BM, Pompei F, Blot I, Simpore J, Modiano G, 2008. Haemoglobin S and haemoglobin C: 'quick but costly' versus 'slow but gratis' genetic adaptations to Plasmodium falciparum malaria. *Hum Mol Genet* 17(6): 789-799.

Monsen ER, Hallberg L, Layrisse M, Hegsted DM, Cook JD, Walter M, Finch CA, 1978. Estimation of available dietary iron. *Am J Clin Nutr* 31 : 134-141.

Sowunmi A, Gbotosho GO, Happi CT, Fateye BA, 2010. Factors contributing to anemia after uncomplicated *Plasmodium falciparum* malaria in children. *Acta Trop 113(2):155-61.*

Nemeth E, Rivera S, Gabayan V, Keller C, Taudorf T, Pedersen BK, Ganz T, 2004. IL-6 mediates hypoferremia of inflammation by inducing the synthesis of the iron regulatory hormone hepcidin. *J Clin Invest* 113 : 1271-1276.

Nestel P et le Comité de pilotage de l'INACG, 2002. *Adjusting hemoglobin values in program surveys*. International Nutritional Anemia Consultative Group (INACG), 6 p.

Ngnie-Teta I, Receveur O, Kuate-Defo B, 2007. Risk factors for moderate to severe anemia among children in Benin and Mali: insights from a multilevel analysis. *Food Nutr Bull* 28(1) : 76-89.

Ngnie-Teta I; Kuate-Defo B; Receveur O, 2009. Multilevel modelling of sociodemographic predictors of various levels of anemia among women in Mali. Public Health Nutrition 12(9):1462-9.

Nicolas G, Chauvet C, Viatte L, Danan JL, Bigard X, Devaux I, et al. 2002. The gene encoding the iron regulatory peptide hepcidin is regulated by anemia, hypoxia, and inflammation. *J Clin Invest* 110 : 1037-1044.

Nkuo-Akenji TK, Ajame EA, Achidi EA, 2002. An investigation of symptomatic malaria parasitaemia and anemia in nursery and primary school children in Buea District Cameroon. Central African journal of medicine. 48 (1-2): 1-4

Nuchsongsin F, Chotivanich K, Charunwatthana P et al. 2007. Effects of Malaria Heme Products on Red Blood Cell Deformability. *Am J Trop Med Hyg* 77(4):617–622.

Oppenheimer SJ, 2001. Iron and its relation to immunity and infectious disease. *J Nutr* 131 : 616S-635S.

Osorio MM, Lira PI, Ashworth A, 2004. Factors associated with Hb concentration in children aged 6–59 months in the State of Pernambuco, Brazil. *Br J Nutr* 91 : 307–315.

Pan WH, Habicht JP, 1991. The non-iron-deficiency-related difference in hemoglobin concentration distribution between blacks and whites and between men and women. *Am J Epidemiol* 134(12) : 1410-1416.

Park YK, Diez-Silva M, Popescu G, Lykotrafitis G, Choi W, Feld MS, Suresh S, 2008. Refractive index maps and membrane dynamics of human red blood cells parasitized by *Plasmodium falciparum PNAS* 105(37):13730–13735

Rock E, Gueux E, Mazur A, Motta C, Rayssiguier Y, 1995. Anemia in copper-deficient rats: role of alterations in erythrocyte membrane fluidity and oxidative damage. *Am J Physiol 269(5 Pt 1):C1245-9.*

Phillips RE & Pasvol G, 1992. Anemia of Plasmodium falciparum malaria. *Baillieres Clin Haematol* 5(2):315-30.

Prentice AM, 2008. Iron metabolism, malaria, and other infections: what is all the fuss about? *J Nutr* 138 (12): 2537-2541.

Price RN, Simpson JA, Nosten F, Luxemburger C, Hkirjaroen L, ter Kuile F, Chongsuphajaisiddhi T, White NJ, 2001. Factors contributing to anemia after uncomplicated falciparum malaria. *Am J Trop Med Hyg* 65:614-622.

Reddy RB, Hurrell RF, Cook RD, 2000. Estimation of nonheme-iron bioavailability from meal composition. *Am J Clin Nutr* 71 : 937–943.

Rihet P, Flori L, Tall F, Traore AS, Fumoux F, 2004. Hemoglobin C is associated with reduced Plasmodium falciparum parasitemia and low risk of mild malaria attack. *Hum Mol Gen* 13(1) : 1–6.

Robertson LJ, Crompton DW, Sanjur D, Nesheim MC (1992) Haemoglobin concentrations and concomitant infections of hookworm and Trichuris trichiura in Panamanian primary schoolchildren. *Trans R Soc Trop Med Hyg* 86: 654–656

Sandberg AS, Brune M, Carlsson NG, Hallberg L, Skoglund E, Rossander-Hulthén L, 1999. Inositol phosphates with different numbers of phosphate groups influence iron absorption in humans. *Am J Clin Nutr* 70 : 240–246.

Sanou D, Turgeon-O'Brien H, Desrosiers T, 2008. Prévalence et déterminants non alimentaires de l'anémie et de la carence en fer chez des orphelins et enfants vulnérables d'âge préscolaire du Burkina-Faso. *Nutr Clin Metab* 22 (1) : 10-19.

Sanou D, Turgeon-O'Brien H, Desrosiers T, 2011. Impact of an integrated nutrition intervention on nutrient intakes, morbidity and growth of rural Burkinabe preschool children. *AJFAND* 11:(4) Epub July 2011. http://www.ajfand.net/Volume11/No4/Sanou9895.pdf

Sargent JD, Stukel TA, Dalton MA, Freeman JL, Brown MJ, 1996. Iron deficiency in Massachusetts communities: Socioeconomic and demographic risk factors among children. *Am J Public Health* 86(4):544-50.

Sazawal S, Black RE, Ramsan M, Chwaya HM, Stoltzfus RJ, Dutta A, et al., 2006. Effects of routine prophylactic supplementation with iron and folic acid on admission to hospital and mortality in preschool children in a high malaria transmission setting: community-based, randomised, placebo-controlled trial. *Lancet* 367 : 133-143.

Semba RD, Bloem MW, 2002. The anemia of vitamin A deficiency: epidemiology and pathogenesis. *Eur J Clin Nutr* 56:271-281

Semba RD, Kumwenda N, Taha TE, Mtimavalye L, Broadhead R, Garrett E, et al., 2001. Impact of vitamin A supplementation on anemia and plasma erythropoietin concentrations in pregnant women: a controlled clinical trial. *Eur J Haematol* 66 : 389-395 .

Shaw FJC, Kuate-Defo B, 2005. Socioeconomic inequalities in early childhood malnutrition and morbidity: modification of the household-level effects by the community SES. *Health Place* 11:205-25.

Shaw JG, Friedman JF, 2011. Iron deficiency anemia: Focus on infectious diseases in lesser developed countries *Anemia* 260380. Epub 2011 May 15

Simpore J, Nikiema JB, Sawadogo L, Pignatelli S, Blot I, Bere A, et al., 2003. Prévalence des hémoglobinopathies HbS et HbC au Burkina. *Burkina Medical* 32 : 1-13

Skeletee RW, 2003. Pregnancy, nutrition and parasitic diseases. *J Nutr* 133:1661S-1667S

Soh P, Ferguson EL, McKenzie JE, Homs MY, Gibson RS. Iron deficiency and risk factors for lower iron stores in 6-24-month-old New Zealanders. Eur J Clin Nutr. 2004 Jan;58(1):71-9.

Sommerfelt AE. Comparative analysis of the determinants of children's nutritional status. Demographic and Health Surveys World Conference, vol 2, 981-98. 1991 Washington DC, 722-43

Stoltzfus RJ, Chwaya HM, Montresor A, Albonico M, Savioli L, Tielsch JM, 2000. Malaria, hookworms and recent fever are related to anemia and iron status indicators in 0- to 5-y old Zanzibari children and these relationships change with age. *J Nutr* 130 : 1724–1733.

Talata S, Svanberg U, Mduma B, 1998. Low dietary iron availability is a major cause of anemia: a nutrition survey in the Lindi district of Tanzania. *Am J Clin Nutr* 68 : 171–178.

Taylor-Robinson DC, Jones AP, Garner P, 2007. Deworming drugs for treating soil-transmitted intestinal worms in children: effects on growth and school performance. *Cochrane Database of Systematic Reviews Issue* 4. Art. No.: CD000371.

ter Kuile FO, Terlouw DJ, Kariuki SK, et al. Impact of permethrin-treated bed nets on malaria, anemia, and growth in infants in an area of intense perennial malaria transmission in western Kenya. Am J Trop Med Hyg 2003;68:68-77.

Thorandeniya T, Wickremasinghe R, Ramanyake R, Atukorala S, 2006. Low folic acid status and its association with anemia in urban adolescent girls and women of childbearing age in Sri Lanka. *Brit J Nutr.* 95 (3): 511-516.

Thurlow RA, Winichagoon P, Green T, Wasantwisut E, Pongcharoen T, Bailey KB, Gibson RS, 2005. Only a small proportion of anemia in northeast Thai schoolchildren is associated with iron deficiency. *Am J Clin Nutr* 82 : 380–387.

Tolentino K, Friedman JF, 2007. An update on anemia in less developed countries. *Am J Trop Med Hyg* 77: 44–51.

Tomkins AM. Protein-energy malnutrition and risk of infection. Proc Nutr Soc 1986;45:289-304.

Totin D, Ndugwa C, Mmiro F, Perry RT, Brooks Jackson J, Semba RD, 2002. Iron deficiency anemia is highly prevalent among human immunodeficiency virus-infected and uninfected infants in Uganda. *Jf Nutr*132(3):423–429.

Umar RA, Jiya NM, Ladan MJ, Abubakar MK, Hassan SW, Nata`ala U, 2007. low prevalence of anemia in a cohort of pre-school children with acute uncomplicated *falciparum* malaria in Nigeria. *Trends Med Res 2: 95-101.*

van Bruggen R, Bautista JM, Petropoulou T, de Boer M, van Zwieten R, Gomez-Gallego F, et al., 2002. Deletion of leucine 61 in glucose-6-phosphate dehydrogenase leads to chronic nonspherocytic anemia, granulocyte dysfunction, and increased susceptibility to infections. *Blood* 100(3) : 1026 - 1030.

Verhoef H, West C, Veenemans J, Beguin Y, Kok F, 2002. Stunting may determine the severity of malaria-associated anemia in African children. *Pediatrics* 110:E48

Walker FC, Kordas K, Stoltzfus RJ, Black RE, 2005. Interactive effects of iron and zinc on biochemical and functional outcomes in supplementation trials. *Am J Clin Nutr* 82 : 5-12.

Wander K, Shell-Duncan B, McDade TW, 2009. Evaluation of iron deficiency as a nutritional adaptation to infectious disease: An evolutionary medicine perspective. *American Journal of Human Biology,* 2009; 21(2):172-179.

Weinberg, ED. Iron withholding: a defense against infection and neoplasia. *Physiological Reviews,* 1984; 64:65-102.

Weiss G, Goodnough LT, 2005. Anemia of chronic disease. *N Engl J Med* 352 : 1011-1023.

WHO, Sickle-cell anemia. Report by the Secretariat of the World Health Organization for the fifty-ninth world health assembly. 24 April 2006.

WHO. 2008. Worldwide prevalence of anemia 1993–2005 : WHO global database on anemia / Edited by Bruno de Benoist,

WHO/UNICEF, 2006. *Iron supplementation of young children in regions where malaria transmission is intense and infectious disease highly prevalent.* Joint statement by the World Health Organization and the United Nations Children's Fund. Geneva. 2 p.

WHO/UNICEF, 2006. *Iron supplementation of young children in regions where malaria transmission is intense and infectious disease highly prevalent.* WHO/UNICEF Joint statement. Geneva.

WHO/UNICEF/UNU. *Iron deficiency anemia assessment, prevention and control: a guide for programme managers.* World Health Organization. (WHO/NHD/01.3) Geneva, 2001.

Zimmermann MB, Chaouki N, Hurrell RF, 2005a. Iron deficiency due to consumption of a habitual diet low in bioavailable iron: a longitudinal cohort study in Moroccan children. *Am J Clin Nutr* 81: 115–121.

Permissions

The contributors of this book come from diverse backgrounds, making this book a truly international effort. This book will bring forth new frontiers with its revolutionizing research information and detailed analysis of the nascent developments around the world.

We would like to thank Dr. Donald S. Silverberg, for lending his expertise to make the book truly unique. He has played a crucial role in the development of this book. Without his invaluable contribution this book wouldn't have been possible. He has made vital efforts to compile up to date information on the varied aspects of this subject to make this book a valuable addition to the collection of many professionals and students.

This book was conceptualized with the vision of imparting up-to-date information and advanced data in this field. To ensure the same, a matchless editorial board was set up. Every individual on the board went through rigorous rounds of assessment to prove their worth. After which they invested a large part of their time researching and compiling the most relevant data for our readers. Conferences and sessions were held from time to time between the editorial board and the contributing authors to present the data in the most comprehensible form. The editorial team has worked tirelessly to provide valuable and valid information to help people across the globe.

Every chapter published in this book has been scrutinized by our experts. Their significance has been extensively debated. The topics covered herein carry significant findings which will fuel the growth of the discipline. They may even be implemented as practical applications or may be referred to as a beginning point for another development. Chapters in this book were first published by InTech; hereby published with permission under the Creative Commons Attribution License or equivalent.

The editorial board has been involved in producing this book since its inception. They have spent rigorous hours researching and exploring the diverse topics which have resulted in the successful publishing of this book. They have passed on their knowledge of decades through this book. To expedite this challenging task, the publisher supported the team at every step. A small team of assistant editors was also appointed to further simplify the editing procedure and attain best results for the readers.

Our editorial team has been hand-picked from every corner of the world. Their multi-ethnicity adds dynamic inputs to the discussions which result in innovative outcomes. These outcomes are then further discussed with the researchers and contributors who give their valuable feedback and opinion regarding the same. The feedback is then collaborated with the researches and they are edited in a comprehensive manner to aid the understanding of the subject.

Every chapter published in this book has been scrutinized by our experts. Their significance has been extensively debated. The topics covered herein carry significant findings which will fuel the growth of the discipline. They may even be implemented as practical applications or may be referred to as a beginning point for another development. Chapters in this book were first published by InTech; hereby published with permission under the Creative Commons Attribution License or equivalent.

Apart from the editorial board, the designing team has also invested a significant amount of their time in understanding the subject and creating the most relevant covers. They scrutinized every image to scout for the most suitable representation of the subject and create an appropriate cover for the book.

The publishing team has been involved in this book since its early stages. They were actively engaged in every process, be it collecting the data, connecting with the contributors or procuring relevant information. The team has been an ardent support to the editorial, designing and production team. Their endless efforts to recruit the best for this project, has resulted in the accomplishment of this book. They are a veteran in the field of academics and their pool of knowledge is as vast as their experience in printing. Their expertise and guidance has proved useful at every step. Their uncompromising quality standards have made this book an exceptional effort. Their encouragement from time to time has been an inspiration for everyone.

The publisher and the editorial board hope that this book will prove to be a valuable piece of knowledge for researchers, students, practitioners and scholars across the globe.

List of Contributors

Yoshihito Iuchi
Yamaguchi University, Japan

Oluyomi Stephen Adeyemi
Redeemer's University, Department of Chemical Sciences, Mowe, Nigeria

Adenike Faoziyat Sulaiman and Musbau Adewumi Akanji
University of Ilorin, Department of Biochemistry, Ilorin, Nigeria

Fawzia Ahmed Habib, Intessar Sultan and Shaista Salman
Taibah University-College of Medicine-Al Madinah Al Munawara, Kingdom of Saudi Arabia

Daniela Vittori, Daiana Vota and Alcira Nesse
Department of Biological Chemistry, School of Sciences, University of Buenos Aires, Argentina   IQUIBICEN - National Council of Scientific and Technical Investigation, Argentina

Vikrant Kale and Abdur Rahmaan Aftab
Gastroenterology Department, St. Luke's Hospital, Kilkenny, Ireland

Eitan Fibach
Hematology, Hadassah – Hebrew, University Medical Center, Jerusalem, Israel

Kayode O. Osungbade and Adeolu O. Oladunjoye
Department of Health Policy and Management, Faculty of Public Health, College of Medicine and University College Hospital, University of Ibadan, Nigeria   Department of Community Medicine, University College Hospital, Ibadan, Nigeria

Anna Blázovics
Department of Pharmacognosy, and II. Department of Medicine, Semmelweis University, Budapest, Hungary

Edit Székely
Department of Pharmacognosy, and II. Department of Medicine, Semmelweis University, Budapest, Hungary

Péter Nyirády, Imre Romics, Miklós Szűcs and András Horváth
Department of Urology, Semmelweis University, Hungary

Ágnes Szilvás
Saint John Hospital, Budapest, Hungary

Klára Szentmihályi
Institute of Materials and Environmental Chemistry, CRC, Hungarian Academy of Sciences, Budapest, Hungary

Gabriella Bekő
Central Laboratory Pest, Semmelweis University, Hungary

Éva Sárdi
Corvinus University, Budapest, Hungary

Alhossain A. Khallafallah
Launceston General Hospital, Launceston, Tasmania, Australia School of Human Life Sciences, University of Tasmania, Australia

Muhajir Mohamed
Launceston General Hospital, Launceston, Tasmania, Australia

Frank T. Wieringa, Jacques Berger and Marjoleine A. Dijkhuizen
NutriPass – UMR204, Institute for Research for Development (IRD), IRD-UM2-UM1, Montpellier, France Department of Human Nutrition, Copenhagen University, Denmark

Michele Magoni, Ghassam Zaqout, Omar Ahmmed Mady, Reema Ibraheem Al Haj Abed and Davide Amurri
Terre des Hommes, Italy

Teresa M. Kemmer
Health and Nutritional Sciences, SDSU Extension and Agricultural Experiment Station South Dakota State University, Brookings, USA

Preston S. Omer
U.S. Army, U.S. Army Medical Command, Fort Riley, USA

Vinod K. Gidvani-Diaz
U.S. Air Force San Antonio Uniformed Services Health Education Consortium, Pediatric Residency San Antonio, USA

Miguel Coello
U.S. Medical Element, Joint Task Force-Bravo, Soto Cano Air Base, Honduras

Dia Sanou
Interdisciplinary School of Health Sciences, Faculty of Health Sciences, University of Ottawa, Canada

Ismael Ngnie-Teta
UNICEF – Haiti and Adjunct Professor, Program of Nutrition, University of Ottawa, Canada